AF712558

Potential Health Benefits of Citrus

ACS SYMPOSIUM SERIES **936**

Potential Health Benefits of Citrus

Bhimanagouda S. Patil, Editor
Texas A&M University

Nancy D. Turner, Editor
Texas A&M University

Edward G. Miller, Editor
Baylor University

Jennifer S. Brodbelt, Editor
University of Texas

Sponsored by the
ACS Division of Agricultural and Food Chemistry, Inc.

American Chemical Society, Washington, DC

Library of Congress Cataloging-in-Publication Data

Potential health benefits of citrus / Bhimanagouda S. Patil, editor ... [et al.] ; sponsored by the ACS Division of Agricultural and Food Chemistry, Inc.

p. cm.—(ACS symposium series ; 936)

"Developed from a symposium sponsored by the Division of Agricultural and Food Chemistry, Inc. at the 228th National Meeting of the American Chemical Society, Philadelphia, Pennsylvania, August 23–26, 2004"—T.p. verso

Includes bibliographical references and index.

ISBN-13: 978–0–8412–3957–9 (alk. paper)
ISBN-10: 0–8412–3957–6

1. Citrus fruits—Analysis—Congresses. 2. Citrus fruits—Health aspects—Congresses. 3. Citrus fruits in human nutrition—Congresses.

I. Patil, Bhimanagouda S., 1962- II. American Chemical Society. Meeting (228th : 2004 : Philadelphia, Pa.) III. Division of Agricultural and Food Chemistry, Inc. IV. Series.

QP144.C58P68 2006
612.3′9—dc22 2006042710

The paper used in this publication meets the minimum requirements of American National Standard for Information Sciences—Permanence of Paper for Printed Library Materials, ANSI Z39.48–1984.

Distributed by Oxford University Press

PRINTED IN THE UNITED STATES OF AMERICA

Foreword

The ACS Symposium Series was first published in 1974 to provide a mechanism for publishing symposia quickly in book form. The purpose of the series is to publish timely, comprehensive books developed from ACS sponsored symposia based on current scientific research. Occasionally, books are developed from symposia sponsored by other organizations when the topic is of keen interest to the chemistry audience.

Before agreeing to publish a book, the proposed table of contents is reviewed for appropriate and comprehensive coverage and for interest to the audience. Some papers may be excluded to better focus the book; others may be added to provide comprehensiveness. When appropriate, overview or introductory chapters are added. Drafts of chapters are peer-reviewed prior to final acceptance or rejection, and manuscripts are prepared in camera-ready format.

As a rule, only original research papers and original review papers are included in the volumes. Verbatim reproductions of previously published papers are not accepted.

ACS Books Department

Contents

Preface xi

1. **Potential Health Benefits of Citrus: An Overview** 1
   Bhimanagouda S. Patil, Jennifer S. Brodbelt, Edward G. Miller, and Nancy D. Turner

Isolation and Characterization of Citrus Bioactive Compounds

2. **Citrus Bioactive Limonoids and Flavonoids Extraction by Supercritical Fluids** 18
   Bhimanagouda S. Patil, Jun Yu, Deepak V. Dandekar, Romeo T. Toledo, Rakesh K. Singh, and Leonard M. Pike

3. **Methods for the Separation of Limonoids from Citrus** 34
   Guddadarangavvanahally K. Jayaprakasha, Jennifer S. Brodbelt, Narayan G. Bhat, and Bhimanagouda S. Patil

4. **Characterization of Flavonoids by Tandem Mass Spectrometry and Metal Complexation Strategies** 52
   Jennifer S. Brodbelt, Junmei Zhang, Michael Pikulski, Barry D. Davis, Basavaraj Girennavar, Guddadarangavvanahally K. Jayaprakasha, and Bhimanagouda S. Patil

5. **Powerful Analytical Tools for Citrus Characterization: LC/MS and LC/NMR Characterization of Polymethoxylated Flavones** 70
   Claus O. Schmidt, Gerhard E. Krammer, Berthold Weber, Detlef Stöckigt, Stefan Brennecke, Günter Kindel, and Heinz-Jürgen Bertram

Bioavailability and Toxicity of Limonoids

6. **Long-Term Screening Study on the Potential Toxicity of Limonoids** **82**
Edward G. Miller, Reed P. Gibbins, Samuel E. Taylor, Jame E. McIntosh, and Bhimanagouda S. Patil

7. **Citrus Limonoid Bioavailability in Humans** **95**
Andrew P. Breksa III, Gary D. Manners, Robert A. Jacob, and Shin Hasegawa

Health Properties of Bioactive Compounds in Citrus

8. **Citrus Flavonoid Nobiletin Suppresses Azoxymethane-Induced Rat Colon Tumorigenesis** **104**
Rikako Suzuki, Hiroyuki Kohno, Shigeyuki Sugie, Akira Murakami, Masamichi Yano, Hajime Ohigashi, and Takuji Tanaka

9. **Comparison of the Chemoprotection Conferred by Grapefruit and Isolated Bioactive Compounds against Colon Cancer** **121**
Nancy D. Turner, Jairam Vanamala, Tety Leonardi, Bhimanagouda S. Patil, Mary E. Murphy, Yingxue C. Liu, Naisyin Wang, Leonard M. Pike, Robert S. Chapkin, and Joanne R. Lupton

10. **Citrus Limonoids and Flavonoids: Enhancement of Phase II Detoxification Enzymes and Their Potential in Chemoprevention** **130**
Hassan Ahmad, Jiaxing Li, Maria Polson, Kimberly Mackie, Walter Quiroga, and Bhimanagouda S. Patil

11. **Prevention of Drug-Induced Programmed and Unprogrammed Cell Death by Citrus Flavonoids** **144**
Sidhartha D. Ray, Daniel Zinkovsky, Ellida Bulku, and Bhimanagouda S. Patil

12. **Antioxidant Effects of Citrus Flavonoid Consumption** **161**
John R. Burgess and Juan E. Andrade

13. ***Citrus* sp.: A Source of Flavonoids of Pharmaceutical Interest** **175**
Ana Ortuño, Pedro Gómez, Ana Báidez, Víctor Frías, and José A. Del Río

14. **Modulation of Cholesterol and Triacylglycerol Biosynthesis by Citrus Polymethoxylated Flavones: Cholesterol-Lowering Properties of Citrus Flavonoids**....186
John A. Manthey and Elzbieta M. Kurowska

15. **The Health Benefits of Modified Citrus Pectin**....199
Isaac Eliaz, John Guardino, and Kerry Hughes

16. **Obesity, Metabolic Syndrome, and the Benefits of Citrus**....211
Ken Fujioka and Michael W. Lee

17. **Whither Grapefruit and Drug Interaction?**....219
Basavaraj Girennavar, Shibu M. Poulose, Jennifer S. Brodbelt, Guddadarangavvanahally K. Jayaprakasha, Narayan G. Bhat, and Bhimanagouda S. Patil

18. **Grapefruit and Cancer: A Review**....235
Kristine Cuthrell and Loïc Le Marchand

Consumer Trends

19. **Trends in Consumer Attitudes toward Food and Health: from Food Biotechnology to Personalized Nutrition**....254
David B. Schmidt

Indexes

Author Index....263

Subject Index....265

Preface

In addition to being one of the most widely available and popular types of fruit, citrus is a storehouse of biological active compounds. Vitamin C is perhaps the most universally recognized nutrient found in citrus, but other classes of compounds, such as flavonoids and limonoids, are gaining recognition for their impressive chemopreventive properties. Their anticancer properties, among others, have prompted an increasing array of studies that are aimed at elucidating the health benefits of citrus, resolving mechanisms of action, and mapping the compounds responsible for the chemopreventive actions.

The concept of this book stemmed from a symposium that was held in 2004 at the 228th American Chemical Society National Meeting in Philadelphia, Pennsylvania. The symposium brought together a diverse group of scientists, ranging from horticulturists to biologists to biochemists, and the significant interchange of both basic information and cutting-edge results spurred interest in collecting and expanding the material into a book. The book is divided into five sections: the first provides a broad overview of the health benefits of citrus. The second section focuses on the separation and characterization of bioactive compounds in citrus, with chapters on the isolation of limonoids and flavonoids from citrus, in addition to the structural characterization of flavonoids by various analytical methods. The third section covers the toxicity and bioavailability of limonoids. The fourth section discusses numerous documented health benefits of citrus, including chapters reporting that nobiletin, a citrus flavonoid, acts as a chemopreventive against colon cancer; the induction of detoxification enzymes by limonoids and flavonoids; and the abilities of two flavonoids to minimize oxidative stress in heptatotoxicity and nephrotoxicity. The effects of citrus consumption on lipid oxidation are described as well as the antifungal properties of flavonoids, the impact of furocoumarins in grapefruit on the bioavailabilities of certain drugs, the inhibition of certain CYP enzymes by citrus compounds, the modulation of the biosynthesis of cholesterol and triacylglycerols by polymethoxylated flavones, the reduction of metastasis and angiogenesis in cancer by citrus pectins, and the potential influence of citrus consumption on metabolic syndrome. The final section of the book describes consumer awareness of the benefits of citrus in the diet and provides some context for attaining consumer acceptance of the promising scientific results about citrus.

Bhimanagouda S. Patil
Vegetable and Fruit Improvement Center
Department of Horticultural Sciences
Mail Stop 2119
Texas A&M University
College Station, TX 77845

Jennifer S. Brodbelt
Department of Chemistry and Biochemistry
University of Texas
Austin, TX 78712–1167

Edward G. Miller
Baylor College of Dentistry
Vegetable and Fruit Improvement Center
Texas A&M University System Health Science Center
3302 Gaston Avenue
Dallas, TX 75246

Nancy D. Turner
Vegetable and Fruit Improvement Center
Department of Nutrition and Food Science
Texas A&M University
2471 TAMU,
College Station, TX 77843

Potential Health Benefits of Citrus

Chapter 1

Potential Health Benefits of Citrus: An Overview

Bhimanagouda S. Patil[1], Jennifer S. Brodbelt[2,3], Edward G. Miller[2,4], and Nancy D. Turner[2,5]

[1]Vegetable and Fruit Improvement Center, Department of Horticultural Sciences, Mail Code 2119, Texas A&M University, College Station, TX 77843
[2]Vegetable and Fruit Improvement Center, Mail Code 2119, Texas A&M University, College Station, TX 77843
[3]Department of Chemistry and Biochemistry, University of Texas, Austin, TX 78712
[4]Baylor College of Dentistry, Texas A&M University Health Science Center, 3302 Gaston Avenue, Dallas, TX 75246
[5]Faculty of Nutrition, Mail Stop 2471, Texas A&M University, College Station, TX 77843

Recent studies have documented a number of health benefits associated with the consumption of citrus, largely due to the natural phytochemicals found in these fruits, such as flavonoids, limonoids, furocoumarins, and pectins. Interest in the chemopreventive properties of phytochemicals has led to more detailed studies to determine the mechanisms of action of these compounds in animal models and humans, to optimize the levels of the phytochemicals in citrus based on agricultural and processing factors, and to develop better analytical methods for identifying and quantifying phytochemicals in complex mixtures. This chapter provides an overview of the many aspects of citrus and its health benefits that will be described in more detail in chapters throughout this book.

Introduction

Citrus is a major fruit crop on a global level with a significant economic impact on countries in which citrus is grown on a large acreage. For example, the annual on-tree value in the U.S. (before harvesting, packing and processing) is approximately $2.66 billion which equates to over $20 billion in retail sales. The U.S. is the world's largest citrus producer after Brazil. For many years anecdotal reports have implied that fruits and vegetables protect us from human ailments. The health promoting properties of citrus have been known for quite some time; however, only in the last decade have citrus and their products been consumed consistently in greater quantities, largely because of the awareness of the health promoting properties of vitamin C. Recent studies have demonstrated that part of the human health benefits of citrus may be derived from phytochemicals other than vitamin C. During the last decade, scientific data available in the literature suggest that citrus contain plant-derived bioactive molecules such as carotenoids (lycopene, lutein and zeaxanthin, and cryptoxanthin), limonoids, flavonoids (naringin and hesperidin, tangeretin and nobiletin), vitamin C (ascorbic acid plus dehydroascorbic acid), pectin, glutarate, furocoumarins and folate, among others. Some of the bioactive compounds are specific to certain groups of citrus. For example, oranges contain lutein, zeaxanthin, and hesperidin, and grapefruit contain lycopene and naringin. Only recently have many of the bioactive compounds been investigated to determine their effects in chemoprevention and anticarcinogenesis studies. Recent reviews of epidemiological and clinical studies (*1-4*) are providing strong evidence that these bioactive compounds are responsible for a chemopreventive and therapeutic role in human health, as demonstrated in large cohort and case-control studies of cancer, heart disease, and many other diseases. For example, recent studies have demonstrated that flavonoids may also have potential as neuro-protective agents (*5,6*). The National Cancer Institute (NCI) initiated a five-year research program on diet and cancer that was designed to study, assess, and develop "Designer Foods" from a host of 40 food classes and 14 biologically active phytochemicals (*7*). Citrus was one of the food classes targeted along with four biologically active citrus phytochemicals. Two of the classes of phytochemicals in citrus that have generated the most interest due to their wide-sweeping benefits on human health are limonoids and flavonoids, as summarized in the next sections.

Beneficial Roles of Citrus Limonoids: From Insect Control to Animal Studies

Early research on citrus phytochemicals concentrated on chemical structure, metabolism, and potential relevance, either positive or negative, to the citrus industry. Today researchers are starting to focus on the role that some of these chemicals might have in insect management and on the health of the consumer. Up to this time most of the work has centered on the citrus limonoids and flavonoids.

Research with azadirachtin, a limonoid from the Indian neem tree, has shown that this compound can act as an antifeedant and inhibitor of development in several insect species (*8-10*). This work led to similar studies with citrus limonoids. Several citrus limonoids, primarily limonin, nomilin and obacunone, have been reported (*11-14*) to have antifeedant activity against a variety of insect pests including the corn earworm (*Helicoverpa zea*), the fall armyworm (*Spodoptera frugiperda*), the Colorado potato beetle (*Leptinotarsa decemlineata*), and the spruce budworm (*Lepidoptera tortricidae*). Limonoids have also been found (*15*) to increase mortality and reduce adult emergence in the mosquito (*Culex quinquefasciatus*).

A considerable amount of research has been done on the effectiveness of limonoids in the management of the Colorado potato beetle. Research (*16,17*) involving a variety of different naturally occurring and synthetic limonoids demonstrated that an intact D ring and furan ring were essential for antifeedant activity. The epoxide group on the D ring was also needed for full biological activity. By comparison, changes in the A ring of the limonoid nucleus did not diminish antifeedant activity. Long-term exposure to limonoids delayed the development of the Colorado potato beetle larvae and increased mortality (*18,19*). In addition, the limonoids acted as a repellent to the Colorado potato beetle adults even when applied to the outer margins of the field (*20*). Studies (*21,22*) with a variety of insecticides (*B. thuringiensis* toxin, azinphosmethyl, endosulfan, esfenvalerate, and oxamyl) used in Colorado potato beetle management consistently showed that prior exposure to limonoids increased the susceptibility of the Colorado potato beetle larvae to the treatment with the insecticide. No phytotoxicity was observed on the potato foliage at concentrations as high as 100 $\mu g/cm^2$. It is estimated (*20*) that 300 metric tons of citrus limonoids could be extracted annually from by-products (seeds, peel, etc.) of juice processing plants in the United States. This increases the potential for these compounds for the management of insects.

Work with animals has primarily focused on the cancer chemopreventive activity of citrus limonoids. Limonin, nomilin and in one case obacunone have demonstrated antineoplastic activity in a model for benz[a]pyrene-induced forestomach tumors in ICR/Ha mice (*23*), 7,12-dimethylbenz[a]anthracene (DMBA)-induced oral tumors in Syrian hamsters (*24*), benz[a]pyrene-induced lung tumors in A/J mice (25), a two-stage model for DMBA-induced skin tumors in SENCAR mice (*26*), 4-(methylnitrosamino)-1-(3-pyridyl)-1-butanone (NNK)-

induced lung tumors in A/J mice (*27*), and azoxymethane-induced colon tumors in male F344 rats (*28*). Some of the early studies also indicated that nomilin and obacunone are blocking agents that can induce higher levels of glutathione S-transferase activity in a variety of different tissues in ICR/Ha mice (*29*). By comparison limonin was ineffective in these assays. The possibility of separate mechanisms of action, one for nomilin and obacunone and a second for limonin, is also supported by the data form the two-stage study on DMBA-induced skin tumors (*26*). Nomilin proved to be more effective during the initiation stage of carcinogenesis, and limonin was more effective during the promotional stage of carcinogenesis. In the hamster cheek pouch model for DMBA-induced oral tumors 13 limonoids, 12 naturally occurring and one synthetic limonoid, were tested for anticancer activity (*24,30-33*). Unlike the earlier work on insect antifeedant activity (*16,17*), the data showed that major changes could be made to the D ring of the limonoid nucleus without any apparent loss of anticancer activity. In addition, changes to the A and B ring usually led to a compound that was inactive.

Human cell culture studies have mainly concentrated on the possible use of limonoids in the treatment of cancer. Initial studies (*34*) showed that a variety of limonoids, including nomilin, a mixture of limonoid glucosides, limonin methoxime, deacetylnomilin, obacunone, isoobacunoic acid, and nomilin 17-β-D-glucoside were potent inhibitors of proliferation of estrogen receptor-negative (MDA-MB-435) and receptor–positive (MCF-7) human breast cancer cells. In a second study (*35*), it was found that limonoids at high doses could induce apoptosis in a human breast cancer cell line (MCF-7). This research plus earlier studies (*36*) also showed that limonoids were not toxic to a variety of other human cancer cell lines or to normal human cells grown in culture. More recently (*37*) it was found that a variety of different limonoid glucosides demonstrated cytotoxicity to neuroblastoma cells, SH-SY5Y cells, grown in culture. At low concentrations, 1-50 μmol/L, the limonoids induced apoptosis. Cytotoxicity was directly related to a time-dependent increase in caspase 3/7 activity. A caspase inhibitor, Ac-DEVD-CHO, blocked limonin 17-β-D-glucopyranoside-induced cytotoxicity. In another study, citrus extract showed induction of apoptosis through caspase-3 pathway in human gastric cancer cells (*38*).

Results from other laboratories indicate that limonoids may have other potential health benefits. In one study (*39*), it was found that limonin, methyl deoxylimonate, and nomilin substantially lowered the lipoprotein-associated apo B in the media over HepG2 cells. Further research with limonin showed that the exposure to this compound had no affect on the synthesis of free cholesterol,

cholesterol esters, or triglycerides in the treated HepG2 cells. Recently (*40*), it was also found that limonin and nomilin can inhibit HIV-1 replication in fresh phytohaemoglutin-activated peripheral blood mononuclear cells from healthy donors and HIV-1 infected patients. Inhibition was also observed in cultures of monocytes/macrophages. Limonin and nomilin also inhibited *in vitro* HIV-1 protease activity. The relevance of all of these potential health benefits is increased by a recent discovery that limonin 17-β-D-glucopyranoside was absorbed from the gastrointestinal tract of human volunteers (*41*). Following consumption of a 200 ml drink containing 0.25-2.0 g of limonoid glucoside, blood was collected and analyzed for the presence of limonoids. In each case, the presence of the aglycone, limonin, was observed. The mean time to maximum concentration was 6 h. No ill effects among the test subjects were detected.

Beneficial Roles of Citrus Flavonoids: From Cell Assays to Animal Studies

Much of the early work on citrus flavonoids focused on tangeretin and nobiletin, two polymethoxylated flavonoids primarily found in the peels of tangerines and oranges. Research with tangeretin and nobiletin has shown that these chemicals can inhibit, *in vitro*, the proliferation of cancer cells (*42-44*) including a human squamous cell carcinoma (HTB43), a gliosarcoma (9L) and two melanoma cell lines (B16F10 and SK-MEL-1). Tangeretin was also found to inhibit the microsome-catalyzed binding of benzo[a]pyrene to DNA (*45*) and the binding of aflatoxin B1 to DNA (*46*).

Work with the polymethoxylated flavonoids primarily has centered on the possible effects of these compounds on the final phase of carcinogenesis, progression. Early studies (*47-49*) using a chick heart assay for measuring the potential for invasion and metastasis showed that tangeretin and to a lesser extent nobiletin inhibited the movement of mouse MO4 cells (Kirsten murine sarcoma virus transformed fetal mouse cells) and MCF-7/6 cells (human breast cancer cell line) into the embryonic chick heart fragments. Research (*49,50*) with the breast cancer cell line showed that tangeretin was upregulating the function of the E-cadherin/catenin complex leading to greater cell-cell adhesion. Since tamoxifen exhibits similar inhibitory effects on the growth and invasive properties of mammary cancer cells *in vitro*, studies were conducted to see if this citrus flavonoid might increase tamoxifen's therapeutic effect *in vivo* (*51*). Unfortunately, the results showed that tangeretin essentially neutralized tamoxifen's inhibitory effect, possibly because tangeretin had downregulated a receptor on T-lymphocytes and natural killer cells (*50,51*).

A couple of investigators have also looked at the potential health-promoting activity of two flavonoids, hesperetin and neohesperidin, that are commonly found in high concentrations in orange juice. Neohesperidin has been shown to have highly significant alkylperoxyl radical-scavenging activity (*52*). These lipid peroxyl-radicals have been shown to enhance colon carcinogenesis in rats treated with carcinogens (*53*). The results of a second paper, however, suggest that neohesperidin is not a strong antioxidant (*54*). Other studies suggest that citrus flavonoids might be used to prevent heart disease. In rats it was found that blood cholesterol levels were reduced by feeding diets supplemented with citrus flavonoids, primarily a mixture of hesperetin and naringin (*55*). Further research with HepG2 cells (*39,56*) showed that a mixture of hesperetin and naringenin significantly reduced, in a dose-dependent fashion, the secretion of apolipoprotein B. In addition, ^{14}C-acetate labeling studies showed a reduction in cholesterol ester synthesis in the presence of these compounds. Tangeretin produced a similar effect (*57*). More recently (*58*) the cholesterol-lowering potential of tangeretin and a mixture of naringin and hesperetin were compared. In a hamster model, tangeretin proved to be the more effective cholesterol- and triacylglycerol-lowering agent.

The predominant flavonoids in grapefruit and grapefruit juice are naringin and naringenin. The combined concentration in grapefruit juice usually exceeds 1,000 ppm (*59*). As already indicated, combinations of naringin and hesperetin have been shown to be cholesterol- and triacylglycerol-lowering agents (*39,55,56,58*). In another study (*60*) using rabbits (New Zealand White rabbits) consuming high-cholesterol diets, it was shown that diets containing naringin (0.1%) and naringenin (0.05%) had no apparent affect on plasma lipoprotein, total cholesterol, triglyceride, and high-density lipoprotein levels. However, the aortic fatty streak areas were significantly lowered in the groups receiving the diets containing naringin and naringenin. In an eight-week feeding trial with humans (normal and hypercholesterolemic subjects), it was found that naringin supplementation (400 mg/capsule/day) lowered plasma total cholesterol by 14% and low-density lipoprotein cholesterol by 17% in the hypercholesterolemic patients (*61*). The plasma triglyceride and the high-density lipoprotein concentrations were not affected. Naringin supplementation had no affect on the lipid plasma profiles in the normal subjects.

The data from a number of different studies suggest that naringin and naringenin possess cancer chemopreventive potential. Naringenin and to a lesser extent naringin have been shown to inhibit the α-hydroxylation pathway in the microsomes that converts the tobacco-specific nitrosamine, NNK, into the ultimate carcinogen (*62*). Both compounds produced a similar effect on the microsomal pathway that converts heterocyclic amines into active carcingens (*63*). Recently, it was also reported that various doses (0.5-8.0 mg/kg body weight) of naringin protected mouse bone marrow cells against radiation-induced

DNA damage (*64*). The naringin was administered forty-five minutes before the exposure to the γ-irradiation. In addition, naringenin and naringin have also demonstrated antineoplastic activity in a number of different animal models for carcinogen-induced neoplasia. In one experiment (*65*), it was found that a naringin-supplemented diet (0.5%) reduced DMBA-induced mammary tumor burden by approximately 20%. A naringenin-supplemented diet (0.25%) proved to be ineffective. Recently, it was reported that both naringin and naringenin inhibited the development of DMBA-induced oral tumors in Syrian hamsters (*66*) and azoxymethane-induced aberrant crypt foci in Sprague Dawley rats (*67,68*). In the hamster cheek pouch model, naringin again proved to be more effective. The treatments with naringin reduced average tumor burden by 70%, while the treatments with naringenin lowered average tumor burden by 30%. Additional evidence supporting the possible use of naringin and naringenin as cancer chemopreventive agents can be found in the results of an epidemiological study (*69*). In-person interviews were used to assess smoking history and the intake of 242 food items for 582 patients with incident lung cancer and 582 matched controls. A statistically significant inverse association was found between lung cancer risk and the intake of white grapefruit.

Research with naringenin has shown that this compound can inhibit the growth of a variety of different human cancer cell lines. Early studies with MDA-MB-435 human breast cancer cells showed that naringenin could inhibit cell proliferation by 50%, IC_{50}, at a concentration of 18 μg/ml (*65*). Naringenin-induced cytotoxicity has now been demonstrated in a wide variety of human cell lines derived from cancers of the breast, stomach, leukemia, colon, pancreas, liver, and cervix (*70*). Naringenin also inhibited tumor growth in sarcoma S-180 implanted mice (70). Naringin was also effective in this mouse model when given by peroral injection (70).

Citrus and Drug Interactions

During the last decade one species of citrus, grapefruit (*Citrus paradisi* Macf) was identified as having an effect on the availability of certain medications. Alternatively, it may be possible to administer the affected drugs in lower dosages when taken along with grapefruit juice, which may prolong availability making the drug more effective. Unlike other citrus species, grapefruit contain large quantities of naringin and small quantities of certain furocoumarins. These bioactive compounds increase the bioavailabilities of certain medications by specifically inhibiting CYP3A activity in the gastrointestinal tract (*71*). However, these bioactive compounds have other positive health benefits. For example, grapefruit juice has been shown to protect against aflatoxin- (a potent hepatocarcinogen) induced damage to liver DNA (*72*). Future directions and challenges relative to drug interactions are discussed in Chapter 17.

Other Health Benefits of Citrus

During the last decade, grapefruit has been suggested to promote weight reduction. However, no scientific evidence was available to justify this observation until several recent investigations. Grapefruit has long been thought to possess weight loss properties. Scientific evidence to support this commonly held belief is now starting to appear. In a recent study at the Scripps Clinic Nutrition and Metabolic Research Center in San Diego, fresh grapefruit intake before meals was associated with a 1.6 kilogram weight loss in obese patients over a 12-week period. Grapefruit consumption also improved insulin levels in patients with a cardiovascular risk factor known as metabolic syndrome (*73*). These intriguing findings are discussed in greater detail by Drs. Fujioka and Lee in Chapter 16.

There also exists some evidence that citrus pectin has the potential to reduce weight along with possessing other health promoting properties. Citrus pectin inhibits the binding of fibroblast growth factor (FGF) with its corresponding receptor, and since the FGF signal pathway has been linked to cholesterol metabolism, citrus pectin may possibly affect cholesterol metabolism (*74*).

While clinical indications and the effectiveness of citrus pectin and modified citrus pectin (MCP), a low molecular pectin, are still being studied, research results suggest that both citrus pectin and MCP have significant health benefits (75-78). In vitro investigations and animal studies have demonstrated the potential of pectins to prevent and treat cancer based on reducing solid tumor growth, metastasis, and angiogenesis (*79*). Recent research has also indicated that MCP may play an important therapeutic role as a chelator of heavy metals (79). Questions related to the size of pectin molecules that can enter the bloodstream and play a therapeutic role remain unanswered. The health benefits, including clinical indications, preclinical research, clinical data, dosage and safety, of MCP are discussed in Chapter 15.

Other citrus components, including carotenoids, limonoids, vitamin C, flavonoids, furocoumarins, folate, and d-limonene (a terpenoid) also possess anticarcinogenic activity. Some of these constituents are discussed in detail in Chapters 6,8,9,10,11,12 and 18.

Optimization of Bioactive Compounds Through Pre- and Postharvest Factors

Awareness of the health benefits of natural phytochemicals has prompted the exploration of preharvest and postharvest factor effects on the levels of phytochemicals. Pre- and postharvest factors can be exploited to achieve an optimal phytochemical content and minimize phytochemical degradation. For example, the concentration of bioactive compounds can be enhanced through the optimum use of nitrogen (*81*) and potassium (*82*), as well as growth regulators (*83,84*). Many studies on citrus trees have been conducted that examine the impact of agricultural factors on only a single bioactive compound, vitamin C. Likewise, in many studies more than one macro-and/or micro-nutrient were applied to the trees simultaneously to monitor their effect on the level of any given phytochemical (*85*), which makes identification of the specific beneficial nutrient effect difficult.

A number of important preharvest and postharvest factors have been identified. Accumulating evidences suggest that auxins may affect positively the limonoids and vitamin C content in citrus fruits (*86-88*). Gibberellic acid application showed positive effects on limonin and naringin (*89*). Very little information is available on the effect of preharvest factors on storage potential and changes in levels of citrus bioactive compounds. It has been suggested that higher storage temperatures after the harvested grapefruit was treated with 2-(4-Chlorophenylthio)-triethylamine hydrochloride leads to increased lycopene accumulation (*90*). Nagy reported that citrus fruits lose vitamin C when stored at temperatures above 5 ^{0}C; the degree of loss depends on temperature and type of the fruit (*91*). A decline of lycopene during storage of grapefruit juice for 12 months was reported (*92*). A significant decrease in the concentration of carotenoids occurred when citrus fruits were stored for 1 year at 4 ^{0}C compared to -80 ^{0}C (*93*). Previous reviews provide information on the impact of several processing factors on the variability in vitamin C content of citrus fruits and their products (*91*). Many of the vitamin C data were collected 25 years ago before major changes occurred in processing techniques and packing materials. Lee and Coates (*94*) conducted an extensive research on the variation of vitamin C content in processed Florida citrus juice products over the last ten years. It was concluded that vitamin C retention can vary markedly depending the type of container used. Our recent results demonstrated that total flavanone and carotenoid levels were changed during storage when different grapefruit juice cartons (100% pure fresh juice and not from concentrate), cans (100% juice from concentrate), and cocktails (35% juice from concentrate) were stored. However, no specific trend was observed. When cocktail in polyethylene toluene (PET) containers were stored at room temperature, the levels of vitamin C were significantly decreased; however, limonin glucoside and lycopene levels were increased. It seems that the functional components in grapefruit juice change during storage depending on the container used (*95*). Our recent results suggest that postharvest irradiation and freeze drying have significant effects on the bioactive components of grapefruit (*96-98*). Thus, it is important to take postharvest processing into consideration when fruit- and vegetable-based dietary supplements are being developed. In order to accurately assess results for the chemopreventive ability of fruit and vegetable components, it is essential to use suitable methods for preservation of bioactive compounds. More investigations are needed to fully evaluate the effect of pre- and postharvest storage potential and level of bioactive compounds.

The Analytical Challenges and Opportunities of Bioactive Compounds in Citrus and Human Tissues

The identification and quantification of bioactive compounds in citrus and related biotransformation products in plasma, urine, and tissue presents both an enormous analytical challenge and a significant opportunity for the development of new methods and strategies. The scope of the analytical challenges can be appreciated by considering some of the complex issues related to investigations of phytochemicals and their health benefits, as discussed in many of the chapters presented in this book. For example, the structures of the sub-groups of each class of bioactive compound and their resulting biotransformation products may have great diversity, therefore making their analysis a complicated and intricate problem. Since many phytochemicals exist as glycosides in plants, the site of glycosylation and identification of the attached sugars are important structural aspects. Likewise, many phytochemicals are hydrolyzed upon consumption, thus increasing the number of chemical forms that must be considered in any type of pharmacokinetics or biotransformation study. Moreover, the bioactivities of compounds may change greatly depending on subtle structural variations, and plants frequently produce isomers that further increase the complexity of structural differentiation. The levels of bioactive compounds in citrus and in urine, plasma or tissue may vary over several orders of magnitude, adding another degree of difficulty in quantitative analysis. An ideal analytical method would offer both the specificity, sensitivity, and dynamic range for the confident identification and quantification of phytochemicals and their metabolites in both citrus matrices and biological samples (urine, plasma, tissue, etc.).

For the most comprehensive and detailed studies of phytochemicals, a strategy involving complementary analytical methods is typically warranted. For example, the capabilities of NMR spectroscopy for detailed structural identification or confirmation of structures are unsurpassed, yet the amount of sample necessary is relatively high, and the applicability for on-line analysis of compounds following chromatographic separation is limited. UV-Vis absorption spectroscopy affords far better detection limits than NMR methods, yet the level of structural information obtained is insufficient for differentiation of some classes of isomers or elucidation of many structural details. Mass spectrometry offers an excellent blend of structural information and utility as a detector for chromatographic separations, in addition to affording very good detection limits. In general, a combination of several analytical methods provides the best framework for addressing both quantitative and qualitative aspects for studies of phytochemicals, whether in citrus, biological samples, or both.

Although these well-established analytical methods have been very useful for numerous applications related to structural identification and quantification of bioactive compounds (*99,100*), there is an ongoing need for new methods that offer improved sensitivity, both in terms of detection limits and the ability to differentiate subtle structural details. For example, new separation strategies, including capillary electrophoresis and capillary liquid chromatography, offer advantages for minimization of sample consumption or improvement in absolute detection limits. New tandem mass spectrometric methods afford more structural information and have shown promise for isomer distinction. Some of these methods and developments will be described later in Chapter 4, but there remains considerable opportunity for further development, optimization and validation of analytical methods to address the complex types of problems described throughout this book. This is expected to be an active and essential area of research activity in the coming decade.

References

1. Potter, J.D.; Steinmetz, K. IARC Sci Publi. **1996**, *139*, 61-90.
2. Nishino, H. *J. Cell Biochem Suppl. 1997; 27*, 86-91.
3. Clinton, S.K. *Nutr. Rev.* **1998,** *56*, 35-51.
4. Silalahi, J. *Asia Pacific J. Clin. Nutr.* **2002**, *11*, 79-84.
5. Youdim K.A.; Spencer J.P.E.; Schroeter H.; Evans, R. C., *Biol. Chem.* **2002,** *383*, 503-519.
6. Youdim K.A.; Michael S.D.; Gunter, K.; Proteggente, A.R.; Abbott, N.J.; Rice-Evans, C. **2003**. *J. Neurochem.* **2003,** *85*, 180-192.
7. Caragay, A.B. *Food Tech.* **1992**, *46,* 65-68.
8. Nakanishi, K. *Recent Adv. Phytochem.* **1975**, *9*, 283-289.
9. Gaaboub, I.A.; Hayes, D.K. *Environ. Entomol.* **1984**, *13*, 803-810.
10. Arnason, J.T.; Philogene, B.J.R.; Donskov, N.; Hudon, M.; McDougall, C.; Fortier, G.; Morand, P.; Gardner, D.; Lambert, J.; Morris, C.; Nozolillo, C. *Entomol. Exp. Appl.* **1985**, *38*, 29-35.
11. Klocke, J.A.; Kubo, I. *Entomol. Exp. Appl.* **1982**, *32*, 299-301.

12. Alford, A.R.; Bentley, M.D. *J. Econ. Entomol.* **1986**, *79*, 35-38.
13. Alford, A.R.; Cullen, J.A.; Storch, R.H.; Bentley, M.D. *J. Econ. Entomol.* **1987**, *80*, 575-578.
14. Ruberto, G.; Renda, A.; Tringali, C.; Napoli, E.M.; Simmonds, M.S. *J. Agric. Food Chem.* **2002**, *50*, 6766-6774.
15. Jayaprakasha, G.K.; Singh, R.P.; Pereira, J.; Sakariah, K.K. *Phytochemistry* **1997**, *44*, 843-846.
16. Bentley, M.D.; Rajab, M.S.; Alford, A.R.; Mendel, M.J.; Hassanali, A. *Entomol. Exp. Appl.* **1988**, *49*, 189-193.
17. Liu, Y.B.; Alford, A.R.; Bentley, M.D. *J. Econ. Entomol.* **1991**, *84*, 1154-1157.
18. Murray, K.D.; Groden, E.; Drummond, F.A.; Alford A.R.; Conley, S.; Storch, R.H.; Bentley, M.D. *Environ. Entomol.* **1995**, *24*, 1275-1283.
19. Murray, K.D.; Groden, E.; Drummond, F.A.; Alford, A.R.; Storch, R.H.; Bentley, M.D. *Entomol. Exp. Appl.* **1996**, *80*, 503-510.
20. Alford, A.R.; Murray, K.D. *Citrus Limonoids Functional Chemicals in Agriculture and Food*; American Chemical Society: Washington, DC, **2000**; pp 201-211.
21. Murray, K.D.; Alford, A.R.; Groden, E.; Drummond, F.A.; Storch, R.H.; Bentley, M.D.; Sugathapala, P.M. *J. Econ. Entomol.* **1993**, *85*, 1793-1801.
22. Alford, A.R. *Advances in Potato Pest Biology and Management*; APS Press: St. Paul, MN, **1994**; pp 342-356.
23. Lam, L.K.T.; Hasegawa, S. *Nutr. Cancer* **1989**, *12*, 43-47.
24. Miller, E.G.; Fanous, R.; Rivera-Hidalgo, F.; Binnie, W.H.; Hasegawa, S.; Lam, L.K.T. *Carcinogenesis* **1989**, *10*, 1535-1537.
25. Lam, L.K.T.; Zhang, J.; Hasegawa, S. *Food Technol.* **1994**, *48*, 104-109.
26. Lam, L.K.T.; Zhang, J.; Hasegawa, S.; Schut, H.A.J. *Food Phytochemicals for Cancer Prevention I. Fruits and Vegetables*; American Chemical Society: Washington, DC, **1994**; pp 209-219.
27. Lam, L.K.T.; Hasegawa, S.; Bergstrom, C.; Lam, S.H.; Kenney, P. *Citrus Limonoids Functional Chemicals in Agriculture and Foods*; American Chemical Society: Washington, DC, **2000**; pp 185-200.
28. Tanaka, T.; Maeda, M.; Kohno, H.; Murakami, M.; Kagami, S.; Miyake, M.; Wada, K. *Carcinogenesis* **2001**, *22*, 193-198.
29. Lam, L.K.T.; Li, Y.; Hasegawa, S. *J. Agric. Food Chem.* **1989**, *37*, 878-880.
30. Miller, E.G.; Gonzales-Sanders, A.P.; Couvillon, A.M.; Wright, J.M.; Hasegawa, S.; Lam, L.K.T. *Nutr. Cancer* **1992**, *17*, 1-17.
31. Miller, E.G.; Gonzales-Sanders, A.P.; Couvillon, A.M.; Binnie, W.H.; Hasegawa, S.; Lam, L.K.T. *Food Technol.* **1994**, *48*, 110-114.
32. Miller, E.G.; Porter-Wright, J.L.; Binnie, W.H.; Guo, I.Y.; Hasegawa, S. *Hypernutritious Foods*; AGSCIENCE Inc.: Auburndale, FL, **1996**; pp 191-204.

33. Miller, E.G.; Porter, J.L.; Binnie, W.H.; Guo, I.Y.; Hasegawa, S. *J. Agric. Food Chem.* **2004**, *52*, 4808-4813.
34. Guthrie, N.; Morley, K.; Hasegawa, S.; Manners, G.D.; Vandenberg, T. *Citrus Limonoids Functional Chemicals in Agriculture and Foods*; American Chemical Society: Washington, DC, **2000**; pp 164-174.
35. Tian, Q.G.; Miller, E.G.; Ahmad, H.; Tang, L.; Patil, B.S. *Nutr. Cancer* **2001**, *40*, 180-184.
36. Miller, E.G.; Taylor, S.E.; Berry, C.W.; Zimmerman, J.A.; Hasegawa, S. *Citrus Limonoids Functional Chemicals in Agriculture and Foods*; American Chemical Society: Washington, DC, **2000**; pp 132-144.
37. Poulose, S.M.; Harris, E.D.; Patil, B.S. *J. Nutr.* **2005,** *135*, 870-877.
38. Kim, Mi-Ja; Park, H.J.; Hong, M.S.; Park, H.J.; Kim, M.S.; Leem, K.H.; Kim, J.B.; Kim, Y.J.; Kim, H.K. *Nutr. Cancr.* **2005**, 51, 78-82.
39. Kurowska, E.M.; Banh, C.; Hasegawa, S.; Manners, G.D. *Citrus Limonoids Functional Chemicals in Agriculture and Foods*; American Chemical Society: Washington, DC, **2000**; pp 175-184.
40. Battinelli, L.; Mengoni, F.; Lichtner, M.; Mazzanti, G.; Saija, A.; Mastroianni, C.M.; Vullo, V. *Planta Med.* **2003**, *69*, 910-912.
41. Manners, G.D.; Jacob, R.A.; Breksa, A.P.; Schoch, T.K.; Hasegawa, S. *J. Agric. Food Chem.* **2003**, *51*, 4156-4161.
42. Kandaswami, C.; Perkins, E.; Soloniuk, D.S.; Drzewiecki, G.; Middleton, E. *Cancer Lett.* **1991**, *56*, 147-152.
43. Kandaswami, C.; Perkins, E.; Drzewiecki, G.; Soloniuk, D.S.; Middleton, E. *Anticancer Drugs* **1992**, *3*, 525-ending page number.
44. Rodriguez, J.; Yanez, J.; Vicente, V.; Alcaraz, M.; Benawente-Garcia, O.; Castillo, J.; Lorente, J.; Lozano, J.A. *Melanoma Res.* **2002**, *12*, 99-107.
45. Le Bon, A.M.; Siess, M.H.; Suschetet, M. *Chem. Biol. Interact.* **1992**, *83*, 65-71.
46. Siess, M.H.; Le Bon, A.M.; Canivenc-Lavier, M-C.; Suschetet, M. *Biofactors* **2000**, *12*, 193-199.
47. Bracke, M.; Vyncke, B.M.; Van Larebeke, N.A.; Bruyneel, E.A.; De Bruyne, G.K.; De Pestel, G.H.; De Coster, W.J.; Espeel, M.F.; Mareel, M.M. *Clin. Exp. Metastasis* **1989**, *7*, 283-286.
48. Bracke, M.; Vyncke, B.; Opdenakker, G.; Foidart, J.M.; De Pestle, G.; Mareel, M.M. *Clin. Exp. Metastasis* **1991**, *9*, 13-ending page number.
49. Bracke, M.E.; Bruyneel, E.A.; Vermeulen, S.J.; Vennekens, K.; Van Marck, V.; Mareel, M.M. *Food Technol.* **1994**, *48*, 121-125.
50. Bracke, M.E.; Boterberg, T.; Depypere, H.T.; Stove, C.; Leclercq, G.; Mareel, M. M. *Adv. Exp. Med. Biol.* **2002**, *505*, 135-141.
51. Bracke, M.E.; Depypere, H.T.; Boterberg, T.; Van Marck, V.L.; Vennekens, K.M.; Vanluchene, E.; Nuytinck, M.; Serreyn, R.; Mareel, M.M. *J. Natl. Cancer Inst.* **1999**, *91*, 354-360.

52. Sawa, T.; Nakao, M.; Akaike, T.; Ono, K.; Maeda, H. *J. Agric. Food Chem.* **1999**, *47*, 397-402.
53. Sawa, T.; Akaike, T.; Kida, K.; Fukushima, Y.; Takagi, K.; Maeda, H. *Cancer Epidemiol. Biomarkers Prev.* **1998**, *7*, 1007-1011.
54. Yu, J.; Wang, L.; Walzem, R.L.; Miller, E.G.; Pike, L.M.; Patil, B.S. *J. Agric. Food Chem.* **2005**, *53*, 2009-2014.
55. Bok, S-H.; Lee, S-H.; Park, Y-B.; Bae, K-H.; Son, K-H.; Jeong, T-S.; Choi, M-S. *J. Nutr.* **1999**, *129*, 1182-1185.
56. Borradaile, N.M.; Carroll, K.K.; Kurowska, E.M. *Lipids* **1999**, *34*, 591-598.
57. Kurowska, E.M.; Manthey, J.A.; Casaschi, A.; Theriault, A.G. *Lipids* **2004**, *39*, 143-151.
58. Kurowska, E.M.; Manthey, J.A. *J. Agric. Food Chem.* **2004**, *52*, 2879-2886.
59. Patil, B.S. *Proc. Intl. Soc. Citricult. IX Congr.* **2000**, *volume II*, 1184-1187.
60. Lee, C.H.; Jeong, T.S.; Choi, Y.K.; Hyun, B.H.; Oh, G.T.; Kim, E.H.; Kim, J.R.; Han, J.I.; Bok, S.H. *Biochem. Biophys. Res. Commun.* **2001**, *284*, 681-688.
61. Jung, U.J.; Kim, H.J.; Lee, J.S; Lee, M.K.; Kim, H.O.; Park, E.J.; Kim, H.K.; Jeong, T.S.; Choi, M.S. *Clin. Nutr.* **2003**, *22*, 561-568.
62. Bear, W.L.; Teel, R.W. *Anticancer Res.* **2000**, *20*, 3323-3330.
63. Bear, W.L.; Teel, R.W. *Anticancer Res.* **2000**, *20*, 3609-3614.
64. Jagetia, G.C.; Reddy, T.K. *Mutat. Res.* **2002**, *519*, 37-48.
65. So, F.V.; Guthrie, N.; Chambers, A.F.; Moussa, M.; Carroll, K.K. *Nutr. Cancer* **1996**, *26*, 167-172.
66. Miller, E.G.; Peacock, J.J.; Taylor, S.E.; Wright, J.M.; Patil, B.S. *HortScience* **2004**, *39*, 742.
67. Leonardi, T.; Vanamala, J.; Taddeo, S.S.; Murphy, M.E.; Patil, B.S.; Wang, N.; Chapkin, R.S.; Lupton, J.R.; Turner, N.D. FASEB J. **2004,** 18:A477.
68. Vanamala, J.; Leonardi, T.; Murphy, M.E.; Taddeo, S.S; Patil, B.S.: Pike, L.M.; Chapkin, R.S.; Lupton, J.R.; Turner, N.D. FASEB J. **2004,** 18:A894.
69. Le Marchand, L.; Murphy, S.P.; Hankin, J.H.; Wilkens, L.R.; Kolonel, L.N. *J. Natl. Cancer Inst.* **2000**, *92*, 154-ending page number.
70. Kanno, S.; Tomizawa, A.; Hiura, T.; Osanai, Y.; Shouji, A.; Ujibe, M.; Ohtake, T.; Kimura, K.; Ishikawa, M. *Biol. Pharm. Bull.* **2005**, *28*, 527-532.
71. Bailey, D.G.; Spence, J.D.; Munoz, C.; Arnold, J.M. Lancet **1991**, 337:268-269.
72. Miyata M.; Takano, H.;. Guo, L.; Nagata, K.; Yamazoe, Y. *Carcinogenesis.* **2004,** 25, 203- 209.
73. Fujioka, K.; Greenway, F.; Sheard, J.; Ying, Y. The effects of grapefruit on weight and insulin resistance: relationship to the metabolic syndrome. *J Med Food* **2005** (in press).

74. Yu, C.; Wang, F.; Kan, M.; Jin, C.; Jones, R. B.; Weinstein, M.; Deng, C.; McKeehan, W. L. *J. Biol. Chem.* **2000**, *275*, 15482–15489.
75. Pienta, K.J.; Naik, H.; Akhtar, A.; Yamazaki, K.; Replogle, T.S.; Lehr, J.; Donat, T.L.; Tait, L.; Hogan, V.; Raz, A. *J. Natl. Cancer Inst.* **1995**, *87*, 348–353.
76. Liu, Y.; Ahmad, H.; Luo, Y.; Gardiner, D.T.; McKeehan, W.; Patil, B.P. *J. Agri. Food Chem.*, **2001**, *49,* 3051-3057.
77. Liu, Y.; Ahmad, H.; Luo, Y.; Gardiner, D.T.; McKeehan, W.; Gunasekara, R.S.; Patil, B.S. *J. Sci. Food Agri.* **2002**, *82*, 469-477.
78. Eliaz, I. *Clinical applications of modified citrus pectin.* Abstracts of Papers, 229th ACS National Meeting, San Diego, CA, United States, March 13-17, **2005**, CELL-148.
79. Nangia-Makker P, Hogan V, Honjo Y, Baccarini S, Tait L, Bresalier R, and Raz A. *J Natl Cancer Inst.* **2002**, *94*, 1854-1862
80. Eliaz, I. Modified citrus pectin (MCP) in the treatment of cancer. Paper presented at: *The American Chemical Society Annual Meeting:* August 23, **2004**; Philadelphia, PA.
81. Patil, B.S.; Pike, L.M.; Hamilton, B.K *New Phytologist* **1995,** *130*, 349-355.
82. Trudel, M.J.; Ozbun, J.L. *J. Amer. Soc. Hort. Sci.* **1971,** *96,* 763-765.
83. Hasegawa, S.; Herman, Z. *Phytochemistry* **1986**, *25*, 2523-2524.
84. Hasegawa, S.; Herman, Z.; Orme, E.; Ou, P. *Phytochemistry* **1986**, *25*, 2783-2785.
85. Mozafer, A. J. Plant Nutr. **1993,** *16*, 2479-2506.
86. Hasegawa, S.; Maier, V.P.; Herman, Z.; Ou, P. *Phytochemistry* **1986**, *25*, 1323-1325.
87. Hasegawa, S.; Herman, Z.; Ou, P. *Phytochemistry* **1986**, *25*, 542-543.
88. Orme, E.D.; Hasegawa, S. *J. Agric. and Food Chem.* **1987**, *4*, 512-513.
89. Shaw, P.E.; Calkins, C.O.; McDonald, R.E.; Greany, P.D.; Webb, J.C.; Nisperos-Carriedo, M.O.; Barros, S.M. *Phytochemistry* **1991**, *30*, 3215-3219.
90. Coggins, C.W. Jr.; Hall, A.E.; Jones, W.W. *J. Amer. Soc. Hort. Sci.* **1981,** *106*:251-254.
91. Nagy, S. *J.Agric. Food Chem.* **1980,** *28*, 8-18.
92. Stein, E.R.; Brown, H.E.; Cruse, R.R. *J. Food Sci.* **1986,** *51*, 574-587.
93. Craft, N.E.; Wise, S.A.; Soares, J.H., Jr. *J. Agric.Food Chem.* **1993**, *41*, 208-213.
94. Lee, H.S.; Coates, G.A. *J. Agric. Food Chem.* **1997,** *45*, 2550-2555.
95. Patil, B.S. Functional Components in Citrus Beverages. *In:* Nutraceutical Beverages, Chemistry, Nutrition and Health Effects, Editors: Shahidi, F and Weerasinghe. *American Chemical Society Symposium Series 871.* Washington, D.C. **2004**, pp 103-122
96. Patil, B.S. Irradiation applications to improve functional components of fruits and vegetables. *American Chemical Society Symposium Series 875.*

In: "Irradiation of Food and Packaging: Recent Developments." Editors: V. Komolprasert. **2004**, pp 117-137.

97. Patil, B.S., Vanamala, J.; Hallman, G. *Postharvest Biology and Technology* **2004,** *34,* 53-64.
98. Vanamala, J., Cobb, G.; Turner, N.D.; Lupton, J.R.; Yoo, K.S.; Pike, L.M.; Patil, B.S. *Journal of Agri. Food Chem.* **2005**, *53*, 3980-3985.
99. Stecher, G.; Huck, C.W.; Stoggl, W.M.; Guggenbichler, W.; Bakry, R.; Bonn, G.K. *Phytochem. Rev.* **2002**, *1*, 413-426.
100. van Elswijk, D.A.; Irth, H. *Phytochem. Rev.*, **2003**, *1*, 427-439.

Isolation and Characterization of Citrus Bioactive Compounds

Chapter 2

Citrus Bioactive Limonoids and Flavonoids Extraction by Supercritical Fluids

Bhimanagouda S. Patil[1], Jun Yu[1], Deepak V. Dandekar[1], Romeo T. Toledo[2], Rakesh K. Singh[2], and Leonard M. Pike[1]

[1]Vegetable and Fruit Improvement Center, Department of Horticultural Sciences, Mail Code 2119, Texas A&M University, College Station, TX 77843
[2]Department of Food Science and Technology, University of Georgia, Athens, GA 30602

The increasing use of organic solvents for extraction of bioactive compounds is a significant environmental concern. In the present report, limonoids and flavonoids were extracted from grapefruit (*Citrus paradisi Macf.*) seeds by an environmentally-friendly supercritical CO_2 extraction (SC-CO_2) technique. Optimum conditions for extraction of limonoid aglycones, such as pressure, temperature, extraction time, CO_2 flow rate and the feeding modes of CO_2, were determined. The highest yield of limonin was 6.3 mg/g seeds at 48.3 MPa, 50°C and 60 min with CO_2 flow rate of approximately 5.0 l/min being fed from the top of the column. The highest extraction yield of limonin glycoside was 0.62 mg/g defatted seeds which was obtained at 48.3 MPa, 50°C and 30% ethanol in 40 min with flow rate of SC-CO_2 of 5.0 l/min and fed from the top of the column. Furthermore, the maximum extraction of naringin (0.2 mg/g defatted seeds) was obtained under the conditions of 41.4 MPa, 50°C, 20% ethanol, 40 min with CO_2 flow rate of approx. 5.0 l/min. The results demonstrated practical commercial application of SC-CO_2 extraction of limonoids and flavonoids from grapefruit seeds.

Introduction: Citrus Limonoids and Flavonoids

Citrus fruits are very popular foods in the world. Limonoids and flavonoids are important constituents of citrus fruits, which provide beneficial effects on human health. Citrus flavonoids have been the subject of intense biochemical investigation in past years (*1-5*). Flavonoids are one of the most diverse groups of plant secondary metabolites from both structural and functional points of view. Limonoids, on the other hand, are a rare natural product group with highly oxygenated triterpenoid backbones. The biological activities, and both food and commercial applications of these compounds have been investigated, and there is increased interest in limonoids for their potential cancer prevention properties (*6-12*).

With the growing interest in the health promoting properties of citrus limonoids, the demand for these chemicals has increased significantly. Various methods and techniques have been investigated for efficient extraction and purification of these compounds from various citrus species (*13*). Different methods of extraction have their own advantages and limitations. But all of them have certain common goals described as follows:

- To obtain the product in its original form, it is important that the damage done to the product during processing should be minimal and the product should be free from undesirable impurities.
- The final yield of the product should be maximum and the method of extraction must be economical.

The main challenge in extraction technology thus lies in selectively transferring the potential compounds present inside cells to the bulk extract.

In recent years, supercritical fluid-based extraction has gained commercial importance as an efficient method of extraction for natural products. Supercritical fluid extraction is a clean technology providing acceptable yields and purity (*14, 15*).

Why Super Critical Fluids (SCF) are useful in Natural Product Extraction?

Any pure compound goes through various phases depending on pressure and temperature conditions. Near absolute zero temperature most of the compounds remain in the solid phase with very low vapor pressure. As temperature increases with constant pressure (isobaric condition), the phase changes from solid to liquid to gas. Similarly, when pressure increases with constant temperature (isothermal condition) the phase changes from gas to liquid. When temperature against pressure is plotted for a compound, a typical diagram shows solid-liquid-gas phases, triple point and critical point (Figure 1). It is important to define 'critical point' to understand supercritical condition.

Critical point for a compound can be simplified by resolving it into two aspects.

- Critical Temperature: Beyond this temperature, any increase in pressure will not turn gas into liquid. The density may increase to approach that of a liquid but there is no latent heat associated with the change as there is no change in phase.
- Critical Pressure: Beyond this pressure, any increase in temperature will not turn liquid into gas.

If a fluid is subjected to conditions beyond both the critical temperature and critical pressure, then it will be neither gas nor liquid. It will have the density and solvation properties of a liquid but the viscosity and diffusivity will be those of a gas. This kind of resonating phase or hybrid phase gives the fluid characteristics of both liquid and gas combining advantages of high solvation capacity of a liquid with faster diffusion of a gas. Thus, while searching for better solvents for more efficient extraction, scientists have been using supercritical fluids that possess both gas- and liquid-like characters.

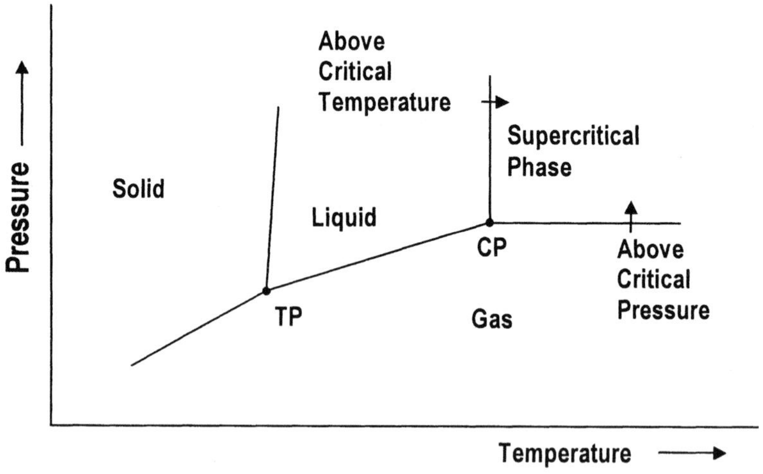

Figure 1: Pressure-temperature diagram for pure compound

To improve efficiency of the extraction process, selectivity is an important characteristic along with diffusion. Selectivity can be defined as the higher solvation capacity of the solvent towards one compound over another. The solvation capacity of the solvent towards any compound or group of compounds changes directly as a function of pressure and temperature. This gives a possibility of manipulating selectivity by pressure and temperature adjustments. It is possible that changing the range of pressure or temperature or both will lead to extraction of completely different compounds or groups of compounds from the same raw material. Improving selectivity thus involves selecting temperature and pressure parameters such that solubility of impurities is at a minimum and solubility of the solute is maximized.

A typical solubility isotherm in the supercritical region demonstrates a sigmoidal curve (Figure 2). This suggests an exponential increase in solvent capacity towards a particular solute with respect to pressure at a constant temperature. These conditions increase the possibility of extracting certain compounds or groups of compounds by selecting temperatures and pressures where the solubilities of these compounds is maximized. Changing these conditions will change the selectivity for different compounds or groups of compounds.

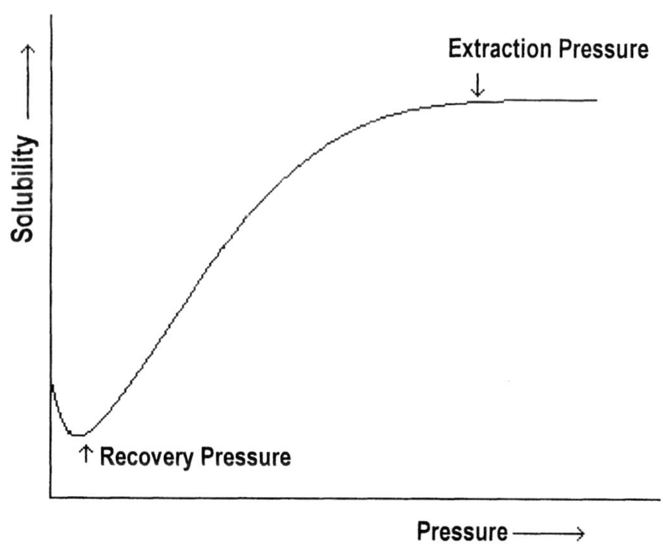

Figure 2: Solubility of solute with respect to pressure at constant temperature

The sigmoidal behavior of solubility enables easy recovery of the dissolved compounds. Close to the critical point, the latent heat of vaporization is very low; i.e. separation of the product from the extract is simple and consumes very little energy. A drop in pressure should be sufficient to recover the extract from the solvent phase.

One strategy entails completion of the extraction at high pressure i.e. at the upper part of the pressure isotherm (Figure 2). At these conditions, the thermodynamic stability of the dissolved solute in the supercritical solvent is high which can be defined as a high solvent capacity for the solute. After the first step, the extract should be separated from the raw material at the same temperature and pressure. Then the pressure is reduced, keeping the temperature constant until the lower side of the curve is reached where solubility is less or negligible (Figure 2). The compound will be precipitated from the extract, as gaseous phase of solvent cannot retain it any longer. No residual solvent will remain in the precipitated solute to cause undesirable health effects.

Carbon dioxide: an ideal SCF solvent

Carbon dioxide (CO_2) is a readily available gas with favourable properties as a supercritical fluid (*14*). When CO_2 attains its supercritical state, its solvating capacity increases exponentially but its viscosity remains like a gas phase. Its diffusivity increases, which allows rapid transfer of the solute from the solid to the solvent phase. The high solvent diffusivity reduces the cycle time for extraction and minimizes the volume of the extraction vessel. CO_2, being gaseous at ambient temperature, can flow in and out of the extraction vessel easily and in its supercritical state can dissolve desired compounds on par with low polar solvents. Recovery of products is very easy. The critical temperature of carbon dioxide is 31° C, which makes it suitable solvent for heat sensitive compounds. Furthermore use of CO_2 makes the conditions anaerobic for highly unsaturated compounds. From the process point of view, handling CO_2 is safe and there is no residual solvent problem in the final products.

When the chemical structure and orientation of atoms in CO_2 molecule is considered, it has two oxygen atoms attached to a carbon but in a perfectly symmetrical manner, which makes supercritical CO_2 a non polar solvent which can be used to extract non polar solutes. To increase the polarity of the supercritical CO_2 often a co-solvent or entrainer is mixed in a very small concentration (1 to 5 mol%). The co-solvent system is in a supercritical state when the pressure and temperature are above the critical pressure and temperature, which are usually not very different from critical values of pure CO_2. The entrainer also gives specific interactions with the solute, which helps in extraction (*15*)

$SC-CO_2$ has been studied extensively for extraction of potential natural compounds from various sources. Many methods and procedures are patented and scaled up for production purposes. Decaffination of coffee and tea using $SC-CO_2$ is widely employed in the food processing industry. Different processes were studied for extraction of different functional compounds/groups from natural products such as flavours and fragrances from flowers and fruits, oils and flavours from spices, natural antioxidants and other potential medicinal compounds from herbs, natural food colours, plant and animal lipids, natural pesticides etc (*14-25*).

Recent studies of the extraction of citrus using $SC-CO_2$ have reported that limonoids and flavonoids could be extracted from citrus seed and byproducts (*26*). During fruit maturation, the glucosidation of the monolactones occurs in the seeds. Three processes are triggered simultaneously in seeds, viz. lactonization of monolactones, aglycone synthesis and the glucosidation of aglycones (*6*). Therefore seeds can be considered as the best source for limonoid aglycones as well as for limonoid glucosides. However, very little information is available on the application of co-solvent, operating parameters and other factors influencing the extraction from seeds. We present here a case study of the process development for extraction of citrus limonoids (both aglycones and glycosides simultaneously) and flavonoids from grapefruit (*Citrus paradisi* Macf) seeds using $SC-CO_2$ and a suitable entrainer. We have studied the extraction of naringin along with limonin and limonin glucoside (LG), and the results are modeled to optimize the best extraction conditions.

Experimental

Grapefruit seeds were obtained from fruits harvested at the Texas A&M University-Kingsville Citrus Center, Weslaco, TX. Seeds were dried under shade, ground, mixed, and preserved at -20°C. All solvents were HPLC grade (Fisher Scientific, Atlanta, GA). High purity CO_2 was used for supercritical fluid extraction (SFE). SFE schematics are illustrated in Figure 3. Analysis of all the SFE extracts was completed using HPLC-UV2000 (Thermo Hypersil-Keystone Company, USA) equipped with a reversed C18 Waters Spherisorb ODS column (250mm x 4.6mm). Analysis conditions were used as described by Yu et al. and Raman et al., as modified for current study (*27, 28*). Limonoid aglycones were eluted from a column using an isocratic mobile phase, water:methanol (6:4) with a flow rate of 1.0 ml/min, with elution of all limonoids achieved after 70 min. Individual limonoids were analyzed in 20 μl of sample with elution of individual peaks being monitored at 210 nm. Limonoid glucosides were separated using the same column and a linear gradient with flow rate of 1.0 ml/min which had a starting composition of 10% acetonitrile in 0.03 mM phosphoric acid and a final composition of 24% acetonitrile in 0.03 mM phosphoric acid. Elution of limonoid glucosides within 20 μl aliquots were completed in 80 min, and elution time of individual eluates were determined by monitoring at 210 nm. Citrus flavonoids were separated by HPLC using the same C18 Waters Spherisorb ODS column eluted with a mobile phase comprised of water:acetonitrile:acetic acid (81.5:18:0.5) flowing at a rate of 1.0 ml/min for 45min. Injection volumes of 20 μl were used, with the elution of individual flavonoid compounds being monitored at 284 nm.

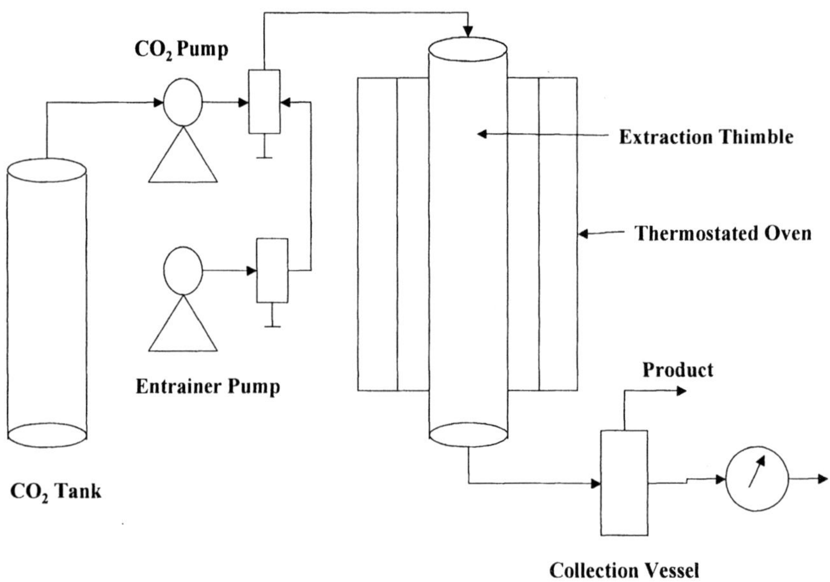

Figure 3: Schematic diagram of SC-CO_2 extraction

To optimize the process for SC-CO_2 extraction, different parameters were altered and the yield of desired compounds was evaluated as a function of specific parameters. Furthermore, the effect of changes in one parameter on other parameters and their combined effects on the total yield were studied. The data was collected in a manner such that the maximum possible information could be obtained from the minimum number of experiments.

Design of Experiment (DOE)

Box-Behnken design was used to achieve maximum information about the process from minimum possible experiments (Figure 4). In the above process three variables (from among pressure, temperature, time of extraction, and percent of entrainer were selected for each set of experiments while keeping the flow rate constant through all the experiments (5.0 l/min). The Box-Behnken design is an independent quadratic design in which the treatment combinations are at the midpoint of the edge of the process space and the center. This design has limited capability for orthogonal blocking compared to Central Composite Designs (CCD) but for three factors, Box-Behnken design requires fewer numbers of runs than CCD.

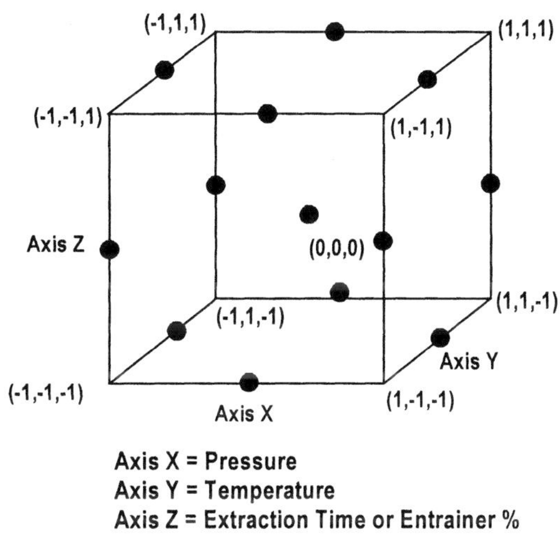

Figure 4: DOE Box Behnken

In general, extraction from grapefruit seeds was completed in two stages as shown in the process flow diagram (Figure 5). In stage one, pure SC-CO_2 was passed over raw material to target extraction of limonoid aglycones. After stage one, the second stage extraction was done using a SC-CO_2 ethanol system to target extraction of limonoid glucosides and flavonoids.

To determine the optimum conditions for SC-CO_2 extraction of limonoids and flavonoids, the yields of prominent limonoids such as limonin (from the limonoid aglycone group), limonin glucoside (LG) (from the limonoid glucoside group) and naringin (from the flavonoid group) were determined (Figure 6). The analysis of the extract was completed at various time intervals to determine the extraction kinetics (data not included here) and at the end the total yield was determined. Since compounds in each group are closely related having the same basic structure, it was assumed that the same optimum conditions (with similar variation) should be reasonable for other compounds in the group.

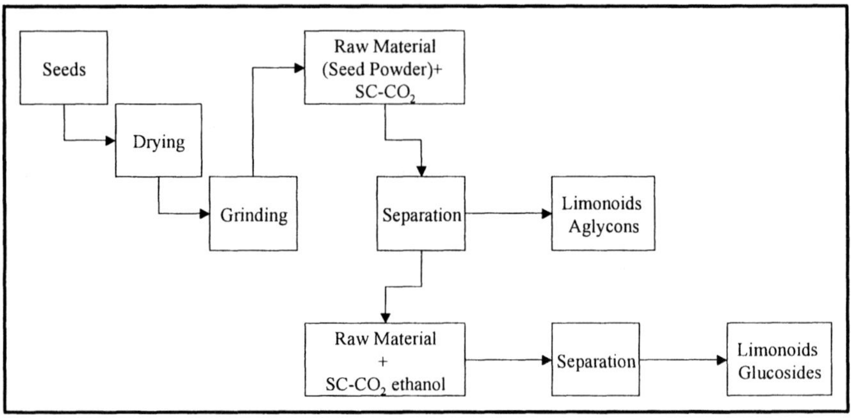

Figure 5: Process Flow Diagram

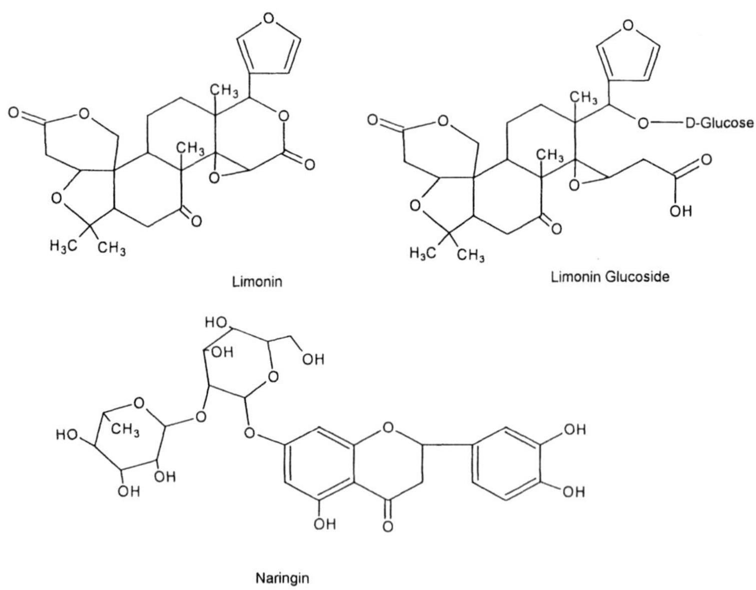

Figure 6: Structures of limonin, LG and naringin

Previous work using SC-CO_2 demonstrated that the time required for complete extraction was a function of the CO_2 flow rate (*14*). High flow rates resulted in fast extraction but reduced the solute yield per liter of SC-CO_2, and low flow rates required prolonged extraction time before maximal solute extraction was achieved. Therefore, considering the practical requirements such as the extraction yield and operation cost, in the present study we chose a SC-CO_2 flow rate of 5.0 l/min.

The challenges in SC-CO_2 extraction of limonoids and flavonoids process

The main challenge in extraction technology lies in selectively transferring the potential compounds present inside cells to the bulk extract. Understanding the mass transfer behavior helps in the process design for SC-CO_2 extraction from citrus seeds. Since the feed is a solid in this study, it makes the raw material a fixed bed on which SC-CO_2 or SC-CO_2 ethanol mixed system flows as a continuous flow solvent phase. However, the mechanism of mass transfer is also dependent on the botanical nature of citrus seeds compared to only the flow characteristics of the SC-CO_2 or SC-CO_2 ethanol mix system.

During extraction of seeds, solvent diffuses through different layers of cells, dissolves limonoids, and brings them into bulk. Grinding the seeds increases the surface area and helps in removing the diffusion resistance, however, using very fine particles of raw material causes processing problems such as clogging the inlet/outlet, high back pressures, formation of a cake of raw material, increased impurities, etc. Therefore, it is possible that the particle size of raw material in the process will be a limiting factor. Even after grinding into finer particles, the solvent still needs to be able to diffuse through the cell walls, reach the desired compounds, and dissolve them. Thus, the rate of mass transfer was determined by the time taken for solvent diffusion and the dissolution of desired compounds. The specific interactions between solvent and solute determine selectivity in extraction. SC-CO_2, being non-polar, selectively dissolves limonoid aglycones while the polar entrainer (ethanol in this case) dissolves limonoid glucosides and naringin.

Results and Discussion

SFE using SC-CO_2 is a solid-liquid type extraction, which is usually done in batches where solids are loaded in the extractor through which SC-CO_2 is passed at a constant flow rate. The mobile phase can be passed either in an upward or downward direction depending on the convenience of handling; however, usually an upward flow eliminates any channeling effect and gives a more even distribution of mobile phase through the extraction vessel. In the present study both upward flow and downward flows were compared to optimize the efficiency of the process while keeping all other parameters same. Table I gives the parameters and results of this study.

Table I: Effect of feeding mode on extraction

Mode of Feeding	*Average yield* of limonin*	*Average yield* of LG*
Top	4.5	0.51
Bottom	5.3	0.43

* (mg/gm of dry seeds)

It was found that when pure SC-CO_2 was passed to target limonoid aglycones, it gave better results when the mobile phase was introduced from the bottom. In the case of the SC-CO_2 ethanol system, to our surprise a top-feeding mode gave a better yield of LG than a bottom feeding mode. It is difficult to explain this result as the nature of mass transfer kinetics depends on where and how the solute is bound to the cellulose matrix and its mechanism of release and transport within the solid matrix, in addition to the pressure and temperature conditions and specific interactions between the solvent and solute.

Response surface analysis (RSA) was completed for the yield data from a number of runs. Due to instrument handling and analytical limitations, performing all the runs in very short time was not possible. This long experimental scheme was stretched over a period of two weeks. Seeds were collected, dried, ground, mixed and preserved at -20°C to make the process variation due to seed composition negligible. Furthermore, the minute deviations due to instrument conditions were beyond control and were considered as noise.

During stage one of all the experiments, the variables selected were pressure, temperature and time of extraction. The yield of limonin obtained from each experiment was studied as a function of these three variables. The extraction conditions that gave the maximum yield of limonin (6.3 mg/g dried seeds) consisted of 48.3 MPa, 50°C and 60 min with SC-CO_2 fed from the bottom.

Response surface analysis of the data demonstrates that the relationship between limonin yield and pressure, temperature and time of extraction was a quadratic with very good regression coefficients (R^2=0.99). RSA shows that the yield goes through maxima with varying pressure and temperature (Figure 7). The density of SC-CO_2 varies with pressure and temperature, and a higher density dissolves more solute. Yield with respect to time of extraction shows a steady increase before a plateau is reached, indicating depletion of solute in the raw material. Finally, a maximum predicted yield of 6.8 mg/g dry seeds was determined by RSA under the conditions, 46 MPa, 43°C and 90 min. This yield is slightly higher than the actually obtained yield of 6.3 mg/g of dry seeds with pressure and temperature conditions almost similar. However, the extraction time required is 50% greater, which may be a critical point in deciding the process conditions.

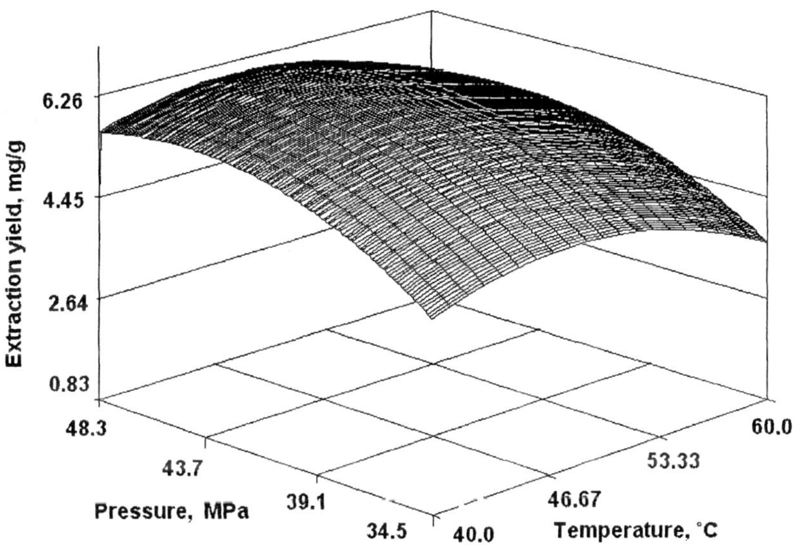

Figure 7: RSA limonin

During stage two of all the runs, the variables selected were pressure, temperature and percent of ethanol. The yield of LG and naringin obtained from each run was then studied independently as a function of these three variables. The extraction conditions that gave the maximum yield of LG (0.62 mg/g dried seeds) consisted of 48.3 MPa, 50°C and 30% ethanol with SC-CO_2 and top feeding. In the case of naringin, the maximum yield of naringin (0.2 mg/g dried seeds) was obtained under the conditions of 41.4 MPa, 50°C, 20% ethanol.

RSA of yield data for LG yielded a quadratic relationship between LG yield and pressure, temperature and percent of ethanol with very good regression coefficients (R^2=0.99). It illustrates that all three parameters studied are critical for extraction yield of LG. The model predicted that the yield of 0.73 mg of LG/g defatted seeds can be achieved by setting conditions at 42 MPa, 52°C and 45% ethanol with top feeding (Figure 8).

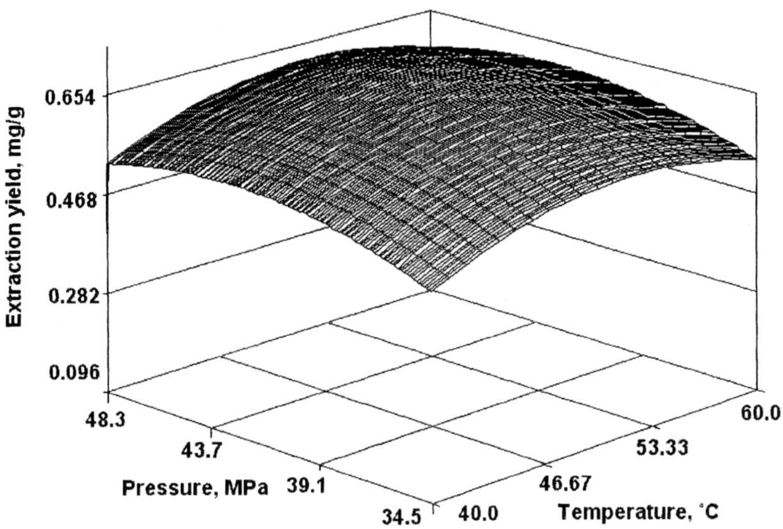

Figure 8: RSA LG

The results indicated that the region selected for extraction in this experimental design is more appropriate for limonin and LG than naringin. Giannuzzo et al. (*26*) studied the extraction conditions for extraction of naringin from peels of *Citrus paradisi.* They showed that within a temperature range of 40-60°C and an ethanol range of 5-15%, the pressure of 9.5 MPa gives very good yield of naringin. In the present study, the pressure conditions were too high for naringin extraction, and naringin at these conditions is thus considered a byproduct.

Conclusion

The SC-CO_2 extraction provides a very good strategy for extraction of limonoids and flavonoids from grapefruit seeds. The same process can be easily extended and modified for extraction of limonoids and flavonoids from different species of citrus and from citrus juice, peels, albedo, flavedo or seeds. The optimum conditions can provide limonoids aglycones, limonoids glucosides and flavonoids free from each other. The operating conditions are non-intensive and easy to set and run. The process can be easily scaled up for all the three important groups of compounds and can be run as a continuous process with appropriate instrumentation modifications.

Acknowledgements

Funded by USDA 2001-52102-11257 and ATP 003658-0359c-2001

References

1. Benavente-Garcy'a, O.; Castillo, J.; Marin, F. R.; Ortuno, A.; Del Rio, J. A. *J. Agric. Food Chem.* **1997,** *45*, 4505-4515.
2. Scambia, G.; Ranelletti, F. O.; Benedetti-Panici, P.; De Vincenzo, R.; Bonanno, G.; Ferrandina, G.; Piantelli, M.; Bussa, S.; Rumi, C.; Cianfriglia, M. *Cancer Chemother. Pharmacol.* **1994,** *34*, 459-464.
3. Bronner, W. E.' Beecher, G. R. *J. Chromatogr. A.* **1995,** *705*, 247-256.
4. Hollmam, P. C. H.; Hertog, M. G. L.; Katan, M. B. *Biochem. Soc. Trans.* **1996,** *24*, 785-789.
5. Soares, N. F. F.; Hotchikiss, J. H. *J. Food Sci.* **1998,** *63*, 61-65.
6. Hasegawa, S.; Berhow, M. A.; Manner, G. D.; Citrus limonoids research: an overview, in: M.A. Berhow, S. Hasegawa and G.D. Manner, (Eds.), *Citrus Limonoids: Functional Chemicals in Agriculture and Foods*, American Chemical Society, Washington, DC **2000,** p 1-8.
7. Lam, L. K. T.; Li, Y.; Hasegawa, S.; *J. Agric. Food Chem.* **1989,** *37*, 878-880.
8. Lam, L. K. T.; Hasegawa, S.; Bergstorm, C.; Lam, S. H.; Kenney, P.; Limonin and nomilin inhibitory effects on chemical-induced tumorigenesis, in: M.A. Berhow, S. Hasegawa and G.D. Manner, (Eds.), *Citrus Limonoids: Functional Chemicals in Agriculture and Foods*, American Chemical Society, Washington, DC **2000,** p 185-200.

9. Miller, E. G.; Taylor, S. E.; Berry, C. W.; Zimmerman, J. A.; Hasegawa, S.; Citrus limonoids: increasing importance as anticancer agents, in: M.A. Berhow, S. Hasegawa and G.D. Manner, (Eds.), *Citrus Limonoids: Functional Chemicals in Agriculture and Foods*, American Chemical Society, Washington, DC **2000,** p 132-144.
10. Tian, Q. G.; Miller, E. G.; Ahmad, H.; Tang, L. L.; Patil, B. S.; *Nutr. Cancer* **2001,** *40*, 180-184.
11. Guthrie, N.; Morley, K.; Hasegawa, S.; Manners, G. D.; Vandenberg, T. S.; Inhibition of human breast cancer cells by citrus limonoids, in: M.A. Berhow, S. Hasegawa and G.D. Manner, (Eds.), *Citrus Limonoids: Functional Chemicals in Agriculture and Foods*, American Chemical Society, Washington, DC **2000,** p 164-174.
12. Kurowska, E. M.; Banh, C.; Hasegawa, S.; Manner, G. D.; Regulation of apo B production in HepG2 cells by citrus limonoids, in: M.A. Berhow, S. Hasegawa and G.D. Manner, (Eds.), *Citrus Limonoids: Functional Chemicals in Agriculture and Foods*, American Chemical Society, Washington, DC 2000a, **2000,** p.185-200.
13. Braddock, R. J.; Cadwallader, K. R.; *Food Technol.* **1992,** *46*, 105-110.
14. Mukhopadhyay, Mamata. *Natural Extraction using supercritical carbon dioxide* CRC Press LLC **2000**
15. Rozzi, N. L.; Singh, R. K. *Comprehensive Rev. Food Sci. Food Safety* **2002,** *1*, 33-44.
16. Sihvonen, M.; Jarvenpaa, E.; Hietaniemi, V.; Huopalahti, R. *Trends Food Sci. Technol.* **1999,** *10*, 217-222.
17. Chouchi, D.; Barth, D.; Nicoud, R. M.. *Proc. 3rd Intl. Symp. SCFs* **1994,** *2*, 183.
18. Randall, J. M.; Schultz, W. G.; Morgan, A. I. *Confructa* **1971,** *16*, 10-19.
19. Calame, J. P.; Stainer, R. *Supercritical extraction of flavours, in Theory and Practice of Supercritical Fluid Technology*, Hirata, M.; Ishikawa, T. Eds., Tokyo Metropolitan Univ. **1987**, p 275.
20. Della Porta, G.; Reverchon, E; Ambrousi, A. *Proc. 5th Meet. SCFs*, France **1998,** *2*, 613.
21. Nguyen, U.; Anstee, M.; Evans, D. A. *Proc. 5th Meet. Super Critical Fluids*, France, 2, Nice, France **1998,** p 523.
22. Then, M.; Daood, H.; Illes, V.; Bertalan, L. *Proc. 5th Meet. Super Critical Fluids*, France **1998,** *2*, 555.
23. Gao, Y.; Simandi, B.; Sass-Kiss, A. Stefanivits, P.; Zs, F.; Czukor, B. *Proc. 4th Intl. Symp. SCFs*, Sendai, Japan, may, **1997**.
24. Jennings, D. W.; Howard, M. D.; Zalkow, L. H.; Teja, A. S. *J. Supercritical Fluids*, 5, No. 1, 1, March **1992**.
25. Kerey, A.; Simandi, B.; Royani, E.; Lemberkovics, E. *Proc. 5th Meet. Supercritical Fluids*, France **1998,** *2*, 561.

26. Giannuzzo, A. N.; Boggetti, II. J.; Nazareno, M. A.; Mishima, H. T. *Phytochemical, Anal.* **2003,** *14*, 221-223.
27. Yu, J.; Wang, L.; Walzem, R. L.; Miller, E. G.; Pike, L. M.; Patil, B. S. *J. Agricultural and Food Chemistry* **2005,** *53* (6), 2009-2014.
28. Raman, G; Jayaprakasha, G. K.; Broadbelt, J.; Cho, M.; Patil, B. S. *Analytical Letters* **2004,** *37* (14), 3005-3016.

Chapter 3

Methods for the Separation of Limonoids from Citrus

Guddadarangavvanahally K. Jayaprakasha[1], Jennifer S. Brodbelt[2], Narayan G. Bhat[3], and Bhimanagouda S. Patil[1]

[1]Vegetable and Fruit Improvement Center, Department of Horticultural Sciences, Mail Code 2119, Texas A&M University, College Station, TX 77843
[2]Department of Chemistry and Biochemistry, University of Texas at Austin, Austin, TX 78712
[3]Department of Chemistry, The University of Texas–Pan American, 1201 West University Drive, Edinburg, TX 78539

Limonoids are naturally occurring triterpenes found in Rutaceae and Meliaceae family plants. Many citrus limonoids have proved to be particularly difficult to purify using conventional methods. This chapter provides an overview of the methods used to extract and purify limonoid aglycones and limonoid glucosides from citrus, including solid liquid extraction, column chromatography, preparative HPLC and flash chromatography. Furthermore, recent literature on analytical methods such as HPLC and LC-MS for the separation and identification of limonoids have been discussed.

Recent studies have demonstrated the natural health promoting properties of fruits and vegetables. Accumulating epidemiological evidence suggests that a strong positive association exists between a diet rich in fresh fruit and vegetables and a decreased risk of cardiovascular diseases and certain forms of cancer (1). It is generally assumed that the active dietary constituents contributing to these protective effects are primarily the antioxidant nutrients. However, more recent work has highlighted the additional role of polyphenolic components in plants (2), which may act not only as antioxidants but also as agents with other mechanisms that contribute to their anticarcinogenic or cardioprotective actions. These bioactive compounds also have potential applications in food stabilization due to their ability to protect against peroxidation of oxygen sensitive foods.

Citrus species are a rich source of several bioactive compounds such as citric acid, ascorbic acid, furocoumarins, folate, carotenoids, limonoids and flavonoids. Determination limonoids and flavonoids in *Citrus* fruits is necessary to understand their biological properties. Limonoids are naturally occurring highly oxygenated triterpenes found in *Rutaceae* family, which include Citrus fruits regularly consumed by humans such as orange, grapefruit, mandarin, lemon and lime. Their basic structure contains a furan ring attached at C-17, oxygen-containing functional groups, a 14,15-epoxide group and a methyl or oxymethylene at C-19. Limonin and nomilin (Figure 1) are the most prevalent of the citrus limonoid aglycones (3).

Until recently, citrus health-promoting properties have always been associated with their content of vitamin C; only in the last decade have studies shown that several bioactive compounds, specifically limonoids and flavonoids play a major role in preventing chronic diseases. Growing evidence seems to suggest that limonoids and flavonoids have different biological functions, including antioxidative, anti-inflammatory, antiallergic, antiviral, antiproliferative, antimutagenic, and anticarcinogenic activities (3-6). Therefore, new Citrus cultivars have been developed for fresh consumption. Furthermore, the particular characteristics of these bioactive compounds have the potential to be used in the pharmacological and food technology area (7, 8).

Structure-function relationship of limonoids

The typical limonoid structure as illustrated in Figure 1 consists of five rings termed as A, A', B, C and D. Limonin differs from nomilin in the absence of the A' ring. Limonin and nomilin has six and seven membered A ring respectively. Nomilin and deacetylnomilin (Figure 1) are similar in structure to obacunone except with changes in the A ring at C-1 and C-2 positions. Maturation of fruit causes glucosidation of the D-ring in limonin resulting in formation of limonin glucoside (9). Previous studies have proven that the intact A ring in limonin, limonin glucoside, nomilin and obacunone (Figure 1) inhibited the average tumor burden in 7,12-dimethylbenz[a]anthracene induced hamster buccal pouch

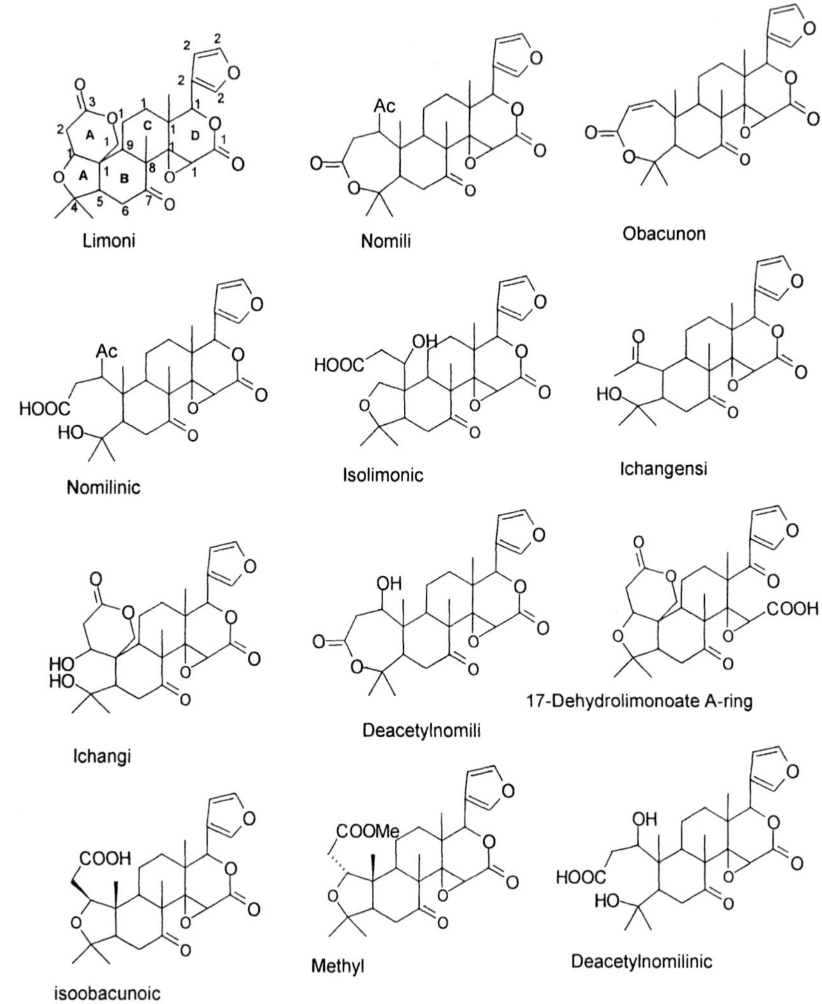

Figure 1. Structures of limonoid aglycones identified from citrus

tumors (10). Nomilin, obacunone and limonin, in decreasing order, have shown to be potent inducers of a detoxifying enzyme system, glutathione S transferase (GST), which may lead to the inhibition of chemically induced carcinogenesis (11). Another study reported obacunone and limonin to be active inhibitors of preneoplastic lesions in rat colon, with an induction of liver GST (12). One of our own recent studies showed that individual limonoid glucosides differ in efficacy as anticancer agents and this difference may reside in structural variations in the A ring of the limonoid molecule (13).

In addition to the human health benefits, citrus limonoids have also been shown to possess several activities in the control of specific insect pests. Obacunone, nomilin, and limonin are found to inhibit moulting in mosquito (*Culex quinquefasciatus*), which suggests their potential utility in formulation of eco-friendly pesticides (14). Another report confirmed the significant antifeedent activity of limonin and obacunone in a study involving *Spodoptera frugiperda* larvae (15).

Extraction and purification of limonoid aglycones

Limonin was first isolated and identified by Bernay in 1841. Later it was obtained from a series of citrus and related *Rutaceae* (16-18) from plant parts, such as fruit, seeds, bark and roots. Emerson (19) reported isolation of limonin from Navel orange juice with benzene. The benzene extracts were concentrated to a minimum volume and limonin was precipitated by the addition of three volumes of petroleum ether. The crude limonin was crystallized by methylene chloride. In another method by the same authors (19), limonin was isolated from Valencia orange seeds. Seed powder was defatted with petroleum ether and extracted with acetone. The acetone extract was concentrated to a thin syrup, diluted with ethanol and concentrated again to obtain most of the limonin. The remaining portion of limonin was secured by the addition of water. Further purification was achieved by crystallization from methylene chloride and alcohol. Nomilin was extracted from the mixture by boiling for a few minutes with a minimum amount of isopropyl alcohol and filtering the hot solution. On cooling nomilin was crystallized. Further purification was accomplished by recrystallization out of methanol from which nomilin separated as slender needles. Emerson (20) also isolated limonoids from raw citrus seed oil. The oil was mixed with petroleum ether and filtered through filter aid such as supercel. The residue was separated, then extracted with acetone and 95% methanol. The crude bitter fraction obtained by concentrating the methanol and acetone extracts was worked up as previously described to obtain limonin and nomilin (19). Obacunone was obtained from the mother liquors of limonin and nomilin. It was separated from limonin due to its greater solubility in isopropyl alcohol and from nomilin because of its greater solubility in hot toluene. Further purification was done by recrystallization from acetone, and then from ethyl acetate. However, this strategy used benzene and toluene, which are now known to be carcinogens.

Since aglycones are compounds of medium polarity, they can be easily extracted with organic solvents. In an another study (21) ground seeds of *P. trifoliata* was extracted with petroleum ether and concentrated to obtain crystalline material which was collected and recrystallized from ethyl acetate-petroleum ether to give deacetyl nomilin (Figure 1). Structure of the compound was confirmed by nuclear magnetic resonance (NMR) (21). The isolation and identification of ichangin from defatted Ichang lemon seeds was completed using acetone (22). The dried fraction was extracted with chloroform and washed with 5% sodium bicarbonate. The solvent was removed from the neutral fraction and the residue was collected in benzene and chromatographed on acid-washed alumina. Elution with benzene gave fractions containing obacunone. Elution with chloroform gave limonin and nomilin. Elution with 10% acetone in chloroform gave fractions containing ichangin; further elution gave deacetylnomilin (Figure 1). The structures of the compounds were identified by NMR studies (22). Bennett (23) reported the separation of five acidic limonoids from grapefruit seeds. Defatted seed powder was extracted with acetone, and the major portion of limonin was removed by crystallization. The leftover mother liquid was partitioned between water and chloroform. The chloroform extract was loaded onto a silica gel column and eluted with dichloromethane and methanol to obtain neutral limonoids. The acidic limonoids were eluted with dichloromethane, methanol and acetic acid. Furthermore, the acidic fraction was methylated with diazomethane in order to facilitate separation of its components by column chromatography to obtain isoobacunoic acid, methyl epi-isoobacunoic acid, nomilinic acid and deacetyl nomilinic acid (Figure 1).

Limonin aglycones can be isolated by conventional open column chromatography using alumina or silica gel as an adsorbent. Hsu et al. (24) reported the extraction of neutral and acidic limonoids from ground tissues of lemon seeds and orange peels using acetone. The dried residue was extracted with chloroform, concentrated and dried. Further, the potassium bicarbonate soluble fraction was extracted with chloroform and pH was adjusted to 2.0 using dilute hydrochloric acid. Acidic limonoids were extracted using chloroform and subjected to methylation and loaded onto silica gel column chromatography to obtain methyl 17-dehydrolimonoate A-ring lactone. Hasegawa et al. (25) used citrus seeds for the extraction of limonoids using tris buffer at pH 8.0 at room temperature. The mixture was incubated at 18 hours to hydrolyze the D ring (soluble acids) by the limonin D-ring lactone hydrolase present naturally in the seeds. The mixture was filtered and acidified to get D ring lactones, and the acidic mixture was extracted with dichloromethane to obtain a mixture of aglycones. Furthermore, individual limonoids were separated on a silica gel column. Bennett and Hasegawa (26) isolated and purified isolimonic acid from *C. aurantium* using Tris buffer at pH 8.2. The extract was filtered through Celite and the filtrate was acidified to pH 2 and extracted with dichloromethane. The residue was separated into acidic and neutral fractions by a method described

(25). The acidic fraction was methylated and separated on a silica gel column via elution with increasing concentrations of ethyl acetate in dichloromethane to obtain methyl isolimonate.

Bennett and Hasegawa (27) extracted defatted grapefruit seed powder with hexane and acetone successively. The acetone extract was fractionated using silica gel column chromatography and eluted with methanol and dichloromethane to get semi-purified fractions containing obacunone, limonin and deacetyl nomilin. These fractions were further subjected to repeated column chromatography to get pure crystallized compounds. Bennett et al. (28) reported the isolation of limonoids from the seeds of *Citrus ichangensis* using tris buffer as mentioned earlier (25). The extract was fractionated by preparative TLC to obtain pure ichangensin. However, the authors have not specified the yield of the pure compound. Three aglycones such as limonin, nomilin and obacunone were purified from *Citrus reticulata* using silica gel column chromatography for the first time (14). More recently, limonin, nomilin, obacunone and deacetyl nomilin were isolated from red Mexican grapefruit seeds for the first time using open column chromatography. The structures of the isolated compounds have been confirmed using spectroscopic studies (29).

Extraction and purification of limonoid glucosides

Since limonoid glucosides are polar compounds (see Figure 2), these compounds can be easily extracted with polar solvents such as water or MeOH. Bennett et al. (30) and Hasegawa et al. (31) extracted grapefruit seed powder with hexane, acetone and methanol. Methanol extract was fractionated twice on amberlite XAD-2 column and eluted with 5% and 65% methanol in water. Fractions containing glucosides were further purified by chromatography on DEAF Sephacel, eluting with dilute hydrochloric acid. Finally, the hydrochloric acid was removed from the glucoside fractions by passing through a C_{18} column adsorbent followed by elution with methanol to obtain limonoid glucosides. Ozaki et al. (32) used 'Yuzu' seed powder for the extraction of limonoids using acidic water (pH 4.0) using pectinase enzyme. The mixture was centrifuged and loaded onto a XAD-2 column. The column was eluted with acetonitrile and concentrated; pH was adjusted to 6.5 and loaded to DEAF sephacel column. The column was first washed with water and glucosides were eluted with dilute sodium chloride. The fractions were desalted and injected onto preparative HPLC to obtain ichangensin glucoside. Several other plants from Rutaceae were used for separation of limonoids. A methanol extract of *Tetradium rutaecarpa* fruit powder was loaded onto a DEAF – Sephacel column. The column was eluted with sodium chloride and the glucoside-containing fractions were pooled and pH was adjusted to 3.5. After repeated fractionation using an XAD-2

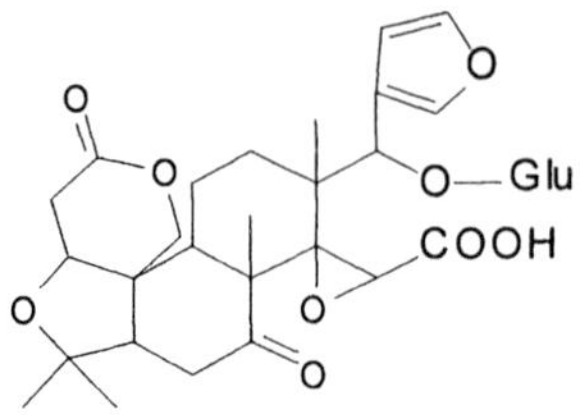

Limonin glucoside

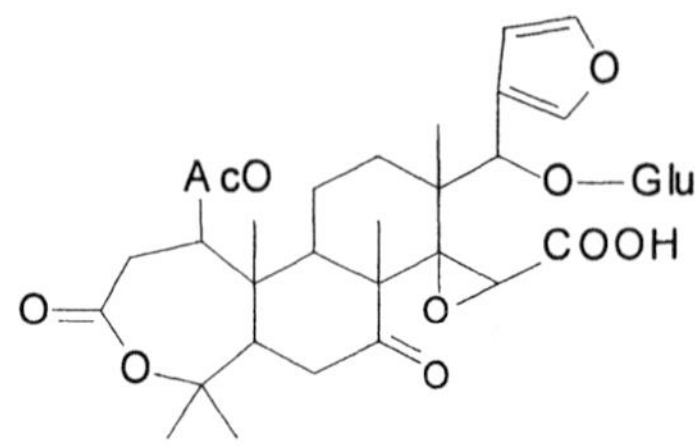

Nomilin glucoside

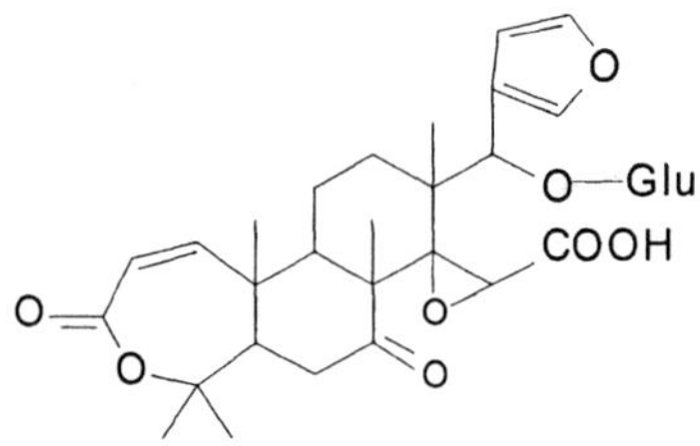

Obacunone glucoside

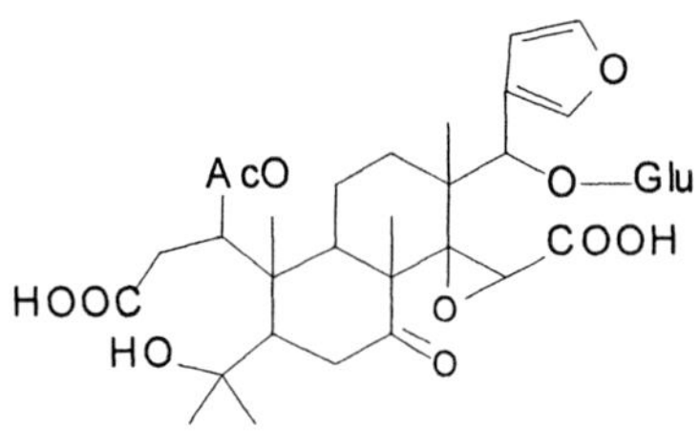

Nomilinic acid glucoside

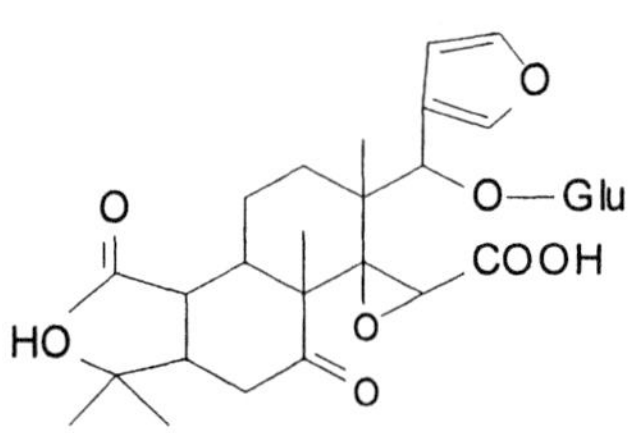

Ichangensin glucoside

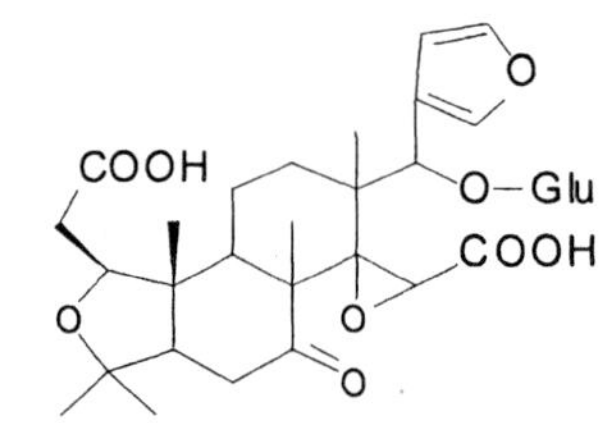

isoobacunoic acid glucoside

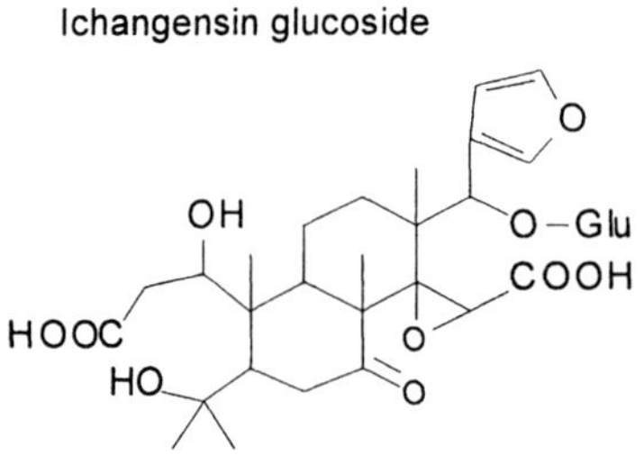

Deacetylnomilinic acid glucoside

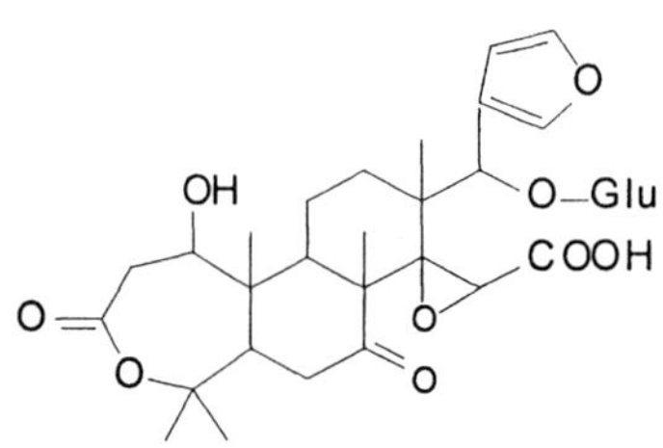

Deacetylnomilin glucoside

Figure 2. Structures of Limonoid Glucosides

column, three glucosides were obtained. However, the procedure required the use of four to five columns, and the authors did not specify the yield of the pure compounds (33). *Citrus aurantium* seed powder was extracted in water at pH 4.0 using pectinase enzyme for 20 h. The mixture was centrifuged and loaded onto an XAD-2 column. The fractions were subjected to preparative HPLC twice to obtain 19-hydroxydeacetylnomilinic acid glucoside, isolimonic acid glucoside and ichangin glucoside. However, the method required several unit operations and preparative HPLC. It is very difficult to obtain large quantities of limonoids using HPLC. The authors have not specified the yield of the pure compounds (34).

Miyake et al. (35) extracted ground citrus seeds with acidic water. The homogenate was stirred with pectinase for 20 h and centrifuged. The clear filtrate was loaded onto the top of an XAD-2 column, and the column was thoroughly washed with water. Then limonoid glucosides were eluted with MeOH and subjected to C-18 reversed-phase preparative HPLC to obtain four glucosides. Generally, it is more laborious to obtain multi-gram quantities of compounds using preparative HPLC methods. Sawabe et al. (36) reported the extraction of three limonoid glucosides from *C. unshiu* peels. Dried peel powder was homogenized with hot water and filtered. The filtrate was loaded onto an amberlite XAD-2 column and washed with a water and water: MeOH mixture. The fraction eluted with water:MeOH (1:1) was separated over neutral alumina. The column was eluted with MeOH:water to obtain mixtures of limonoid glucosides. Finally, this fraction was further purified using silica gel column chromatography to get nomilinic acid 17-*O*-β-D-glucopyranoside, methyl nomilinate 17-*O*-β-D-glucopyranoside and obacunone 17-*O*-β-D-glucopyranoside. Recently, Schoch et al. (37) isolated limonoid glucosides from Citrus molasses. Molasses was diluted with methanol and centrifuged. The clear solution was loaded onto a Dowex-50 column, and the eluate was passed through a SP-70 column which was eluted with ethanol and evaporated to a minimal volume. The partially purified mixture was loaded onto a Q-Sepharose column and the column was eluted with sodium chloride. Limonoid-containing fractions were pooled and passed through a Dowex-50 column coupled to a SP-70 column for the removal of salt. Finally the limonoid glucoside mixture was eluted from the SP-70 column using 80-100% ethanol. However, the method provided a mixture of limonoid glucosides, not individual compounds.

A summary of the limonoids isolated from various varieties of citrus is presented in Table 1.

Table 1. Limonoid aglycones and glucosides isolated from different varieties of citrus.

Source / Citrus varieties used for the extraction	*Compounds isolated*	*Ref.*
C. ichangensis	Ichangensin	28
C.reticulata	Limonin, nomilin, obacunone	14
C. reticulata var. *austera* X *Fortunella* sp. (Calamondin)	17-β-D-glucopyranosides of calamin, methyl deacetylnomilinic acid, 6-keto-7β-deacetylnomilol, nomilinic acid, deacetylnomilinic acid	35
C. aurantium (sour orange)	17-β-D-Glucopyranosides of limonin, obacunone, deacetylnomilin, nomilin, deacctylnomilinic acid, nomilinic acid, isolimonic acid, ichangin, 19-hydroxydeacetylnomilinic acid.	34
	Iso-limonic acid, Methyl isolimonate	26
	Deacetyl nomilinic acid glucoside	38, 39
C. unshiu peels	Nomilinic acid 17-O-β-D-glucopyranoside, methyl nomilinate 17-O-β-D-glucopyranoside, obacunone 17-O-β-D-glucopyranoside.	36
C. paradisi (Grapefruit)	Limonin, obacunone, deacetyl nomilin	27
	Limonin, isoobacunoic acid, methyl epi-isoobacunoic acid, nomilinic acid, deacetyl nomilinic acid	23
	Iso-obacunoic acid glucoside, limonin glucoside	38, 39
	Limonin 17-β-D-glucopyranoside, nomilin 17-β-D-glucopyranoside, deacetylnomilin 17-β- D-glucopyranoside, obacunone 17-β-D-glucopyranoside	30

Table 1. *Continued.*

Source / Citrus varieties used for the extraction	*Compounds isolated*	*Ref.*
C. paradisi (Grapefruit) *(continued)*	17-β-D-glucopyranosides of nomilmic acid, deacetylnomilinic acid, iso-obacunoic acid, epi-isobacunoic acid, obacunoic acid, trans-obacunoic acid	31
C. junos (Yuzu), *C. sudachi* (Sudachi), *C. sphaerocarpu* (Kabosu)	Ichangensin 17-β-D-glucopyranoside, 17-β-D-glucopyranosides of deacetylnomilin, nomilin, nomilinic acid, obacunone, limonin, deacetylnomilinic acid.	32
Ichang lemon seeds	Limonin, nomilin, obacunone, ichangin	22
Lemon seeds and oranges peels	Methyl-17-dehydrolimonate A ring lactone	24
Molasses	Mixtures of limonoids glucosides	37
Navel oranges	Limonin, nomilin	19
P. trifoliate	Deacetyl nomilin	21
Red Mexican grapefruit	Limonin, nomilin, obacunone, deacetyl nomilin	29
	Limonin glucoside	38, 39
Seed oil	Limonin, nomilin, obacunone	20
Tetradium rutaecarpa fruit	Limonin 17-β-D-glucopyranoside, limonin diosphenol 17-β-D –glucopyranoside, 6-hydroxy-5-epilimonin 17-β-D -glucopyranoside.	33

Considering the potential biological activities and lack of information on yield of purified limonoids, there continues to be a need to develop rapid separation methods for limonoids. More recently, Jayaprakasha et al. (38, 39) isolated and identified limonin glucoside, iso-obacunoic acid glucoside, and deacetyl nomilinic acid glucoside from different varieties of citrus seeds in gram levels. The method involved Soxhlet extraction of seed powder of sour orange, grape fruit and red Mexican grapefruit with hexane for the removal of fatty matter. Then, the defatted powder was extracted with ethanol and concentrated to obtain a viscous liquid, and it was loaded onto ion-exchange and non-ionic resins successively (Scheme 1). Finally, the non-ionic resin column was eluted with different polar solvents. The fractions obtained from the column was analyzed by TLC and HPLC. Fractions containing the same peaks were pooled, concentrated and crystallized to obtain deacetyl nomilinic acid glucoside, iso-obacunoic acid glucoside and limonin glucoside.

Defatted seed powder

↓

Extracted with EtOH

↓

Cation Exchange resin, washed

↓

Water extract loaded onto synthetic adsorbents (non-ionic resin)

↓

Eluted (0 - 100%) aq. Polar solvent

↓

Concentrated and crystallized

↓

Limonin glucoside, iso-obacunoic acid glucoside and deacetyl nomilinic acid glucoside

Scheme 1. Isolation and purification of limonoid glucosides from citrus seeds

The yields of limonoids glucosides from various citrus fruit based on the method shown in Scheme 1 are presented in Table 2.

Table 2. Yield of limonoid glucosides

Citrus varieties	*Major compounds isolated*	*Yield (g)*
Sour orange (4.4 Kg)	Deacetyl nomilinic acid glucoside	9.50
Grapefruit (4.4 Kg)	Iso-obacunoic acid glucoside and Limonin glucoside	0.40 and 1.50
Mexican Red (4.4 Kg)	Limonin glucoside	4.90

Identification and analysis of limonoids

Previous sections focused on the isolation of limonoids, but methods for confirming the identities of the isolated compounds are also important in this process. Compound identities have been confirmed based on retention times from thin layer chromatography (TLC) or LC-UV-Vis absorption with comparison to standards, by NMR methods, and by mass spectrometry. For example, limonoids have been identified using TLC on silica gel plates (40, 41). The plates were sprayed with Ehrlich's reagent (2% N, N-dimethyl amino benzaldehyde in ethanol) and developed in an HCl gas chamber. Typical pink/reddish colored spots were obtained for limonoids. Isolated compounds were identified by comparing R_f values with authentic standards (42). However, quantification of limonoids was not possible using this method.

HPLC is the most widely used technique for the determination of limonin levels in citrus juice and processed products since it is very accurate and reliable. Ohta et al. (43) developed a reversed-phase high-performance liquid chromatography method for the separation of limonoids with UV absorption at 215 nm. A number of HPLC methods have been developed for quantification of limonoids (44-48). Ozaki et al. (32, 33) analyzed limonoids by HPLC using a C_{18} reversed-phase column (4.6 × 250 mm) and eluted isocratically with water, MeOH, and acetonitrile (49:41:10) at a flow rate of 1 ml/min. Limonoids were detected by UV absorption with 210 nm and identified based on comparison of the retention time of standards.

TLC and HPLC with UV-Vis absorption detection have been the most commonly used techniques for identification and quantification of limonoids. However, limited availability of standards and lack of characteristic UV/visible spectra have often made the positive identification of limonoids by TLC and HPLC difficult. NMR spectroscopy has often been employed for identification of citrus limonoids, requiring extensive and laborious purification to obtain sufficient pure quantities.

Mass spectrometry and tandem mass spectrometry are powerful techniques for identification and structural elucidation of limonoids by providing not only molecular weight, but also important fragmentation information which may assist in identifying unknown compounds (49). Tian and Ding (50) reported the application of liquid chromatography/electrospray ionization mass spectrometry (LC/ESI-MS) for screening of limonoid glucosides in citrus and electron ionization mass spectrometry of limonoid aglycones (51). ESI-MS and atmospheric pressure chemical ionization mass spectrometry were also recently used for quantification of limonoid glucosides and aglycones in citrus fruits, respectively (52). More recently, collisionally activated dissociation tandem mass spectrometry for characterization and structural elucidation of several limonoid aglycones and glucosides was reported (51). These mass spectrometric techniques allowed positive identification of limonoids in complex matrices. Fragmentation patterns observed in the EI spectra also can be used as important references for the positive characterization of limonoid aglycones (53).

More recently, we have reported the identification of limonoids by electrospray ionization mass spectrometry using a ThermoFinnigan LCQ Duo ion trap mass spectrometer operated in the negative electrospray ionization mode. Purified limonoids were diluted in methanol and infused at a flow rate of 5 μl/min. The lens and octapole voltages, sheath gas flow rate, and capillary voltage were optimized for maximum abundances of the ions of interest. In the negative ESI mode, the ion corresponding to $[L - H]^-$ was optimized, where L is the limonoid. The structures of the isolated compounds such as nomilin 17-β-D-glucopyranoside and nomilinic acid 17-β-D-glucopyranoside were confirmed based on the molecular weights of the deprotonated species and fragmentation patterns obtained by collisional activated dissociation of the deprotonated parent species (54).

Flash Chromatography

In 1978 Clark Steel demonstrated that purification in glass columns could be carried out at high flow rates (5 ml/min), and it was named flash chromatography. As a result, purification became much faster. Today flash chromatography is widely used for purification of low molecular weight compounds and products of organic synthetic reactions. Modern flash techniques include the use of convenient disposable flash cartridges instead of glass columns. Flash purification systems allow users to speed up the purification process for quicker results. It has been used for the isolation and purification of compounds from reaction mixtures and natural product extraction (55). It has also been used successfully for the separation of gingerols and shogaols from ginger (56). Continuous gradient purification of closely related drug intermediates of oxazoline analogs has been reported by flash chromatography (57). Furthermore, flavanone glucosides such as naringin and narirutin were separated successfully using flash chromatography (58). This technique has been used extensively by organic chemists for drug discovery and development. Separation using flash chromatography offers the advantages of speed and high loading capacity, which are ideal for large-scale separations.

Purification of limonoids by flash chromatography

Several citrus limonoid glucosides have proved to be particularly difficult to purify using conventional techniques like column chromatography or liquid extractions. Thus, a reversed-phase flash chromatographic technique (Figure 3)

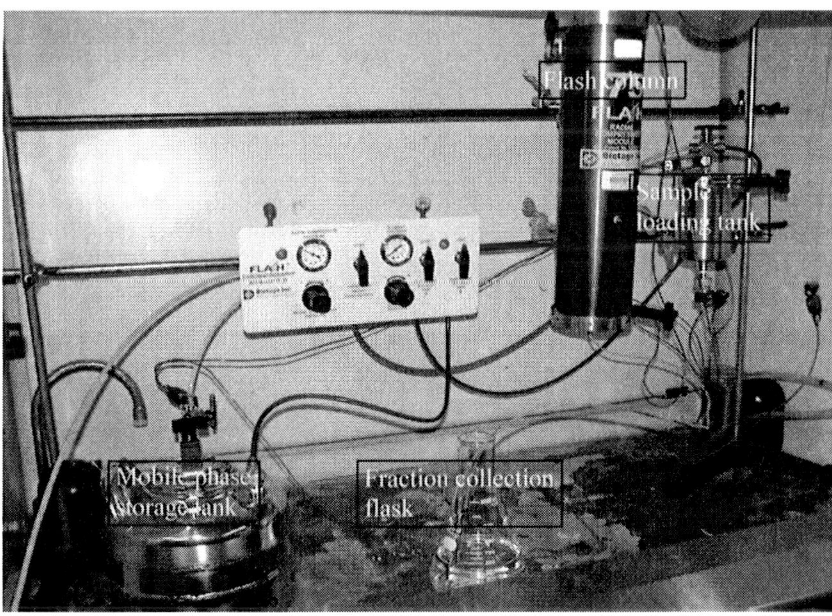

Figure 3. Flash chromatography separation apparatus: mobile phase storage tank, flash column, sample loading tank, fraction collection flask.

was developed for the separation and purification of two closely related limonoid glucosides, including nomilin 17-β-D-glucopyranoside and nomilinic acid 17-β-D-glucopyranoside, with confirmation by electrospray ionization mass spectrometry (54).

The scaling column proved to be one of the simplest method development tools for selecting the mobile phase composition for flash chromatography. The optimization method using 12 mm ID cartridges was finalized with minimum consumption of the sample and solvents. This optimized method was readily applied to scaled-up purification. The apparatus is presented in Figure 3. Our reversed-phase flash chromatographic method yielded relatively pure compounds such as nomilin 17-β-D-glucopyranoside and nomilinic acid 17-β-D-glucopyranoside (Figure 2) and allowed the other glucosides to be semi-purified with fewer contaminants, thereby increasing their ease of separation (54).

Conclusions

Isolation and purification of limonoids has been an important step in understanding the biological properties of citrus limonoids. Bioassays, animal studies, and human studies require availability of the purified compounds, and isolation of such compounds requires development of robust and reliable extraction and purification methods, as outlined in this chapter. Column chromatography, liquid extraction, and flash chromatography have played key roles in the development of rapid and efficient methods for separation of bioactive compounds from citrus. Further work is needed to purify minor limonoids present in citrus seeds/peels using new techniques.

Acknowledgements

This work was supported by the USDA-IFAFS (2001-52102-11527) and USDA-CSREES-Special grant # 2004-34402-14768.

References

1. Salah, N.; Miller, N. J.; Paganga, G.; Tijburg, L.; Bolwell, G. P.; Rice-Evans, C. *Arch. Biochem. Biophys.* **1995**, *2*, 339-346.
2. Hertog, M. G. L.; Feskeens, E. J. M.; Hollman, C. H.; Katan, M. B.; Kromhout, D. *Lancet* **1993**, *342*, 1007-1011.
3. Hasegawa, S.; Miyake, M. *Food Rev. Int.* **1996**, *12*, 413-435.
4. Benavente-Garcý, O.; Castillo, J.; Marý′, J. R.; Ortun, A.; Del Rý, J. A. *J. Agric. Food Chem.* **1997**, *45*, 4505–4515.

5. Middleton, E. J.; Kandaswami, C. *Biochemistry and Pharmacology,* **1992,** *43*, 1167–1179.
6. Rice-Evans, C. A.; Miller, N. J.; Paganda, G. *Trends in Plant Science,* **1997,** *2,* 152– 159.
7. Del Rý, J. A.; Fuster, M. D.; Sabater, F.; Porras, I.; Garcý, Lido, A.; Ortun, A. *Food Chemistry*, **1997,** *59*, 433–437.
8. Ortuno, A.; Reynaldo, I.; Fuster, M. D.; Botý, J. M.; Garcý, Puig, D.; Sabater, F.; Garcý′ a-Lido, A.; Porras, I.; Del Rý′ J. A. *Scientia Horticulturae* **1997,** *68*, 231–236.
9. Hasegawa, S.; Berhow, M. Analysis of limonoids by thin layer chromatography. *In citrus limonoids functional chemicals in agriculture and foods*; Berhow, M., Hasegawa, S., Manners, G., Eds., American chemical society: Washington, DC, 2000; pp 31
10. Miller, E. G.; Fanous, R.; Rivera-Hidalgo, F.; Binnie, W.H.; Hasegawa, S. *Carcinogenisis* **1989,** *10*: 1535-1537.
11. Lam, L. K. T.; Hasegawa, S. *Nutrition and Cancer*, **1989,** *12,* 43-47.
12. Tanaka, T.; Makita, H.; Mori, H. *Carcinogenesis*, **1996**, 1167–1170
13. Poulose, S.M., Harris, E.D.; Patil, B.S. *J. Nutrition* **2005,** *135*, 870-877.
14. Jayaprakasha, G. K.; Singh, R. P.; Pereira, J.; Sakariah, K. K. *Phytochemistry*, **1997**, *44*, 843-846.
15. Ruberto, G.; Renda, A.; Tringali, C.; Napoli, E.M.; Simmonds, M.S.J. *Agric. Food Chem*, **2002,** *50,* 6766-6770.
16. Schechter,; Haller, J. *J. Am. J. Chem. Soc.* **1940,** *69,* 1307-1311.
17. Mookerjee, *J. Indian Chem. Soc..* **1940,** *17*, 593-597.
18. Seshadri. T. R.; Veeraragavia. *Proc. Indian Acad. Sci.* **1940,** 505.
19. Emerson, O. H. *J. Am. Chem. Soc.* **1948,** 70, 545-547.
20. Emerson, O. H. *J. Am. Chemical Soc.* **1951,** 73, 2621- 2624.
21. Dreyer, D. L. *J. Org. Chem.* **1965,** *30*, 749-751.
22. Dreyer, D. L. *J. Org. Chem.* **1966,** *31*, 2279-2281.
23. Bennett, R. D. *Phytochemistry* **1971,** *10*, 3065-3068
24. Hsu, A.C.; Hasegawa, S.; Maier, V.P.; Bennett, R.D. *Phytochemistry,* **1973**. *12*, 663 - 567.
25. Hasegawa, S.; Bennett, R.D.; Verdon, C.P. *J. Agric. Food* Chem. **1980**, *28*, 922-925.
26. Bennett, R.D.; Hasegawa, S. *Phytochemistry*, **1980**, *19*, 2417-2419.
27. Bennett, R. D.; Hasegawa, S. *Phytochemistry,* **1982**, *21*, 2349-2354.
28. Bennett, R.D.; Herman, Z.; Hasegawa, S. *Phytochemistry,* **1988**, *27*, 1543-1545.
29. Mandadi, K. K.; Jayaprakasha, G.K. Narayana Bhat,; Patil, B.S. *Food Chemistry and Toxicology,* **2005** (Communicated).
30. Bennett, R. D.; Hasegawa, S.; Herman, Z. *Phytochemistry*, **1989,** *28*, 2777-2780.

31. Hasegawa S.; Bennet R. D.; Herman, Z.; Fong, C. H.; Ou P. *Phytochemistry* **1989,** *28,* 1717-1720.
32. Ozaki, Y.; Miyake, M.; Maeda, H.; Ifuku, Y.; Bennett, R.D.; Herman, Z.; Fong, C.H.; Hasegawa, S. *Phytochemistry,* **1991,** *30,* 2659-2661.
33. Ozaki, Y.; Fong, C.H.; Herman, Z.; Maeda, H.; Miyake, M.; Ifuku, Y.; Hasegawa, S. *Agric. Biol. Chem.* **1991**, 55, 137-141.
34. Benneta, R.D.; Miyake, M.; Ozaki, Y.; Hasegawa, S. *Phytochemistry,* **1991,** *30,* 3803-3805.
35. Miyake, M.; Ozaki, Y.; Ayano, S.; Bennett, R.D.; Herman, Z.; Hasegawa,S. *Phytochemistry,* **1992,** *31,* 1044 –1046.
36. Sawabe, A.; Morita, M.; Kiso, T.; Kishine, H.; Ohtsubo, Y.; Minematsu, T.; Matsubara, Y.; Okamoto, T. *Carbohydrate Research* **1999,** *315,* 142–147.
37. Schoch, T. K.; Manners, G. D.; Hasegawa, S. *J. Food Sci,* **2002,** *67,* 3159.
38. Jayaprakasha, G.K.; Brodbelt, J.S.; Bhat, N.G.; Patil, B.S. Rapid methods for the separation of bioactive compounds from citrus, Presented during 228th ACS National Meeting, Philadelphia, PA, August 22-26, 2004, Philadelphia, USA.
39. Jayaprakasha, G.K.; Bhat, N.G. Patil, B.S. An improved process for the isolation of limonoid glucosides from citrus, 2005, (Patent submitted).
40. Hasegawa, S.; Bennett, R. D.; Maier, V. P. Biosynthesis of limonoids, *Phytochemistry* **1984**, *28*, 922-925.
41. Bennett, R. D.; Herman, Z.; Hasegawa, S. Ichangensin: a new citrus limonoid. *Phytochemistry* **1988,** *27,* 1543-1545.
42. Hasegawa, S.; Berhow, M.A.; In-*Citrus limonoids, - Functional Chemicals in Agriculture and Foods*, Berhow, M.A.; Hasegawa, S.; Manners, G.D. eds. Oxford University Press: Washington, DC, 2000, pp.31-39.
43. Ohta. H.; Fong, C.H.; Berhow, M.; Hasegawa, S. *J. Chromatogr.* **1993,** *639,* 295-302.
44. Rouseff, R.L.; Fisher, J.F. *Anal. Chem.* **1980,** *52,* 1228-1233.
45. Shaw, P.E.; Wilson, C.W. *J. Food Sci.* **1984,** *49,* 1216-1218.
46. Van Beck, T.A.; Blaakmeer, A. *J. Chromatogr.* **1989,** *464,* 375-386.
47. Haswgawa, S.; Ou P.; Fong, C.H.; Herman, Z.; Coggins, C.W.; Atkin, D.R. *J. Agric. Food Chem.* **1991,** *39,* 262-265.
48. Manners, G.D.; Hasegawa, S.; Bennett, R.D.; Wong, R.Y. In-*Citrus limonoids, - Functional Chemicals in Agriculture and Foods*, Berhow, M.A.; Hasegawa, S.; Manners, G.D. eds. Oxford University Press: Washington, DC, 2000, pp.40 - 59.
49. Busch, K. L.; Glish, G. L.; McLuckey, S.A.; Mass Spectrometry/Mass Spectrometry: Techniques and Applications of Tandem Mass Spectrometry. VCH: New York, 1988; 1–4.
50. Tian, Q.; Ding, X. *J. Chromatogr. A,* **2000,** *874,* 13-19.
51. Tian, Q.; Schwartz, S. J. *Anal. Chem.* **2003**; *75,* 5451-5457.

52. Manners, G. D.; Breksa, A. P.; Schoch, T. K. Hidalgo, M. B.; *J. Agric. Food Chem.* **2003**; *51,* 3709-3713.
53. Tian, Q.; Li, D.; Barbaci, D.; Schwartz, S.; Patil, B.S. *Rapid Communication in Mass Spectrometry,* **2003,** *17,* 2517-2522.
54. Raman, G.; Cho, M.; Brodbelt, J.S.; Patil, B.S. *Phytochemical Analysis* **2005,** *16,* 155-160.
55. Zarate, R.; Sukrasno, M.M. Yeoman, *J. Chromatogr.* **1992,** *609*, 407-413.
56. Banerjee, S.; Desai, U.R.; Trivedi, G.K. *Synth. Commun.,* **1991**, *21*, 757-770.
57. Abraham, M.H.; Roses, M.; Poole, C.F.; Poole, S. K. *J. Phy. Org. Chem.* **1997,** *10*, 358-368.
58. Raman, G.; Jayaprakasha, G.K.; Brodbelt, J.S.; Minhee Cho.; Patil, B.S. *Analytical Letters,* **2004,** *37*, 3005-3016.

Chapter 4

Characterization of Flavonoids by Tandem Mass Spectrometry and Metal Complexation Strategies

Jennifer S. Brodbelt[1], Junmei Zhang[1,2], Michael Pikulski[1], Barry D. Davis[1], Basavaraj Girennavar[2], Guddadarangavvanahally K. Jayaprakasha[2], and Bhimanagouda S. Patil[2]

[1]Department of Chemistry and Biochemistry, University of Texas at Austin, Austin, TX 78712
[2]Vegetable and Fruit Improvement Center, Department of Horticultural Sciences, Mail Code 2119, Texas A&M University, College Station, TX 77843

Tandem mass spectrometry is a versatile and sensitive strategy for characterizing the structures of phytochemicals. In particular, the differentiation of isomeric flavonoids by tandem mass spectrometry is the focus of this chapter. Metal complexation offers a degree of "tunability" which enhances the identification of flavonoids.

The tremendous growth in the number of studies devoted to mapping the phytochemicals in citrus and understanding their health benefits (1-2), as detailed in many of the other chapters in this book, has spurred the development of more sensitive and versatile analytical methods for characterizing phytochemicals in fruits and vegetables, plasma, and urine (3-7). The analysis of phytochemicals poses a significant challenge for several reasons. First, the structures of phytochemicals are diverse, including potentially thousands of structures even within a single phytochemical class. Second, the levels of phytochemicals and their biotransformation products may vary over several orders of magnitude in fruits and vegetables, and in plasma and urine after consumption. In addition, the matrices in which the phytochemicals or their biotransformation products are found are complex, thus requiring optimization of extraction, isolation or purification methods that are robust and efficient.

There are several categories of phytochemicals found in citrus, including flavonoids (especially flavanones), limonoids, and coumarins, among others. Flavonoids in particular are one of the most widely studied groups of phenolic phytochemicals (8), and they represent an excellent example of the structural diversity that makes the analysis of phytochemicals so challenging. Flavonoids typically exist as glycosides in plants, and the site of glycosylation and identification of the attached sugars are critical structural issues. Three isomeric diglycosyl flavonoids shown in Figure 1 illustrate some of the structural features that must be deciphered for confident identification of flavonoids.

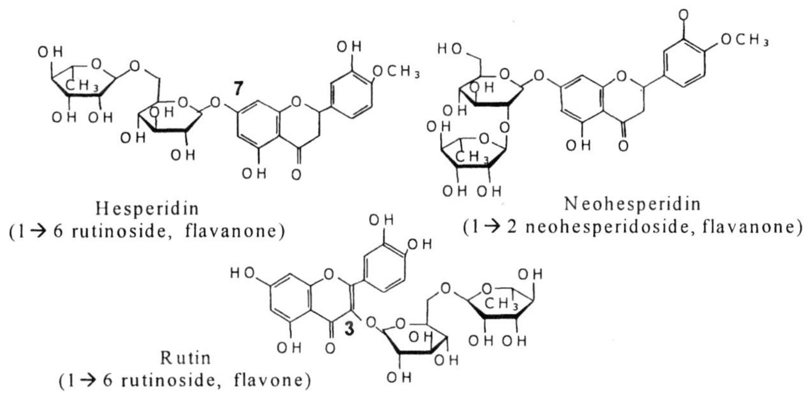

Figure 1. Structures of three isomeric flavonoids with molecular weight 610 Da.

The three vary based on the class of flavonoid aglycon (flavone versus flavanone), the site of diglycoysl attachment (7-O versus 3-O), and the type of intersaccharide linkage (rutinoside is 1 → 6 and neohesperidoside is 1 → 2). Flavonoids are frequently hydrolyzed to aglycons upon consumption, then biotransformed to other species, and the resulting aglycons, metabolites and glycoside forms may be absorbed to different extents and exert different physiological activities, thus making the mapping of pharmacokinetics and bioavailability a complex problem. Biotransformation of the flavonoids may lead to conjugation resulting in glucuronides or sulfates, among others. There exists evidence that the biological activities of flavonoids are affected by subtle structural factors, including changes in the degree of hydroxylation and methoxylation, and the presence or absence of specific double bonds at key positions. These types of structural features must be pinpointed to allow confirmation of structure/activity relationships in human studies.

Few analytical methods offer both the specificity and sensitivity to detect low levels of flavonoids in complex matrices. Some methods, such as UV-Vis and fluorescence spectroscopy, offer excellent detection limits but afford a relatively low degree of specific structural information and are often incapable of differentiating isomers. Other methods, such as infrared absorption spectroscopy or nuclear magnetic resonance spectroscopy, give far more structural information but have less impressive detection limits and are in many cases less suitable for analysis of complex mixtures. Mass spectrometry has established a rich history for the characterization of flavonoids (6,7), including analysis of mixtures by gas chromatography mass spectrometry (GCMS) (9-13) or liquid chromatography mass spectrometry (LCMS) (14-36) and structural elucidation by tandem mass spectrometry (MS/MS) (37-70). Early studies entailed the use of fast atom bombardment, electron ionization or chemical ionization methods to create ions, but electrospray ionization (ESI) (71) has become the current method of choice for ionization of flavonoids and other phytochemicals. A brief inspection of the literature over the past decade reveals the growth in the application of mass spectrometry for analysis of phytochemicals, and its excellent detection limits and structural information have cemented its impact for many years into the future. Our group has focused on the development of mass spectrometric methods for the characterization of phytochemicals and their quantification in mixtures (34-36,61-69), and thus this chapter will focus primarily on this versatile and sensitive analytical strategy for characterization of flavonoids.

Overview of Electrospray Ionization, Tandem Mass Spectrometry and Collisional Activated Dissociation

Electrospray ionization (71) has revolutionized the way that compounds can be analyzed by mass spectrometry. Electrospray ionization entails the formation of analyte ions directly from droplets created by the application of a large voltage to the tip of a capillary or needle through which the analyte solution is sprayed. The process involves electrostatic nebulization in which species in solution are volatized, ionized, and transformed into individual gas-phase ions which can be analyzed after introduction into a mass analyzer. Electrospray ionization is also a convenient interface for uniting high performance liquid chromatography to mass spectrometry because the effluent from the chromatograph can be directly coupled to the electrospray device.

"Tandem mass spectrometry" is a general phrase used to indicate any type of mass spectrometric experiment that involves more than one stage of mass analysis (72-73). Its most common form involves the selection and mass analysis of a specific precursor ion, followed by energization of the precursor ions, and then mass analysis of the resulting fragments. Energization of the precursor ions is most frequently undertaken via gas-phase collisions with inert target gas molecules, such as argon or helium. This process is termed "collisional activated dissociation" (CAD) or more generally "MS/MS". Each collision converts some of the kinetic energy of the precursor ion into internal energy, thus cumulatively "heating" the precursor ions until they dissociate. Interpretation of the ensuing fragment ions provides a structural fingerprint of the initial precursor ions. CAD is an excellent method when combined with electrospray ionization because electrospray ionization is a particularly gentle ionization method that promotes the formation of intact precursor ions, with little or no fragmentation. Thus, the molecular weights of the compounds of interest can be pinpointed based on examination of the electrospray ionization mass spectra, and then additional structural information can be obtained by subsequent CAD experiments. Different fragment ions are formed from protonated molecules versus deprotonated molecules versus metal-cationized molecules, and thus the selection of the specific ionization mode plays a critical role in defining the structural information obtained from CAD, as shown in some of the following examples. All of the examples from this chapter will be drawn from flavonoids to showcase some of the elegant uses of tandem mass spectrometry to probe structural details of compounds, to differentiate isomers, and to allow quantification in mixtures based on high performance liquid chromatographic separation with tandem mass spectrometry.

Electrospray Ionization Mass Spectrometry of Flavonoids

Because flavonoids are phenolic compounds without the presence of basic groups, such as amines, they do not protonate efficiently during electrospray ionization. They undergo deprotonation more effectively due to the presence of one or more hydroxyl groups, and thus flavonoids are often analyzed as negative ions. A comparison of the electrospray ionization mass spectra of rutin in the positive and negative ESI modes is shown in Figure 2. The abundance of deprotonated rutin is nearly thirty times greater than the abundance of protonated rutin, reflecting the greater ionization efficiency of rutin in the negative ionization mode. The absolute ionization efficiency is not the only factor that must be evaluated when developing an analytical strategy for flavonoids. The diagnostic utility of the fragmentation patterns obtained upon collisional activated dissociation of the flavonoid ions is an equally important issue because it determines the ability to differentiate isomeric structures. In some cases, the fragmentation patterns of the deprotonated flavonoids are not sufficient to allow confident structural assignment, as illustrated in the next section. It is this type of problem that spurred our development of metal complexation modes based on addition of metal salts with or without auxiliary ligands to generate abundant metal-cationized flavonoid species.

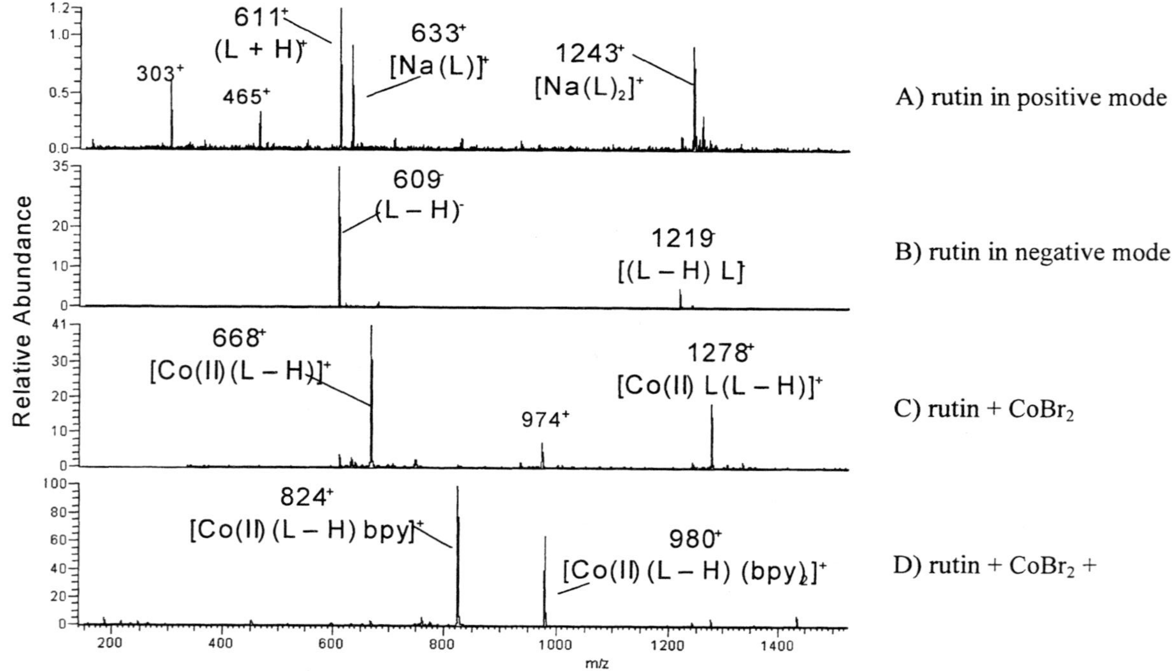

Figure 2. Electrospray ionization mass spectra of rutin obtained in four ionization modes. A) positive mode upon addition of acetic acid, B) negative mode upon addition of ammonium hydroxide, C) cobalt complexation upon addition of $CoBr_2$, and D) cobalt complexation with the auxiliary ligand, 2,2'-bipyridine. The vertical scales reflect the relative abundances.

Such an example is illustrated in Figure 2 for rutin. Rutin readily forms metal complexes of the type [M(II) (flavonoid – H)]$^+$ and [M(II) flavonoid (flavonoid – H)]$^+$ where M(II) represents an alkaline earth or transition metal ion (61). These complexes are formed spontaneously upon addition of a soluble metal salt to the flavonoid solution, producing abundant complexes upon ESI. The ability of flavonoids to coordinate metal ions via binding through oxygen atoms is well known and thus offers a convenient way to form alternative ions for analysis. Complexes of the type [M(II) (flavonoid – H) + auxiliary ligand]$^+$ are formed upon further addition of a suitable auxiliary ligand, typically a chelating agent, to the flavonoid solution. Based on comparison of the relative abundances of the various types of flavonoid ions, as exemplified in Figure 2, the metal complexes that incorporate the auxiliary ligand are typically most abundant, often 10 to 100 times more abundant than protonated flavonoids and three to five times more abundant than deprotonated flavonoids. There is also some "tunability" in the ionization strategy based on the specific metal and auxiliary ligand used which dictate the types and abundances of coordination complexes formed in the ESI process. The fragmentation patterns resulting from these complexes also vary with the nature of the metal ion. Clearly metal complexation strategies can offer the potential for improved detection limits while also affording unique types of ions that give different fragmentation patterns, as discussed in the next sections.

Tandem Mass Spectrometry of Flavonoids

As illustrated in the preceding ESI mass spectra, molecular ions that can be used to elucidate molecular weights are typically observed for the flavonoids, but diagnostic fragment ions are not formed due to the gentle nature of the ESI process. Combining ESI with tandem mass spectrometry is the method of choice for identification of flavonoids (34-36,61-64,66-69). The fragmentation patterns of deprotonated flavonoid glycosides are typically simple with only one or two dissociation routes. Common fragmentation pathways include the loss of sugar moieties, and occasionally cross-ring cleavages which involve breaking of the saccharide ring structures. Two examples of the tandem mass spectra obtained via collisional activated dissociation for deprotonated rhoifolin and isorhoifolin (Figure 3) are shown in Figure 4.

Rhoifolin and isorhoifolin are isomeric diglycosyl flavones which differ only by their intersaccharide linkage. The only significant dissociation route seen in Figure 4 for each isomer is the loss of the disaccharide moiety (loss of 308 Da). This is a characteristic process for many flavonoid glycosides. Although the fragmentation patterns of the deprotonated flavonoids are easily interpreted and are diagnostic for the general class of flavonoid compounds, they do not allow ready differentiation of isomers, thus illustrating the need for other types of ions for structural elucidation of isomeric flavonoids.

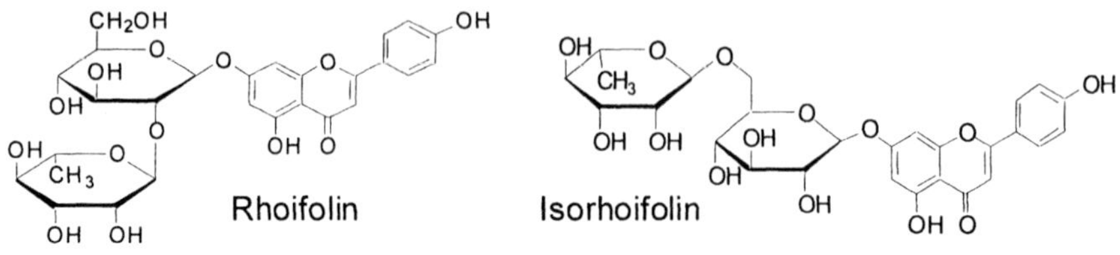

Figure 3. Structures of rhoifolin and isorhoifolin

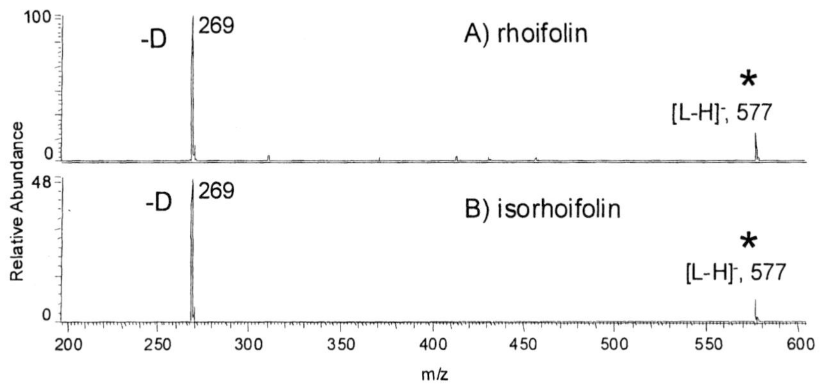

Figure 4. CAD mass spectra for deprotonated A) rhoifolin and B) isorhoifolin. The parent ions are labeled with asterisks. The loss of the disaccharide group is indicated by –D.

Metal complexation, with or without an auxiliary ligand, leads to different types of flavonoid ions that are often more conducive to differentiation by tandem mass spectrometry (36, 61-64, 66-69). For example, the addition of a magnesium salt to flavonoid solutions results in the formation of [Mg(II) flavonoid (flavonoid – H)]$^+$ complexes that allow identification of the site of glycosylation of C- and O-bonded monoglycosyl flavonoids (66). For example, quercetin-3-O-glucoside, quercetin-4'-O-glucoside, and quercetin-7-O-glucoside are three isomeric flavonoids that differ only by the location of the glucose moiety. Collisional activated dissociation of the deprotonated flavonoids results only in the loss of the glucose residue, giving identical product ions for each of the three isomers. The corresponding magnesium complexes, on the other hand, give unique fragmentation patterns that involve one or more of the following processes: loss of the glucose residue, loss of the aglycon portion, loss of two glucose residues, and a cross-ring cleavage reaction. The C- and O-glycosyl flavonoids give specific fragment ions too, thus allowing confident differentiation of isomers. A flow chart that summarizes the determination of the glycosylation site is shown in Scheme 1. Based on a simple tabulation of

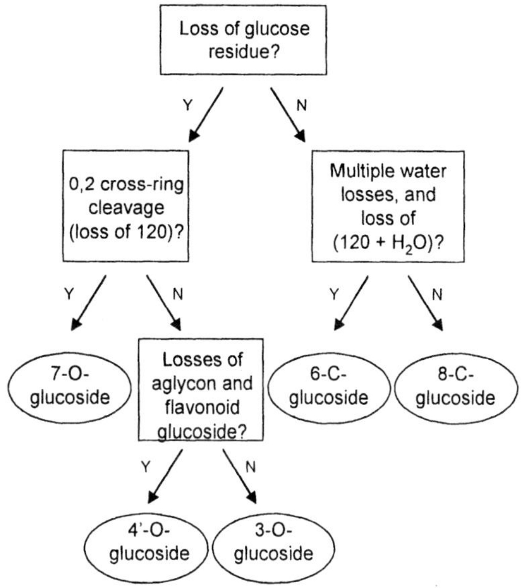

Scheme 1. Determination of glycosylation site based on evaluation of fragmentation patterns of [Mg(II) flavonoid (flavonoid – H)]$^+$ complexes.

the fragment ions observed upon collisional activation of the magnesium complexes, the 3-O, 7-O, 4'-O, 6-C, and 8-C glucosides are distinguished.

A related method that utilizes manganese, rather than magnesium, for metal complexation allows identification of the specific type of sugar residue attached to monoglycosyl flavonoids (36). Based on the diagnostic fragmentation patterns of [Mn(II) flavonoid (flavonoid – H)]$^+$ complexes, the attached sugar can be elucidated as glucose, galactose, arabinose, or xylose.

Silver complexation and tandem mass spectrometry allows structural characterization of eighteen diglycosyl flavonoids from seven isomeric series (68). The fragmentation patterns of the (flavonoid + Ag^+) complexes were used to identify the site of glycosylation, the type of disaccharide (rutinose versus neohesperidose), and the type of aglycon (flavonol versus flavone versus flavanone). Aluminum complexation offers another alternative strategy for differentiation of flavonoid isomers. In this case, complexes of the type [Al(III) (flavonoid – H)$_2$]$^+$ were the key ions (69). Because of the large number of metals available, one can envision many routes for exploiting metal complexation strategies to enhance differentiation of isomers by ESI-MS.

Metal complexation in conjunction with an auxiliary ligand also offers great versatility for the structural characterization of flavonoid isomers (61-64,67). For example, rutin and hesperidin are two isomeric diglycosyl flavonoids (see Figure 1). Despite the fact that rutin is a 3-O-diglycosyl flavonol and hesperidin is a 7-O-diglycosyl flavanone, both yield virtually identical fragmentation patterns for the deprotonated species: each undergoing the loss of the diglycosyl species.

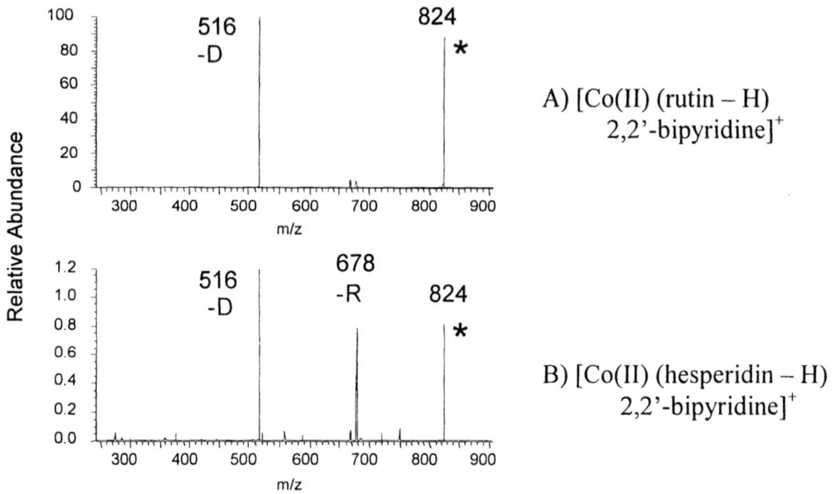

Figure 5. CAD mass spectra of [Co(II) (flavonoid – H) 2,2'-bipyridine]$^+$ complexes for two isomers. The loss of the disaccharide group is indicated by –D; the loss of the rhamnose residue is indicated by –R.

Collisional activated dissociation of the corresponding [Co(II) (flavonoid – H) 2,2'-bipyridine]$^+$ complexes allow differentiation of the two isomers, as shown in Figure 5 (64). The rutin complex still dissociates by loss of the diglycosyl moiety, but the hesperidin complex also dissociates by a unique pathway: the elimination of the terminal sugar residue. These types of transition metal/2,2'-bipyridine/diglycosyl flavonoid complexes typically dissociate by up to four different pathways, thus allowing differentiation of many types of isomers, such as those that differ by the position of glycosyl attachment (i.e. 7-O or 3-O), or those that differ by the type of diglycosyl unit (rutinoside or neohesperidoside). A summary of the four major dissociation routes is shown in Scheme 2.

The fragmentation patterns are also somewhat "tunable" based on the type of metal and auxiliary ligand incorporated into the complexes (62,64). For example, Figure 6 shows the fragmentation patterns of two complexes of rhoifolin, a diglycosyl flavone (64). The fragmentation pattern of the Ni complex shows only the loss of the disaccharide portion, whereas the fragmentation pattern of the corresponding Co complex shows two additional diagnostic ions. These differences are attributed to changes in the bond strengths of the metal ion to the flavonoid and auxiliary ligand, and to possible variations in the coordination geometries of the complexes.

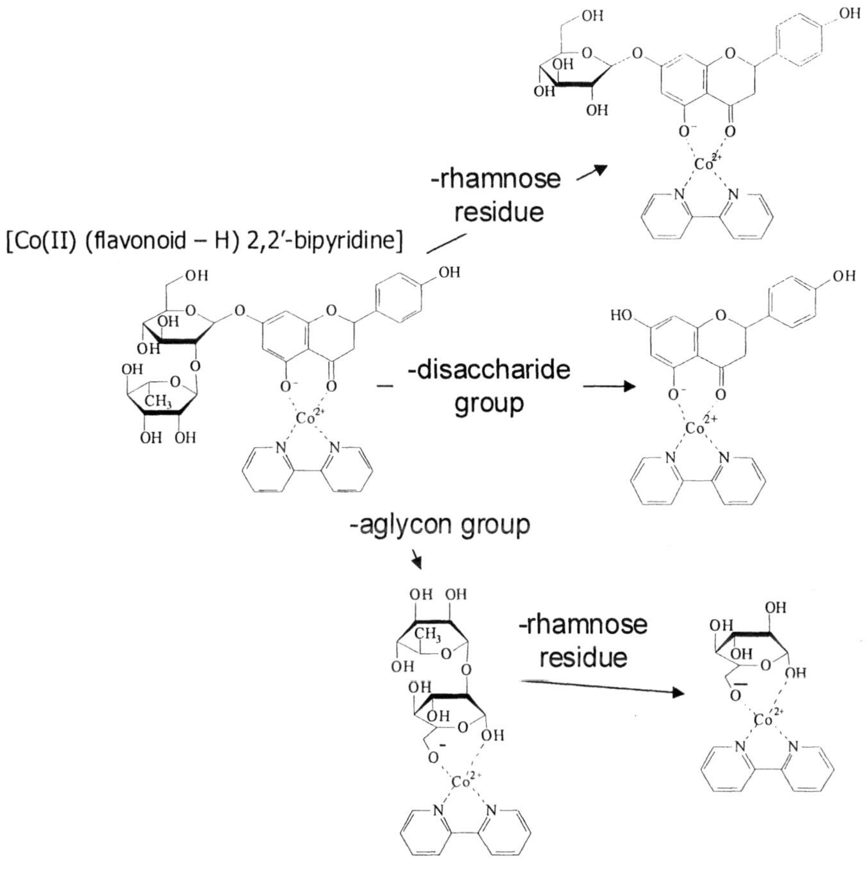

Scheme 2. Dissociation of [M(II) (flavonoid – H) 2,2'-bipyridine]⁺ complexes.

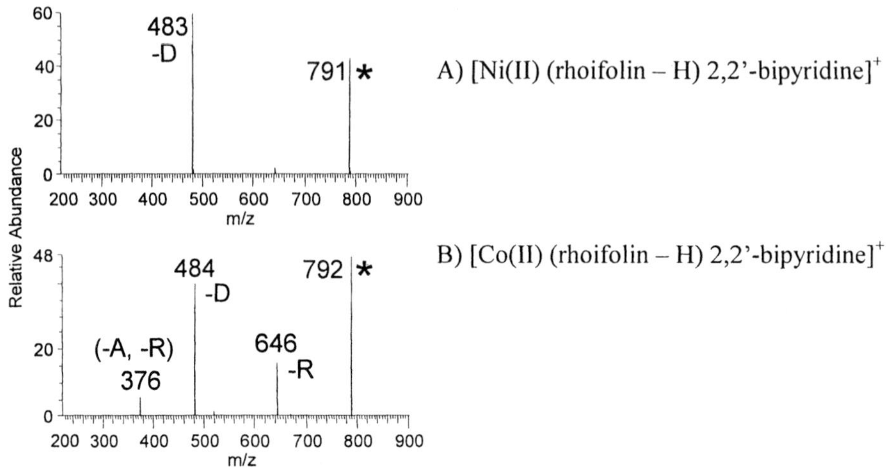

Figure 6. CAD mass spectra for [M(II) (rhoifolin – H) 2,2'-bipyridine]$^+$ complexes. The parent ions are indicated by asterisks. The loss of the aglycon portion is indicated by –A, the loss of the rhamnose residue is indicated by –R, and the loss of the disaccharide moiety is indicated by –D.

An example of the impact of the auxiliary ligand on the dissociation patterns of flavonoid complexes is shown in Figure 7 for a series of complexes containing cobalt and rhoifolin. Depending on the choice of auxiliary ligand, all of which are pyridyl-based ligands that strongly coordinate transition metals through their nitrogen atoms, a notable change in the collisional activated dissociation patterns is observed (64). For the complex containing 2,2':6',2"-terpyridine, a tridentate ligand, only two fragmentation routes are observed, with the dominant one attributed to the loss of the disaccharide moiety. For the other complexes, all of which contain bidentate ligands having varying metal binding strengths, an additional fragmentation pathway due to the loss of both the aglycon portion and one sugar residue is observed. The abundances of the fragment ions vary across the series of complexes, underscoring the influence of the auxiliary ligand based on its binding strength to the metal ion and the resulting changes in electron densities and labilities of the complexes.

The ability to "tune" the fragmentation pattern is particularly useful for differentiation of certain flavonoid isomers that can not be distinguished based on the fragmentation patterns of the deprotonated species. For example, rhoifolin and isorhoifolin (shown in Figure 3) are difficult to differentiate because the deprotonated species dissociate predominantly by only one common pathway, the loss of the disaccharide moiety (see Figure 4). The [Co(II) (isorhoifolin – H) 4,7-diphenyl-1,10-phenanthroline]$^+$ complex dissociates by two routes, including the elimination of the rhamnose residue or the loss of

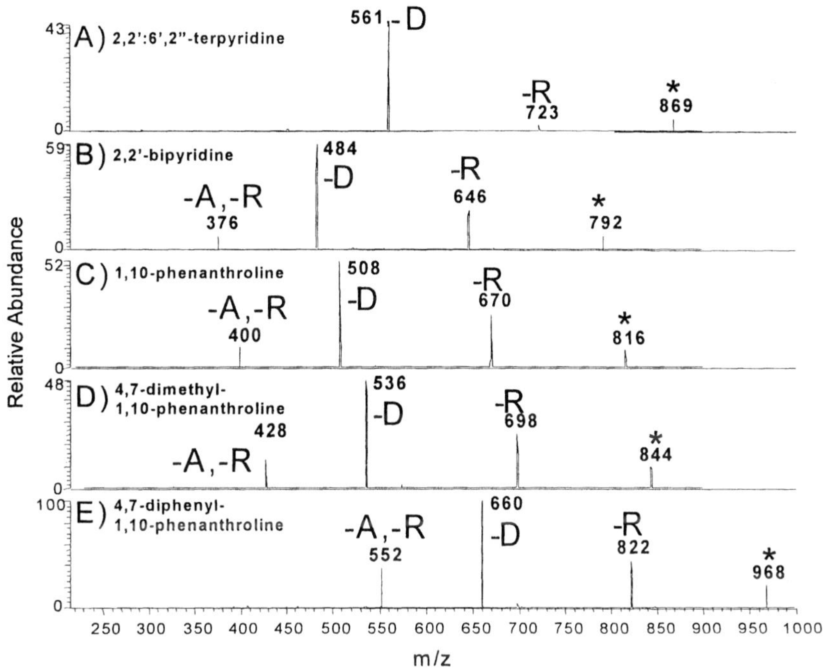

Figure 7. CAD mass spectra of [Co(II) (rhoifolin-H) pyridyl ligand]$^+$ complexes, showing relative fragment ion abundances with the variation of the auxiliary ligand. The parent ion is designated with an asterisk, the loss of the rhamnose residue is designated by -R, the loss of the disaccharide moiety is designated by -D, and the loss of the aglycon group and the rhamnose residue is designated by –A, -R.

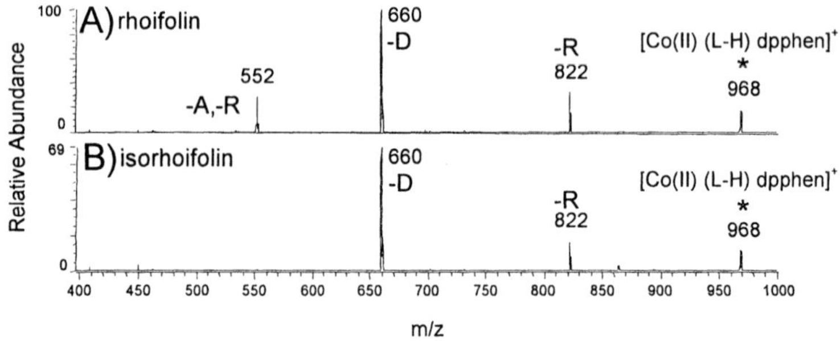

Figure 8. CAD mass spectra of parent [Co(II) (L-H) 4,7-diphenyl-1,10-phenanthroline]$^+$ complexes of A) rhoifolin and B) isorhoifolin. The loss of the disaccharide group is indicated by -D, the loss of the rhamnose residue is indicated by –R, and the loss of the aglycon portion is indicated by –A.

the disaccharide moiety (64). The analogous rhoifolin complex has an additional fragmentation pathway involving the loss of the aglycon portion and the rhamnose residue (see Figure 8). The latter unique pathway makes the differentiation of the two isomers unambiguous and is a convincing example of the versatility of metal complexation strategies for enhancing isomer differentiation of flavonoids.

HPLC-MS/MS Applications

The metal complexation methods described above may also be incorporated into analysis of mixtures via HPLC-ESI-MS/MS. LC-MS has been used extensively for quantification and identification of flavonoids (14-34), usually based on conventional protonation or deprotonation ionization modes. Metal complexation methods are implemented via addition of a suitable metal salt to the chromatographic effluent after the analytes are separated by reversed-phase high performance liquid chromatography. For example, a post-column silver complexation method was developed for the analysis of flavonoids in grapefruit juice (68). Flavonoids were extracted from a commercial grapefruit juice sample as described by Zhang and Brodbelt (35). The flavonoids in the extract were separated using a C_{18} column (2.1 × 50 mm, 3.5 μm) with a guard column (2.1 × 10 mm, 3.5 μm), and a mobile phase composed of solvent A (0.33% formic acid), B (acetonitrile with 0.33% formic acid), and C (isopropanol with 0.33% formic acid) applied in a gradient mode. The HPLC effluent was mixed with 1×10^{-3} M silver nitrate (introduced through a tee by a syringe pump at 20 μL/min) before introduction into the mass spectrometer by electrospray ionization. The CAD spectra for the six flavonoids extracted from grapefruit juice and analyzed by the post-column silver complexation method are shown in Figure 9.

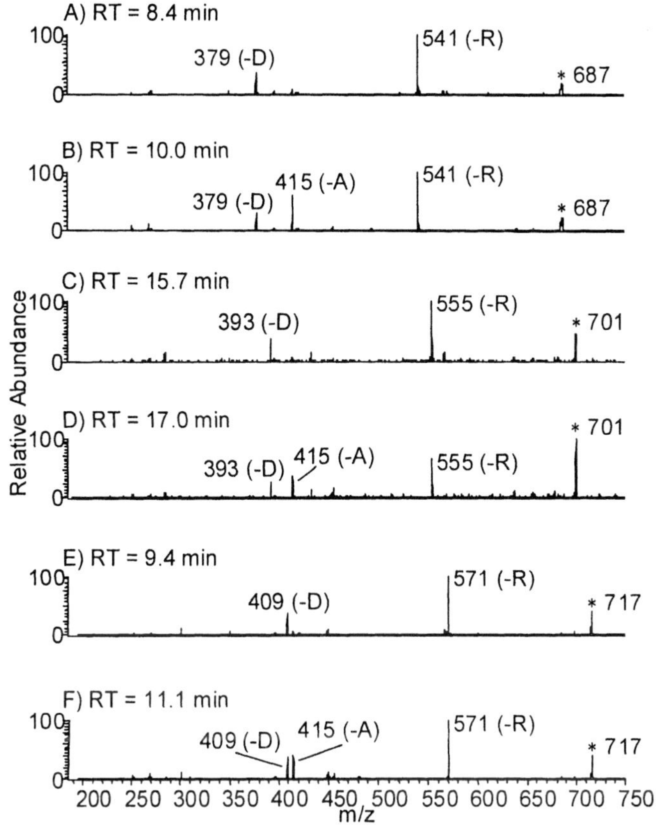

Figure 9. LC/MS/MS analysis of a grapefruit extract after post-column silver complexation, resulting in formation of $(L + Ag)^+$ ions, where L is a flavonoid. The selected parent ions are indicated by asterisks. Loss of the rhamnose residue is indicated by –R, the loss of the aglycon moiety is indicated by –A, and the loss of the disaccharide group is indicated by –D.

The two major flavonoids dissociate via the dominant loss of the rhamnose residue (m/z 541), and by the loss of the disaccharide (m/z 379) and/or the aglycon (m/z 415) residues, indicating that they are both flavanones, narirutin (retention time (RT) = 8.4 min) and naringin (RT = 10.0 min). The four other flavonoids were identified as didymin (RT = 15.7 min), poncirin (RT = 17.0 min), hesperidin (RT = 9.4 min) and neohesperidin (RT = 11.1 min), based on the diagnostic fragmentation patterns of the silver/flavonoid complexes.

Analysis of Flavonoid Biotransformation Products

Tandem mass spectrometry is also useful for characterizing metabolites after consumption of flavonoid-rich foods, such as citrus (35). For example, urine was collected from three human volunteers after consumption of grapefruit juice following an overnight fast. After addition of an internal standard (3,7-dihydroxyflavone), then precipitation of proteins via addition of methanol and centrifugation, the samples were dried completely and then reconstituted in 50% aqueous methanol prior to HPLC-ESI-MS/MS analysis. The metabolites were separated using a C_{18} column (2.1 × 50 mm, 3.5 μm) with a guard column (2.1 × 10 mm, 3.5 μm), and a gradient mobile phase composed of solvent A (0.33% formic acid), B (acetonitrile with 0.33% formic acid), and C (isopropanol with 0.33% formic acid). The dominant metabolites identified in urine by LC-ESI-MS/MS based on their characteristic fragmentation patterns were two different naringenin glucuronides, naringenin-7-O-glucuronide and naringenin-4′-O-glucuronide. Three naringenin sulfate isomers were also identified, along with two naringenin glucuronide sulfates. One naringenin diglucuronide was identified based on its diagnostic losses of one or both of its glucuronyl units upon tandem mass spectrometry. The profiles of the major metabolites were monitored as a function of time after consumption of the grapefruit juice. The highest levels of metabolites for all three volunteers appeared around 4 - 8 hours after grapefruit juice consumption. Little if any metabolites were detectable after 12 hours. The LC-MS/MS strategy offered higher selectivity as well as lower detection limits compared to the conventional LC-UV approach.

Conclusions

Tandem mass spectrometry offers a versatile method for characterization of flavonoids. New metal complexation strategies developed for electrospray ionization give enhanced sensitivity and tunability of fragmentation patterns, allowing differentiation of isomers. These methods are readily incorporated into LCMS strategies, making them viable for analysis of complex mixtures. It is expected that many of these tandem mass spectrometric approaches will be adopted for studies involving bioavailability and pharmacokinetics of flavonoids in future years.

Acknowledgements

This work was supported by the Welch Foundation (F-1155), USDA-IFAFS (2001-52102-11527), and the National Institutes of Health (R01-GM63512).

References

1. Surh, Y.-J., *Nat. Rev. Canc.* **2003**, *3*, 766-780.
2. Cornwell, T., Cohick, W., Raskin, I., *Phytochem.* **2004**, *65*, 995-1016.
3. Robards, K. *J. Chromatogr. A* **2003**, *1000*, 657-691.
4. Stecher, G., Huck, C.W., Stoggl, W.M., Guggenbichler, W., Bakry, R., Bonn, G.K, *Phytochem. Rev.* **2002**, *1*, 413-426.
5. van Elswijk, D.A., Irth, H., *Phytochem. Rev.* **2003**, *1*, 427-439.
6. Cuyckens, F., Claeys, M. *J. Mass Spectrom.* **2004**, *39*, 1-15.
7. Stobiecki, M., *Phytochem.* **2000**, *54*, 237-256.
8. Bohn, B.A., *Introduction to flavonoids.* Harwood Academic Publishers: Singapore, **1998**.
9. Watson, D.G., Pitt, A.R., *Rapid Commun. Mass Spectrom.* **1998**, *12*, 153-162.
10. Soleas, G.J., Diamandis, E.P., Karumanchiri, A., Goldberg, D.M., *Anal. Chem.* **1997**, *69*, 4405-4412.
11. Liggins, J., Bluck, L., Coward, W.A., Bingham, S.A., *Biochem. Soc. Trans.* **1998**, *26*, 87-95.
12. Adlercruetz, H., Fotsis, T., Bannwart, C., Wahala, K., Brunow, G., Hase, T., *Clin. Chim. Acta* **1991**, *199*, 263-269.
13. Stobiecki, M.; Olechnowicz-Stepien, W.; Rzadkowska-Bodalska, H.; Cisowski, W.; Budko, E., *Biomed. Environ. Mass Spectrom.* **1988**, *15*, 589-594.
14. Witig, J., Herderich, M., Graefe, E.U., Veit, M., *J. Chromatogr. B* **2000**, *753*, 237-243.
15. He, X., Lin, L., Lian, L., *J. Chromatogr. A* **1996**, *755*, 127-134.
16. Schroder, E., Merfort, I., *Biol. Mass Spectrom.* **1991**, *20*, 11-17.
17. Wolfender, J., Rodriguez, S., Hostettmann, K., Wagner-Redeker, W., *J. Mass Spectrom.* **1995**, S35-S46.
18. Aramendia, M.A., Garcia, I., Lafont, F., Marina, J.M., *Rapid Commun. Mass Spectrom.* **1995**, *9*, 503-508.
19. Careri, M., Elviri, L., Mangia, A., *Rapid Commun. Mass Spectrom.* **1999**, *13*, 2399-2405.
20. Huck, C.W., Huber, C.G., Ongania, K.-H., Bonn, G.K., *J. Chromatogr. A* **2000**, *870*, 453-362.
21. Doerge, D.R., Chang, H.C., Churchwell, M., Holder, C., *Drug Metab. Disps.* **2000**, *28*, 298-307.
22. Nielson, S.E., Freese, R., Cornett, C., Dragsted, L.O., *Anal. Chem.* **2000**, *72*, 1503-1509.
23. Cuyckens, F.; Claeys, M., *Rapid Commun. Mass Spectrom.* **2002**, *16*, 2341-2348.
24. Fabre, N.; Rustan, I.; de Hoffmann, E.; Quetin-Leclercq, J., *J. Am. Soc. Mass Spectrom.* **2001**, *12*, 707-715.

25. de Rijke, E.; Zappey, H.; Ariese, F.; Gooijer, C.; Brinkman, U.A.T. *J. Chromatogr. A* **2003**, *984*, 45-58.
26. Hvattum, E., *Rapid Commun. Mass Spectrom.* **2002**, *16*, 655-662.
27. Maillard, M.N.; Giampaoli, P.; Cuvelier, M.E. , *Talanta* **1996**, *43*, 339-347.
28. Pietta, P.; Facino, R.M.; Carini, M.; Mauri, P., *J. Chromatogr. A* **1994**, *661*, 121-126.
29. Boue, S.M.; Carter-Wientjes, C.H.; Shih, B.Y.; Cleveland, T.E., *J. Chromatogr. A* **2003**, *991*, 61-68.
30. Sanchez-Rabaneda, F.; Jauregui, O.; Lamuela-Raventos, R.M.; Bastida, J.; Viladomat, F.; Codina, C., *J. Chromatogr. A* **2003**, *1008*, 57-72.
31. Sanchez-Rabaneda, F.; Jauregui, O.; Casals, I.; Andres-Lacueva, C.; Izquierdo-Pulido, M.; Lamuela-Raventos, R.M., *J. Mass Spectrom.* **2003**, *38*, 35-42.
32. Nielsen, S.E.; Freese, R.; Cornett, C.; Dragsted, L.O., *Anal. Chem.* **2000**, *72*, 1503-1509.
33. Satterfield, M., Black, D., Brodbelt, J.S., *J. Chromatogr. A* **2001**, *759*, 33-41.
34. Zhang, J., Satterfield, M., Brodbelt, J.S., Britz, S.J.,Clevidence, B., Novotny, J.A., *Anal. Chem.* **2003**, *75*, 6401-6407.
35. Zhang, J., Brodbelt, J.S., *Analyst* **2004**, *129*, 1227-1233.
36. Davis, B., Brodbelt, J.S., *Anal. Chem.* **2005**, *77*, 1883-1890.
37. Weintraub, R.A., Ameer, B., Johnson, J.V., Yost, R.A., *J. Agric. Food Chem.* **1995**, *43*, 1966-1968.
38. Borges, C.; Martinho, P.; Martins, A.; Rauter, A.P.; Ferreira, M.A.A., *Rapid Commun. Mass Spectrom.* **2001**, *15*, 1760-1767.
39. Ma, Y.L.; Li, Q.M.; Van den Heuvel, H.; Claeys, M., *Rapid Commun. Mass Spectrom.* **1997**, *11*, 1357-1364.
40. Ma, Y.L.; Vedernikova, I.; Van den Heuvel, H.; Claeys, M., *J. Am. Soc. Mass Spectrom.* **2000**, *11*, 136-144.
41. Ma, Y.L.; Van den Heuvel, H.; Claeys, M., *Rapid Commun. Mass Spectrom.* **1999**, *13*, 1932-1942.
42. Cuyckens, F.; Ma, Y.L.; Pocsfalvi, G.; Claeys, M., *Analusis* **2000**, *28*, 888-895.
43. Li, Q.M.; Van den Heuvel, H.; Dillen, L.; Claeys, M., *Biol. Mass Spectrom.* **1992**, *21*, 213-221.
44. Ma, Y.L.; Cuyckens, F.; Van den Heuvel, H.; Claeys, M., *Phytochem. Analysis* **2001**, *12*, 159-165.
45. Cuyckens, F.; Shahat, A.A.; Pieters, L.; Claeys, M., *J. Mass Spectrom.* **2002**, *37*, 1272-1279.
46. Cuyckens, F.; Rozenberg, R.; de Hoffmann, E.; Claeys, M., *J. Mass Spectrom.* **2001**, *36*, 1203-1210.
47. Hughes, R.J.; Croley, T.R.; Metcalfe, C.D.; March, R.E., *Int. J. Mass Spectrom.* **2001**, *210/211*, 371-385.
48. Hvattum, E.; Ekeberg, D., *J. Mass Spectrom.* **2003**, *38*, 43-49.
49. Justesen, U., *J. Mass Spectrom.* **2001**, *36*, 169-178.

50. Prasain, J.K.; Patel, R.; Kirk, M.; Wilson, L.; Botting, N.; Darley-Usmar, V.M.; Barnes, S., *J. Mass Spectrom.* **2003**, *38*, 764-771.
51. Kuhn, F.; Oehme, M.; Romero, F.; Abou-Mansour, E.; Tabacchi, R., *Rapid Commun. Mass Spectrom.* **2003**, *17*, 1941-1949.
52. Wolfender, J.L.; Waridel, P.; Ndjoko, K.; Hobby, K.R.; Major, H.J.; Hostettmann, K., *Analusis* **2000**, *28*, 895-906.
53. Waridel, P.; Wolfender, J.L.; Ndjoko, K.; Hobby, K.R.; Major, H.J.; Hostettmann, K., *J. Chromatogr. A* **2001**, 926, 29-41.
54. Rauha, J.P.; Vuorela, H.; Kostiainen, R., *J. Mass Spectrom.* **2001**, *36*, 1269-1280.
55. Keki, S.; Deak, G.; Zsuga, M., *J. Mass Spectrom.* **2001**, *36*, 1312-1316.
56. Frison-Norrie, S.; Sporns, P., *J. Agric. Food Chem.* **2002,** *50*, 2782-2787.
57. Franski, R.; Bednarek, P.; Wojtaszek, P.; Stobiecki, M., *J. Mass Spectrom.* **1999**, *34*, 486-495.
58. Justesen, U., *J. Chromatogr. A* **2000**, *902*, 369-379.
59. Llorach, R.; Gil-Izquierdo, A.; Ferreres, F.; Tomas-Barberan, F.A., *J. Agric. Food Chem.* **2003**, *51*, 3895-3899.
60. Mauri, P.L.; Iemoli, L.; Gardana, C.; Riso, P.; Simonetti, P.; Porrini, M.; Pietta, P.G., *Rapid Commun. Mass Spectrom.* **1999**, *13*, 924-931.
61. Satterfield, M., J. Brodbelt, J.S., *Anal. Chem.*, **2000**, *72*, 5898-5906.
62. Satterfield, M., Brodbelt, J.S., *J. Am. Soc. Mass Spectrom.* **2001**, *12*, 537-549.
63. Zhang, J., Brodbelt, J.S., *J. Mass Spectrom*, **2003**, *38*, 555-572.
64. Pikulski, M., Brodbelt, J.S., *J. Am. Soc. Mass Spectrom.* **2003**, *14*, 1437-1453.
65. Zhang, J., Brodbelt, J.S., *J. Am. Chem. Soc.* **2004**, *126*, 5906-5919.
66. Davis, B.,Brodbelt, J.S., *J. Am. Soc. Mass Spectrom.* **2004**, *15*, 1287-1299.
67. Zhang, J., Wang, J, Brodbelt, J.S., *J. Am. Soc. Mass Spectrom.* **2005**, *16*, 139-151.
68. Zhang, J., Brodbelt, J.S., *Anal. Chem.* **2005**, *77*, 1761-1770.
69. Zhang, J., Wang, J., Brodbelt, J.S., *J. Mass Spectrom.* **2005**, *40*, 350-363.
70. Cuyckens F. Claeys, M., *J. Mass Spectrom.* **2005**, *40*, 364-372.
71. R.B. Cole, Ed., *Electrospray Ionization Mass Spectrometry: Fundamentals, Instrumentation, and Applications* John Wiley and Sons: New York, **1997**.
72. De Hoffmann, E., *J. Mass Spectrom.* **1996**, *31*, 129-137.
73. McLuckey, S. A., *J. Am. Soc. Mass Spectrom.* **1992**, *2*, 599-614.

Chapter 5

Powerful Analytical Tools for Citrus Characterization: LC/MS and LC/NMR Characterization of Polymethoxylated Flavones

Claus O. Schmidt*, Gerhard E. Krammer, Berthold Weber, Detlef Stöckigt, Stefan Brennecke, Günter Kindel, and Heinz-Jürgen Bertram

Symrise GmbH and Company KG, Mühlenfeldstrasse 1, D–37603 Holzminden, Germany
***Corresponding author: telephone: +49–5531–90–2629; fax: +49–5531–90–49629; email: claus.oliver.schmidt@symrise.com**

Citrus fruits are well known for their unique flavor and their health benefits. Volatile compounds such as terpenes are formed as secondary metabolites in the plant. These volatile compounds mainly contribute to the flavor and scent of the plant. However, other non-volatile metabolites are formed via biosynthesis in citrus. These non-volatile compounds contribute to certain health benefits like anticarcinogenic, antitumor, antiviral or antimicrobial activities. Our goal is to establish efficient analytical technologies to identify and characterize the volatile and non-volatile compounds from citrus plants. For a fast and reliable screening of volatile compounds in citrus flavors, solid phase micro-extraction (SPME) and solid phase dynamic extraction (SPDE) are well known techniques for flavor analysis. Residues obtained from molecular distillation of cold pressed peel oils of oranges and clementines were analyzed using LC/MS and LC/NMR to characterize non-volatile compounds.

Introduction

Oils of citrus fruits obtained by molecular distillation of cold pressed oils are of high importance in the flavoring of food. After pressing the citrus fruits and addition of water, the oil layer separates out from the juice phase. The oil is filtered, centrifuged and then chilled, the latter treatment resulting in precipitation of waxes. This cold pressed oil is subjected to molecular distillation thereby obtaining an almost colorless oil with a sharp sensory profile.

Recently the non-volatiles of lemon peel oils were analyzed using LC/NMR (1). During our work on citrus we extended these studies to the residue obtained from clementine peel oils. These residues were expected to be enriched in polymethoxyflavones which could be confirmed by LC/MS experiments. Further LC/NMR measurements were necessary to actually confirm the structures of the different individual components.

The chromatograms obtained from LC/MS and LC/NMR experiments (detection at 210 nm) are very similar since the same stationary phase was used. In Figure 1 the chromatogram and the total ion current (TIC) from the LC/MS experiment obtained by atmospheric chemical ionization in the positive mode are shown. The retention time interval between 17 and 30 min is occupied by different polymethoxyflavones. Compounds **1** to **6** are indicated as tetra-, penta-, hexa- and heptamethoxy substituted flavones as based on the detected masses of the molecular species, with m/z = 343, 373, 403 and 433, respectively. Compound **7** is a monohydroxylated hexamethoxyflavones with MW = 418.

The two-dimensional plot from the LC/NMR experiment in the on-flow mode (Figure 2) clearly shows the characteristic signal pattern for polymethoxylated flavones due to the aromatic protons between 7 and 9 ppm and also for the methoxy groups around 3.7 to 4.1 ppm. This experiment was repeated in the loop collection mode for a better signal to noise ratio and therefore better identification of the constituents. The substitution pattern of the phenyl residues of the different flavones can easily be deduced. The para-substituted phenyl moieties of compounds **4** and **6** are deduced from two doublets at about 7.92 and 7.06 ppm and a coupling constant of about 9.0 Hz. For both compounds the typical singlet signal of the proton attached to C-3 is observed at about 6.62 ppm. Bearing in mind the remaining four methoxy groups, compound **6** can be unambiguously identified as tangeretin. The identity of compound **4** with three methoxy groups at positions C-5, C-6 and C-7 is deduced as a result of a detailed comparison with recently isolated tetramethylscutellarein (2).

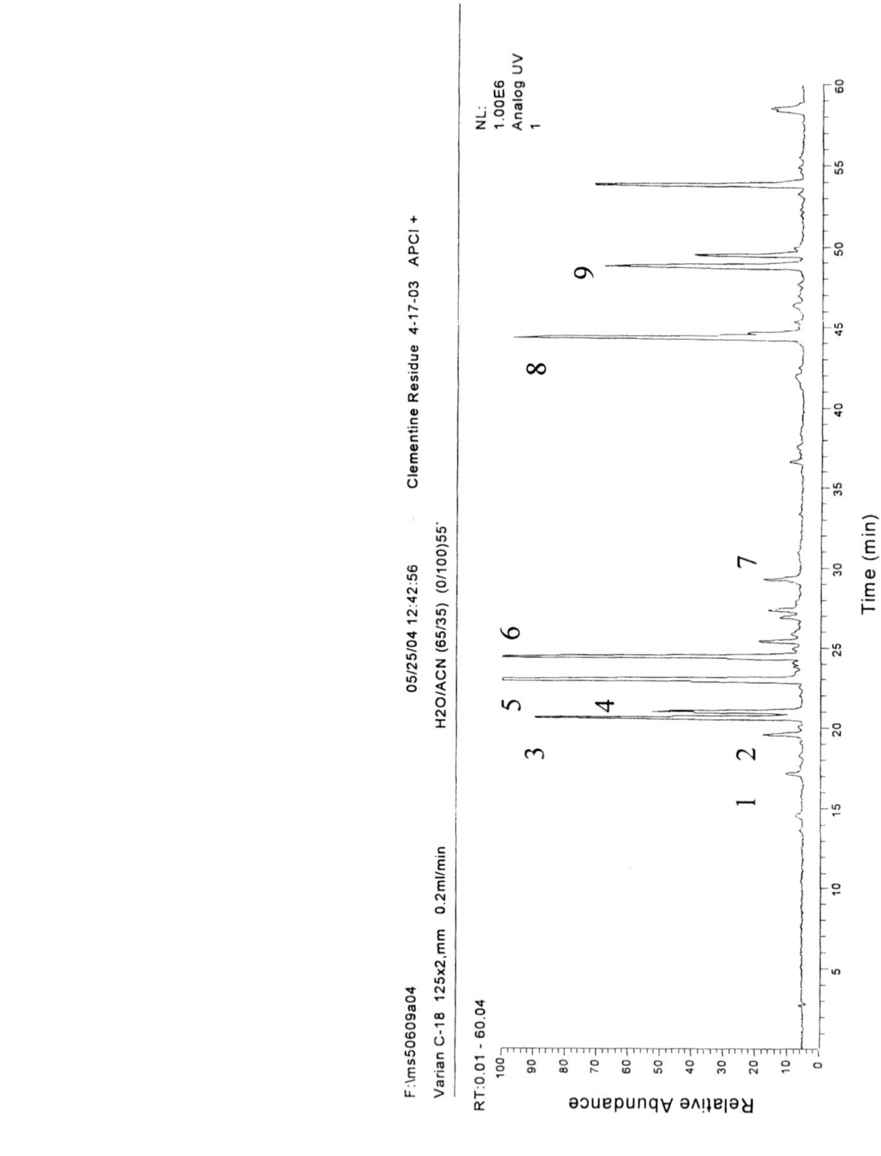
F:\ms50609a04
Varian C-18 125x2,mm 0.2ml/min
05/25/04 12:42:56
H2O/ACN (65/35) (0/100)55'
Clementine Residue 4-17-03 APCI +
RT:0.01 - 60.04
NL:
1.00E6
Analog UV
1
Relative Abundance
Time (min)
1
2
3
4
5
6
7
8
9

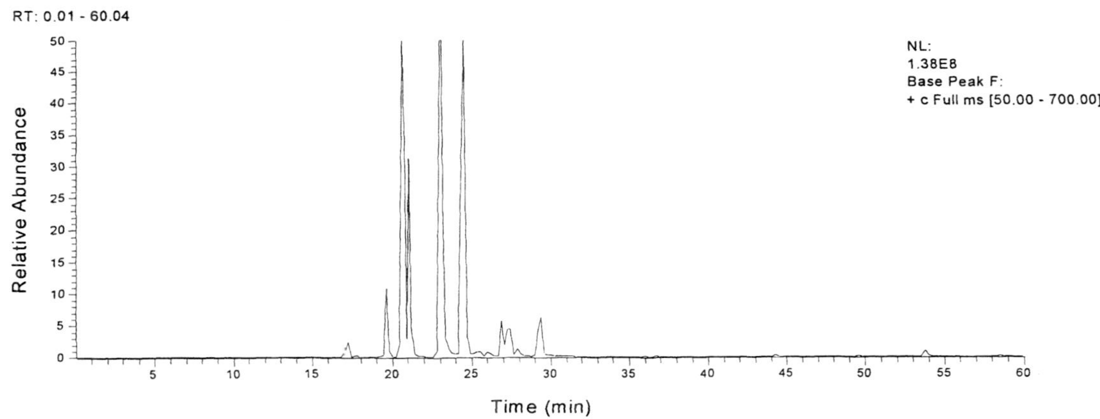

Figure 1. Chromatogram (detection at 210 nm) and TIC originating from LC/MS experiment.

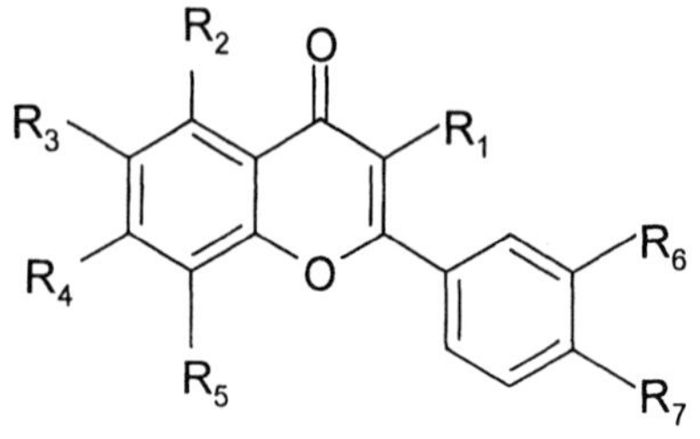

1 - 7

Table I. Structures of detected polymethoxylated flavones

	Name	R_1	R_2	R_3	R_4	R_5	R_6	R_7	MW
1	5,6,7,3',4'-Pentamethoxyflavone (sinensetin)	H	OCH_3	OCH_3	OCH_3	H	OCH_3	OCH_3	372
2	3,5,6,7,3',4'-Hexamethoxyflavone	OCH_3	OCH_3	OCH_3	OCH_3	H	OCH_3	OCH_3	402
3	5,6,7,8,3',4'-Hexamethoxyflavone (nobiletin)	H	OCH_3	OCH_3	OCH_3	OCH_3	OCH_3	OCH_3	402
4	5,6,7,4'-Tetramethoxyflavone (Tetramethyl-scutellarein)	H	OCH_3	OCH_3	OCH_3	H	H	OCH_3	342
5	3,5,6,7,8,3',4'-Heptamethoxyflavone	OCH_3	OCH_3	OCH_3	OCH_3	OCH_3	OCH_3	OCH_3	432
6	5,6,7,8,4' Pentamethoxyflavone (tangeretin)	H	OCH_3	OCH_3	OCH_3	OCH_3	H	OCH_3	372
7	5-Hydroxy-3,6,7,8,3',4'-Hexamethoxyflavone	OCH_3	OH	OCH_3	OCH_3	OCH_3	OCH_3	OCH_3	418

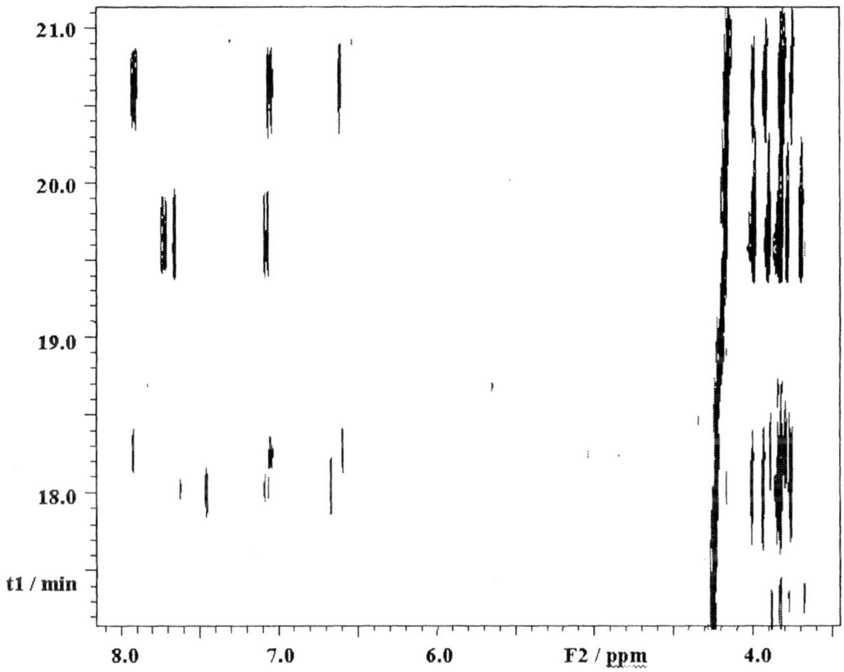

Figure 2. 2D plot of the LC/NMR on-flow experiment.

The phenyl residues of flavones **1**, **2**, **3** and **5** are in fact 1,3,4-substituted isomers as concluded from the double doublet at about 7.6 (**1**,**3**) or 7.7 ppm (**2**,**5**), another doublet around 7.5 (**1**,**3**) or 7.6 ppm (**2**,**5**) and a further doublet at 7.1 ppm with coupling constants of 8.6 and 2.1 Hz. The lack of substitution at C-3 for **1** and **3** is evident as a result of the presence of the signal at 6.6 ppm for the proton. Compound **3** is therefore unambiguously identified as nobiletin (Figure 3) due to the remaining four methoxy groups. Comparison of the chemical shifts of **1** with those of tetramethylscutellarein **4** and especially with respect to the protons at the chromen-4-one system, reveals almost identical shifts leading to the assignment of sinensitin for **1**. For compound **5**, all protons of the chromen-4-one system are substituted by methoxy groups, thus confirming the structure as the trisubstituted phenyl-containing 3,5,6,7,8,3',4'heptamethoxyflavone. The LC/MS experiment indicates compound **2** as hexamethoxyflavone. The absence of the signal in the ^{1}H-NMR spectrum at about 6.6 ppm for the proton at C-3 due to substitution by a methoxy group, raises the question about the substitution pattern on the aromatic ring of the chromen-4-one moiety by the residual methoxy groups. Both 3,5,6,7,3',4'- and 3,5,7,8,3',4'-hexamethoxyflavone have recently been reported from orange peel (3). The experimental NMR data of the former fit better with the published data (4, 5). NMR data in $CDCl_3$ of compound **2** isolated by preparative HPLC are identical to those from literature for 3,5,6,7,3',4'-hexamethoxyflavone (5).

Compound **7** is indicated as hydroxy-hexamethoxyflavone, which is confirmed by the LC/NMR experiments. The 1,2,4-trisubstituted pattern is reflected by the three signals of the aromatic protons as described above. Since the chemical shifts of these protons are almost identical to those of compounds **2** and **5**, three of the six methoxy groups should be attached to C-3, C-3' and C-4'. The exact position of the hydroxyl group could not be determined by the LC/NMR measurements and preparative isolation of the component was performed by HPLC. By comparison of the experimental and published ^{1}H-NMR data (6), compound **7** is identified as being 5-hydroxy-3,6,7,8,3',4'-hexamethoxyflavone.

By comparing the intensities of the UV absorptions and the mass spectrometric total ion current resulting from the less polar constituents, UV absorption appears to be a more favorable detection method for those compounds. Using LC/NMR, compound **8** (44.5 min) can be readily identified as a sinensal isomer and **9** (48.8 min) as limonene.

Experimental

Plant material

Residues from the molecular distillation of cold pressed peel oil of clementines (Citrus reticulata Blanco var. Clementine) were analyzed.

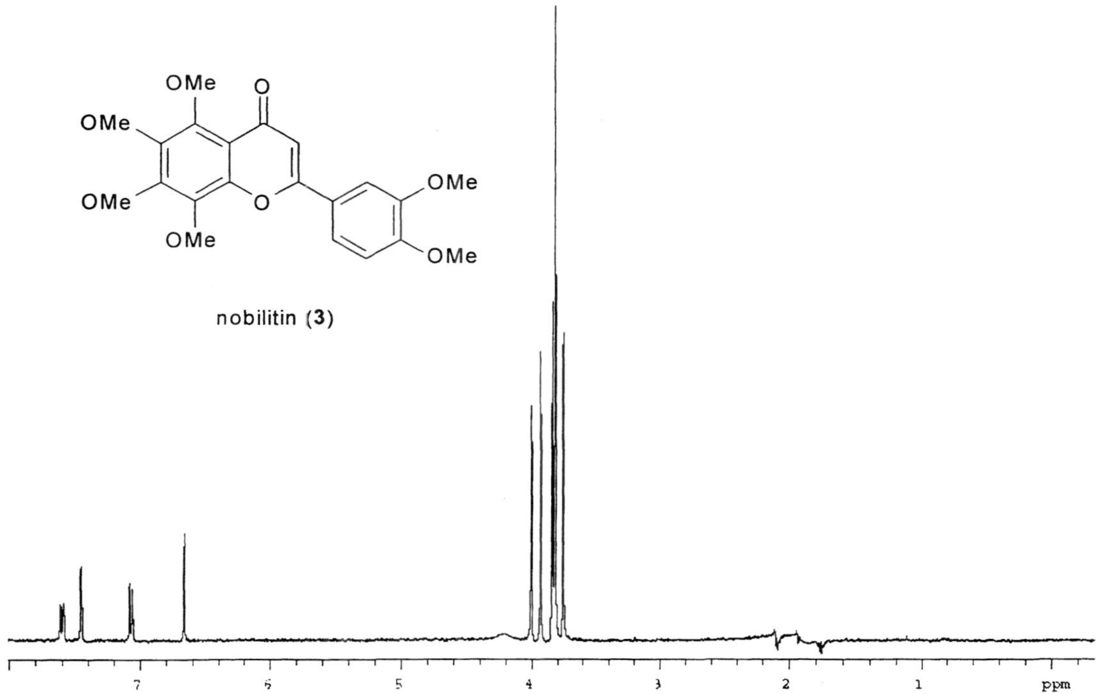

Figure 3. [1]*H-LC/NMR-spectrum of nobilitin* **3** *with solvent suppression around 4.5 (HDO) and 2 ppm (acetonitrile).*

HPLC/MS analyses

LC/MS experiments were performed on a system consisting of a ThermoQuest LCQ mass spectrometer with an APCI interface and a Hewlett Packard HP 1100 HPLC system. APCI experiments were carried out in the positive mode. Nitrogen was used as sheath gas. Gradients with H_2O (containing 0.01% formic acid) and acetonitrile were run with a flow rate of 0.2 ml/min and a Varian C18 column (125 x 2 mm, particle size 3 μm) was used for chromatographic separations.

HPLC/NMR analyses

For LC/NMR measurements D_2O (99,9%) was purchased from Deutero GmbH, Kastellaun, Germany, and acetonitrile (HPLC/NMR grade) was bought from Riedel de Haën, Seelze, Germany.
LC/NMR experiments were performed on the ^{Unity}INOVA system using a $^1H\{^{13}C/^{15}N\}$PFG triple resonance indirect detection microflow LC/NMR probe (IFC probe) with a detection volume of 60 μL at 20 °C. The HPLC system consisted of a ternary Varian ProStar 230 pump, a Varian ProStar 330 Photodiode Array Detector (210 nm) and a Varian ProStar 510 column oven (50 °C). Chromatographic separation was carried out on an OmniSpher C18 column (250 x 4.6 mm, particle size 5 μm) running gradients with acetonitrile and D_2O (containing 0.01% TFA v/v). Solvent suppression was achieved by performing a WET pulse sequence (7). During gradient elution, shapes of selective pulses were automatically calculated on the fly based on a scout scan recorded before each increment. Chemical shifts were referenced to acetonitrile (1.93 ppm). NMR spectra of isolated compounds were also recorded on a Varian ^{Unity}INOVA (400 MHz) spectrometer.

Conclusions

In the past, polymethoxylated flavones were normally identified by comparing MS and UV spectra from LC/MS experiments with isolated reference materials, which is quite time-consuming, or with the aid of published data, which implies a certain tentativeness. HPLC/NMR represents a powerful tool for the identification of constituents without any prior isolation being necessary. The method is somewhat limited when dealing with molecules with only few protons. However, with increasing reported NMR data in the given solvent system D_2O/acetonitrile, identification will become more easy and reliable. In addition, components which possess a strong UV absorption but low mass spectrometric ionization efficiency or vice versa can be readily characterized by LC/NMR.

Acknowledgement

The author are indebted to their colleagues Dr. Ingo Reiss suppling the clementine residues obtained from molecular distillation of the essential oils and Michael Roloff for the preparative HPLC work.

References

1. Sommer, H.; Bertram, H.-J., Krammer, G.; Kindel, G.; Kühnle, T.; Reinders, G.; Reiss, I.; Schmidt, C.O.; Schreiber, K.; Stumpe, W.; Werkhoff, P.; *Perfumer&Flavorist* **2003**, *28,* 18-34.
2. Weber, B.; Hartmann, B. Unpublished results.
3. Malterud, K.E.; Rydland, K.M. *J. Agric. Food Chem.* **2000**, *48*, 5576-5580.
4. Joseph-Nathan, P.; Abramo-Bruno, D; Torres, M. A. *Phytochemistry* **1981**, *20*, 313-318.
5. Machida, K.; Osawa, K. *Chem. Pharm. Bull.* **1989**, *37*(4), 1092-1094.
6. Roitman, J. N.; James, L. F. *Phytochemistry* **1985**, *24*(4), 835-848.
7. Smallcombe, S.H.; Patt, S.L.; Keifer, P.A. *J. Magn. Reson.* Series A **1995,** *117*, 295-303.

Bioavailability and Toxicity of Limonoids

Chapter 6

Long-Term Screening Study on the Potential Toxicity of Limonoids

Edward G. Miller[1,2], Reed P. Gibbins[1], Samuel E. Taylor[1], Jame E. McIntosh[1], and Bhimanagouda S. Patil[2]

[1]Department of Biomedical Sciences, Baylor College of Dentistry, Texas A&M University Health Science Center, 3302 Gaston Avenue, Dallas, TX 75246
[2]Vegetable and Fruit Improvement Center, Department of Horticultural Sciences, Mail Code2119, Texas A&M University, College Station, TX 77843

Twelve pregnant rats were separated into 3 equal groups. Group 1 was fed the standardized rat chow, the AIN93G diet. Groups 2 and 3 were given the same diet supplemented with a 0.25% blend of mixed limonoid glucosides (group 2) or a 0.15% blend of mixed aglycones (group 3). At weaning, 33 pups per group were selected and placed on their mother's diet. Six weeks later 15 young female rats (5/group) were bred to males in the same group. The remaining animals were sacrificed and blood samples were collected. Multiple statistical differences were found in the blood chemistries. At weaning the pups from the 15 litters were sacrificed and autopsied. The male pups from groups 2 and 3 weighed significantly less than the male pups from group 1. For the females, the pups in group 2 weighed significantly less than the pups in group 1. The data consistently showed that at this high level of exposure, that the diets with limonoids caused problems with weight gain.

General Introduction

Limonoids – basic research

Limonoids are a group of structurally related triterpene derivatives. Early research concentrated on the fact that several limonoids are extremely bitter. The primary ones are limonin, which is found in a wide variety of citrus juices, and nomilin, which primarily contributes to bitterness in grapefruit juice. The bitterness threshold for these two limonoids in citrus juice is 3-6 ppm (*1,2*). To minimize the economic impact of this problem a considerable amount of research has focused on the synthesis of these compounds in citrus. Through the use of radioactive tracer techniques, it was found that nomilin is synthesized from acetate and mevalonate, via farnesyl pyrophosphate in the phloem region of the stem (*3*). Once formed nomilin is translocated from the stem to other regions of the plant (leaves, fruit tissue, peels, and seeds) where it is metabolized into the other limonoids (*4*). Four different pathways, the limonin pathway, the calamin pathway, the ichangensin pathway, and the 7-acetate limonoid pathway have been identified for the biosynthesis of the other limonoids (*5*). Research on consumer acceptance has also shown that limonin is the major cause of delayed bitterness (*6*) and that bitterness decreases as fruit maturation progresses (*7*).

Early research on limonoids in citrus tissues and juices usually started with an extraction with a non polar solvent. The aqueous phase was routinely discarded. In 1989, it was reported (*8,9*) that the aqueous phase contains a large number of modified limonoids. NMR analyses showed that in each of these compounds the aglycone was linked with one glucose molecule at C-17 by a β-glycosidic linkage. Unlike the aglycones, which are found in low concentrations in the fruit and juice, the limonoid glucosides are found in high concentrations. Using TLC analyses (*10*) and HPLC (*11*), it was found that the concentration of mixed limonoid glucosides in orange juice averaged 320-330 ppm. The predominant limonoid glucoside accounting for over 50% of the total is limonin 17-β-D-glucopyranoside. Unlike limonin which is bitter limonin 17-β-D-glucopyranoside is essentially tasteless (*8*).

Limonoids – anticancer activity

Starting in 1989 a number of papers have shown that limonoids can inhibit the development of carcinogen-induced tumors in animals. In most of these studies limonin and nomilin were tested for cancer chemopreventive activity.

These two limonoids have exhibited antineoplastic activity in a model for benz[a]pyrene-induced forestomach tumors (*12*) in ICR/Ha mice, in a model for 7,12-dimethylbenz[a]anthracene (DMBA) induced oral tumors in Syrian golden hamsters (*13*), in a model for benz[a]pyrene-induced lung tumors in A/J mice (*14*), in a two-stage model for DMBA-induced skin tumors in SENCAR mice (*15*), in a model for 4-(methylnitrosamino)-1-(3-pyridyl)-1-butanone-induced lung tumors in A/J mice (*16*) and in a model for azoxymethane-induced aberrant crypts in male F344 rats (*17*). One interesting sidelight to the data with the animal models is the apparent agreement with earlier epidemiological evidence on citrus consumption and cancer in humans (*18*). Approximately two dozen epidemiological studies have consistently shown that citrus consumption can significantly reduce an individual's risk for a variety of different cancers including cancers of the oral cavity, stomach, lung, colon, rectum, esophagus, larynx, and pancreas.

In the model for oral carcinogenesis, 12 citrus limonoids have been tested for cancer chemopreventive activity (*13,19-22*). Four (limonin, limonin 17-β-D-glucopyranoside, deoxylimonin, and limonin carboxymethoxime) were found to have significant activity. Each of these limonoids lowered tumor burden by 50-60%. The effect on tumor number was considerably less, a 15-30% inhibition. Three (nomilin, obacunone, and nomilin 17-β-D-glucopyranoside) were classified as having partial activity. With these chemicals there was a 20-30% reduction in tumor number. Since there was no effect on tumor volume, the overall reduction in tumor burden was similar to the reduction in tumor number. The data for the remaining limonoids (limonol, ichangensin, nomilinic acid 17-β-D-glucopyranoside, deoxylimonic acid, and 17,19-didehydrolimonoic acid) showed that these chemicals were inactive. In addition to identifying new limonoids with antineoplastic activity, the data from these experiments indicated that some of the structural features in limonoids could be modified without affecting anticancer activity. One area where major modifications can be made is the D ring in the limonoid nucleus.

Limonoids – other potential health benefits

Data from a number of different laboratories suggest that limonoids may have additional health-promoting properties. In one paper (*23*), it was reported that the substitution of grapefruit juice and orange juice for drinking water significantly lowered cholesterol levels in casein fed rabbits. Experiments with a human liver cell line, HepG2 cells, showed that limonoids were primarily responsible for this effect on LDL cholesterol. In another study, it was shown that a variety of limonoids including deacetylnomilin, obacunone, nomilin, and a mixture of limonoid glucosides were potent inhibitors of proliferation of estrogen receptor-negative (MDA-MB-435 cells) and –positive (MCF-7 cells) human breast cancer cells (*24*). Similar cytotoxic effects were not seen with a variety of other human cancer cell lines (*25*) or with normal human cell lines grown in culture (*26*). It was also shown that limonoids could induce apoptosis in MCF-7 cells (*25*). Finally, in a recent paper limonin and nomilin were found to have anti-HIV activity (*27*). The two limonoids inhibited HIV replication in a variety of different cellular systems. Both of the compounds were also found to inhibit *in vitro* HIV-1 protease activity.

Limonoids – commercial interest

Overall this research on the potential health benefits of citrus limonoids plus the extensive epidemiological evidence (*18*) has led a number of investigators and companies to start work on the production of new products. Early research on the metabolism of limonoids in the plant has led to work on the development of transgenic varieties of citrus that are free of bitter limonoids containing elevated concentrations of mixed limonoid glucosides (*28,29*). Commercial interest in the use of these citrus chemicals in new products has centered on the limonoid glucosides. There are several reasons for this focus. As already indicated one of the primary reasons is that the limonoid glucosides are tasteless (*8*). The fact that limonoid glucosides are polar also increases the potential for product development. These chemicals could easily be incorporated into a wide array of different products as food additives. Another factor is human consumption. The high concentration of mixed limonoid glucosides in citrus fruits and juices indicates that humans may be able to tolerate higher levels of exposure. Finally, research on by-products from juice processing plants has shown that mixed limonoid glucosides can be isolated in large quantities from citrus molasses and seeds (*30-32*). The seeds (30) are also a good source of the aglycones (limonin and nomilin).

Even though the technology is in place to create a wide variety of foods containing elevated concentrations of citrus limonoids, we feel that product formulation at this time is premature. The primary reason is that very little is known about the pharmacokinetics of these chemicals in mammalian systems.

Research is needed to determine how effectively limonoids are absorbed in the GI tract. Once absorbed, how are these chemicals distributed throughout the body? How rapidly are the chemicals metabolized and do any of these metabolites have health-promoting properties? Finally, at higher levels of consumption are there any side effects or toxicity? To start to answer these questions this laboratory has shifted its focus from basic studies on carcinogenesis to research on uptake, distribution, turnover, and toxicity in mammalian systems. The primary objective of this experiment was to provide data on any potential toxicity that might be produced over several generations of rats through long-term systemic exposure.

Experimental Design

First generation

For the experiment, 12 Sprague Dawley rats 10 days into their pregnancies were purchased from Harlan (Indianapolis, IN). At the time of arrival, the rats were separated into 3 equal groups (4 rats/group) and immediately placed on one of the three test diets. The animals in the control group, group 1, were fed the AIN93G diet prepared by Bio-Serv in Frenchtown, NJ. The pregnant rats in groups 2 and 3 were fed the same diet supplemented with a 0.25% mixture of limonoid glucosides (group 2) or a 0.15% mixture of limonoid aglycones. In an earlier short-term feeding trial with hamsters (*33*), 2 groups of animals were fed diets supplemented with mixed limonoid glucosides at a concentration of 0.05% or 0.50%. For this experiment, the concentrations were set between these limits (0.05-0.50%).

The percent composition of the limonoid glucoside mixture isolated from citrus molasses was 35.9% limonin 17-β-D-glucopyranoside, 32.0% nomilinic acid 17-β-D-glucopyranoside, 12.7% nomilin 17-β-D-glucopyranoside, 8.7% deacetylnomilinic acid 17-β-D-glucopyranoside, 6.6% deacetylnomilin 17-β-D-glucopyranoside, and 4.1% obacunone 17-β-D-glucopyranoside (*33*). The aglycone mixture prepared in this laboratory was 90% limonin and 10% nomilin. Limited availability of the two chemicals dictated the reduced concentration (0.15%) and the 9/1 ratio. The limonin and nomilin were prepared from citrus seeds (*30*). During this time and throughout the rest of the experiment the food in powdered form and water were provided *ad libitum*. The animals were housed in solid bottomed plastic cages containing litter and nesting material in a room reserved for breeding. The room was maintained at 22°C with a 14:10 h light-dark cycle.

Second generation

At the time of weaning (32 days later), 33 pups per group were randomly selected and placed in individual stainless steel cages. The pups were moved to a separate room reserved for rats maintained at 22°C with a 12:12 h light-dark cycle. The pups were placed on their mother's diet. Approximately 6 weeks later, 15 female rats (5/group) weighing at least 200 grams were selected and bred to males in the same group but from different litters. The average weights for the females used in this part of the study were 210 g (group 1), 213 g (group 2), and 221 g (group 3). During the six week period weight gain and food intake were monitored. After the pregnancies were established, the remaining animals were sacrificed and blood samples were collected and processed. Serum samples were sent to an outside laboratory (Texas Veterinary Medical Diagnostic Laboratory System in College Station, Texas), where a complete series of blood chemistries were run. The technicians at this facility had no prior knowledge about how the rats had been treated.

Third generation

At day 21, the pups from the 15 litters were sacrificed (carbon dioxide exposure). The sex and weight of the pups were determined. Following an autopsy the heart, a kidney, and the small lobe of the liver were taken. The samples were fixed in 10% neutral-buffered formalin, embedded in paraffin, processed by routine histological techniques, and stained with hematoxylin and eosin. The histologist who examined the slides for abnormalities had no prior knowledge about the treatment assignments..

Experimental Results

Food intake & weight gain

The data for food intake during the six-week period showed that there were some problems for the rats in group 2. The primary problem was seen in the male rats given the diet containing the mixed limonoid glucosides. During three of the first four weeks daily food intake was significantly reduced (two-tailed Student's t-test) by 1.0-2.0 g when compared to the data for the male rats in group 1. During week two a significant reduction (1.5 g) was also seen for the female rats in group 2. Throughout the six-week period the weight gain profile for the male rats in group 2 was significantly less than the weight gain profile for the male rats in group 1. At the end of the six-week period, the average weight for the male rats in the three groups was 349 g (group 1), 318 g (group 2), and 342 g (group 3). For the females, the averages were 219 g (group 1), 209 (group 2), and 214 g (group 3).

Blood chemistries

For the blood assays, the male rats in groups 2 and 3 were compared to the male rats in group 1 and the females in groups 2 and 3 were compared to the females in group 1. For 14 out of the 17 assays, one or more significant differences (two-tailed Student's t-test) were found in these four comparisons. Multiple differences (2-4) were found in 9 of the 17 assays. The data for these nine assays are given in Table I. Overall the results were highly consistent. Significant differences when they occurred were in almost every case in the same direction. For most of the assays, the non-significant results for groups 2 and 3 trended in the same direction as the significant results. For example, if the significant changes for groups 2 and 3 were higher than the corresponding data for group 1, then the non-significant results usually were elevated. This can be seen in the results for creatine kinase, globulins, alanine transaminase, amylase, creatinine, total serum protein, and alkaline phosphatase. The primary exception was the data for blood calcium. A significant decrease in blood calcium levels was seen in the male rats in groups 2 and 3; however, the levels of blood calcium were significantly increased in the female rats in group 3 and slightly elevated in the female rats in group 2.

Even though a large number of numerically significant differences were found the results usually fell within the normal range of values for rats. This was also found to be true for the assays (phosphorus, albumin globulin ratio, glucose, aspartate transaminase, albumin) in which a single significant difference was seen. The exceptions were creatine kinase and amylase. Both sets of values were routinely high in the male and female rats in the three groups. The way in which the animals were sacrificed may have contributed to these two sets of results. To get adequate amounts of blood, the animals were stunned for a limited period of time in CO_2 and decapitated. Muscular movement during this time could have led to the release of creatine kinase. The reason for the extremely high means for the male and female rats in group 1 is not known. The manner in which the blood was collected might have also led to contamination with saliva and the high values for amylase. The values for the female rats in groups 2 and 3 were especially high.

Table I. Blood Assays (Multiple Differences)[a]

Test	Group 1		Group 2		Group 3	
	Males	Females	Males	Females	Males	Females
Creatine kinase	3440	8060	393[d]	716[d]	201[e]	290[c]
Calcium	11.1	10.5	10.4[b]	10.7	10.1[b]	11.2[e]
Globulins	2.18	1.74	2.22	1.93[b]	2.34[b]	2.00[b]
Alanine transaminase	37.3	48.0	34.1	36.4[b]	27.0[e]	35.3[b]
cholesterol	104	94.1	91.6[d]	92.7	88.9[e]	95.9
Amylase	3300	1770	3610	2380[b]	3930	3120[d]
creatinine	0.221	0.286	0.269[d]	0.323	0.295[e]	0.300
serum protein	6.53	5.99	6.54	6.23	6.85[c]	6.48[b]
Alkaline phosphatase	196	194	171	176	153[e]	144[b]

[a] Units for the different assays were mg/dl for calcium, cholesterol, and creatinine; g/dl for total serum protein and globulins; U/l for amylase, alanine transaminase, alkaline phosphatase, and creatine kinase.

[b-e] Indicate that these values are significant (two-tailed Student's t-test) when compared to the corresponding values for group 1 ([b] $p<0.05$, [c] $p<0.01$, [d] $p<0.005$, and [e] $p<0.001$).

The results for cholesterol were also interesting. Here we found a significant reduction of 10-15% for the male rats in groups 2 and 3. The cholesterol means for the male rats in the three groups were 104 mg/dl (group 1), 91.6 mg/dl (group 2), and 88.9 mg/dl (group 3). This effect on blood cholesterol levels supports the results from another study (*23*) suggesting that limonoids are hypocholesterolemic agents. The data, however, were totally unexpected. There were two reasons why we were surprised to see these results. One, rats are a poor species for this type of research. Normal blood cholesterol levels of 90-105 mg/dl are by comparison to humans and many other species low. Two, the AIN93G diet is a standardized chow that is not designed to promote high cholesterol levels in rats. The means for the female rats in the three groups were similar ranging from 92.7-95.9 mg/dl.

Litters (generation three)

The pups at the end of the study were counted on the day of birth and at the time of sacrifice (day 21). During this three-week period, 3 of the 48 pups in group 1, 21 of the 61 pups in group 2, and 8 of the 61 pups in group 3 died. Part of the reason for the poor survival data for group 2 was that one of the mothers killed all of her pups (13). This is not unusual with first-time breeders. If the data for this litter are excluded, then 8 of the 48 pups in group 2 were lost during the 21 day period. Most of the dead pups were cannibalized by their mothers. Dead pups when retrieved were autopsied. No abnormalities were found.

At the time of sacrifice, the pups were weighed. Since litter size can greatly influence final weight, we decided to compare the weights of the animals in large litters (10-15 pups). The average size of the litters used in these comparisons were 12.5 pups in two litters for group 1, 12.3 pups in three litters for group 2, and 11.5 pups in four litters for group 3. The average weights for the male and female pups used in these comparisons are given in Table II. There were 13 male pups in group 1, 16 in group 2, and 20 in group 3. The number of female pups ranged from 12 in group 1, to 21 in group 2, to 26 in group 3. As illustrated, the average weights for the male pups were 54.0 g (group 1), 50.1 g (group 2), and 49.6 g (group 3). The differences between groups 1 and 2, and groups 1 and 3 were significant (two-tailed Student's t-test). For the females, the averages were 52.4 g (group 1), 47.8 g (group 2), and 50.6 g (group 3). The differences between groups 1 and 2 were significant (two-tailed Student's t-test). No signs of abnormalities were found in the tissues (heart, liver, and kidney) taken for histological evaluation.

Table II. Weight Data (Similar Size Litters)

Group	Averge weight in grams[a]	
	Males	Females
1	54.0 ± 0.75	52.4 ± 0.71
2	50.1 ± 1.0[b]	47.8 ± 1.0[c]
3	49.6 ± 1.1[c]	50.6 ± 0.96

[a]Values are means ± SE.
[b]$p < 0.01$ when compared to group 1.
[c]$p < 0.005$ when compared to group 1.

Conclusions

Overall the data from this long-term feeding trial covering 3 generations of rats consistently showed problems with the diets containing limonoids. The problems were mainly associated with the diet containing the highest concentration of limonoids, the limonoid glucoside diet, and were primarily seen in male rats. This was especially true for the data on food intake and weight gain during the six-week period (second generation). The only problems with food intake were restricted to the animals on the 0.25% limonoid glucoside diet and the only problems with weight gain were seen with the male rats in this group. The data at the end of the study with the pups also highlighted problems with the limonoid diets. Excluding the one litter in group 2 the data for percent survival for the three groups were 94% for group 1 (45/48), 83% for group 2 (40/48), and 87% for group 3 (53/61). The average weights for weanlings in litters containing 10-15 pups showed that the male pups in groups 2 and 3 weighed significantly less than the male pups in group 1. The average weight for the female pups in group 2 was also significantly reduced. Finally, the fact that a large number of differences were seen in the blood assays suggests that the diets containing the limonoids might have been altering to some extent the metabolic function of some of the major tissues. One positive result was the significant reduction in blood cholesterol levels in the male rats fed the diets containing the limonoids.

Two earlier studies focused at least to some extent on the systemic effects of limonoids on rodents (*24,33*). In one experiment (*24*), nude mice NCR nu/nu were placed on test diets containing limonin or a limonoid glucoside mixture at concentrations of 0.5%, 1.0%, 2.0%, 4.0%, and 8.0%. During the two week exposures the mice were monitered daily for signs of toxicity. At autopsy, liver samples were taken and examined histologically. Early signs of liver degeneration were found in the mice fed the 4.0% and 8.0% diets containing the limonoid glucoside mixture. Weight loss and signs of inactivity were seen at the 8.0% level with limonin. Liver toxicity was observed at the 4.0% and 8.0% levels with limonin. The authors concluded that the maximum tolerated dose was 2.0% by weight for limonin and 4.0% for the limonoid glucoside mixture. In the second experiment (*33*), performed in our laboratory female Syrian golden hamsters were fed diets containing either 0.05% or 0.50% mixed limonoid glucosides. Compared to the control group that was fed an unmodified AIN76A diet some minor differences in food intake and weight gain were seen. Food intake and weight gain were reduced by 4% and 3% in the hamsters on the 0.05% limonoid glucoside diet and 6% and 7% in the animals fed the 0.50% limonoid glucoside diet. At the end of the 45 day experiment, blood samples were taken. Some variability was found in the data for an abbreviated set of blood chemistries; however, no significant differences or trends were seen.

Unfortunately, it is difficult to compare the data from this experiment to the two earlier studies. This study covered three generations not one. The earlier experiments were short-term feeding trials (14 and 45 days) and this experiment from start to finish lasted 116 days. Another complication was the use of different animals (mice, hamsters, and rats). Finally in this experiment males were compared to males and females to females. Similar comparisons were not done in the earlier studies.

Even though the data clearly show that the diets for group 2 and to some extent group 3 caused problems with weight gain, the level of exposure needs to be put in perspective. Using the weight gain and food intake data for the adult rats (second generation) in groups 2 and 3, it was calculated that on average the animals in group 2 were consuming 313 mg of mixed limonoid glucosides per week and the animals in group 3 were ingesting 189 mg/week of the aglycone mixture. To put the number for the limonoid glucoside mixture in perspective an adult weighing 60 kg would have to consume 130 glasses of orange juice per day for one week to achieve a similar proportional intake. This level of exposure greatly exceeds the supplemental levels currently being considered for product development.

Acknowledgments

Support for this research was provided through a grant from the United States Department of Agriculture (CSREES #2001-52102-11527). The authors would like to thank Jannett Marshall, Jo Taylor, Connie Tillberg, and Priscilla Gillaspie for their technical assistance. The authors would also like to thank Dr. Sandra L. Lovering at the Texas Veterinary Medical Diagnostic Laboratory System in College Station, Texas for her help in the interpretation of the blood data.

References

1. Guadagni, D.G.; Maier, V.P.; Turnbaugh, J.G. *J. Sci. Food Agric.* **1973**, *24*, 1277.
2. Rouseff, R.L.; Matthews, R.F. *J. Food Sci.* **1984**, *49*, 777.
3. Ou, P.; Hasegawa, S.; Herman, Z.; Fong, C.H. *Phytochemistry* **1988**, *27*, 115.
4. Hasegawa, S.; Herman, Z.; Orme, E.; Ou, P. *Phytochemistry* **1986**, *25*, 2743.
5. Hasegawa, S.; Berhow, M.A.; Manners, G.D. *Citrus Limonoids Functional Chemicals in Agriculture and Foods;* American Chemical Society: Washington, DC, **2000**; pp 1-8.
6. Maier, V.P.; Hasegawa, S.; Hera, E. *Phytochemistry* **1969**, *8*, 405.
7. Hasegawa, S.; Ou, P.; Fong, C.H.; Herman, Z.; Coggins, C.W.; Atkin, D.R. *J. Agric. Food Chem.* **1991**, *39*, 262.
8. Hasegawa, S.; Bennett, R.D.; Herman, Z.; Fong, C.H.; Ou, P. *Phytochemistry* **1989**, *28*, 1717.
9. Bennett, R.D.; Hasegawa, S.; Herman, Z. *Phytochemistry* **1989**, *28*, 2777.
10. Fong, C.H.; Hasegawa, S.; Herman, Z.; Ou, P. *J. Food Sci.* **1990**, *54*, 1505.
11. Herman, Z.; Fong, C.H.; Ou, P.; Hasegawa, S. *J. Agric. Food Chem.* **1990**, *38*, 1860.
12. Lam, L.K.T.; Hasegawa, S. *Nutr. Cancer* **1989**, *12*, 43.
13. Miller, E.G.; Fanous, R.; Rivera-Hidalgo, F.; Binnie, W.H.; Hasegawa, S.; Lam, L.K.T. *Carcinogenesis* **1989**, *10*, 1535.
14. Lam, L.K.T.; Zhang, J.; Hasegawa, S. *Food Technol.* **1994**, *48*, 104.
15. Lam, L.K.T.; Zhang, J.; Hasegawa, S.; Schut, H.A.J. *Food Phytochemicals for Cancer Prevention I. Fruits and Vegetables*; American Chemical Society: Washington, DC, **1994**; pp 209-219.
16. Lam, L.K.T.; Hasegawa, S.; Bergstrom, C.; Lam, S.H.; Kenney, P. *Citrus Limonoids Functional Chemicals in Agriculture and Foods*; American Chemical Society: Washington, DC, **2000**; pp 185-200.
17. Tanaka, T.; Kohno, H.; Kawabata, K.; Honjo, S.; Miyake, M.; Wada, K. *Citrus Limonoids Functional Chemicals in Agriculture and Foods*; American Chemical Society: Washington, DC, **2000**; pp 145-163.
18. Block, G. *Am. J. Clin. Nutr.* **1991**, *53*, 270s.
19. Miller, E.G.; Gonzales-Sanders, A.P.; Couvillon, A.M.; Wright, J.M.; Hasegawa, S.; Lam, L.K.T. *Nutr. Cancer* **1992**, *17*, 1.
20. Miller, E.G.; Gonzales-Sanders, A.P.; Couvillon, A.M.; Binnie, W.H.; Hasegawa, S.; Lam, L.K.T. *Food Technol.* **1994**, *48*, 110.
21. Miller, E.G.; Porter-Wright, J.L.; Binnie, W.H.; Guo, I.Y.; Hasegawa, S. *Hypernutritious Foods*; Agscience Inc.: Auburndale, FL, **1996**; pp 191-204.

22. Miller, E.G.; Porter, J.L.; Binnie, W.H.; Guo, I.Y.; Hasegawa, S. *J. Agric. Food Chem.* **2004**, *52*, 4908.
23. Kuroska, E.M.; Hasegawa, S.; Manners, G. *Citrus Limonoids Functional Chemicals in Agriculture and Foods*; American Chemical Society: Washington, DC, **2000**; pp 175-184.
24. Guthrie, N.; Hasegawa, S.; Manners, G.; Carroll, K.K. *Citrus Limonoids Functional Chemicals in Agriculture and Foods*; American Chemical Society: Washington, DC, **2000**; pp 164-174.
25. Tian, Q.G.; Miller, E.G.; Ahmad, H.; Tang, L.; Patil, B.S. *Nutr. Cancer* **2001**, *40*, 180.
26. Miller, E.G.; Taylor, S.E.; Berry, C.W.; Zimmermann, J.A.; Hasegawa, S. *Citrus Limonoids Functional Chemicals in Agriculture and Foods*; American Chemical Society: Washington, DC, **2000**; pp 132-144.
27. Battinelli, L.; Mengoni, F.; Lichtner, M.; Mazzanti, G.; Saija, A.; Mastroianni, C.M.; Vullo, V. *Planta Med.* **2003**, *69*, 910.
28. Hasegawa, S.; Lam, L.K.T.; Miller, E.G. *Phytochemicals and Phytopharmaceuticals*; AOCS Press: Champaign, IL, **2000**; pp 79-94.
29. Omura, M.; Kita, M.; Endo-Inagaki, T.; Moriguchi, T.; Matsumoto, R.; Suhayda, C.; Hasegawa, S. *Citrus Limonoids Functional Chemicals in Agriculture and Foods*; American Chemical Society: Washington, DC, **2000**; pp 230-237.
30. Ozaki, Y.; Fong, C.H.; Herman, Z.; Maeda, H.; Miyake, M.; Ifuku, Y. Hasegawa, S. *Agric. Biol. Chem.* **1991**, *55*, 137.
31. Ozaki, Y.; Ayano, S.; Inaba, N.; Miyake, M.; Berhow, M.; Hasegawa, S. *J. Food Sci.* **1996**, *60*, 186.
32. Hasegawa, S.; Fong, C.H.; Miyake, M.; Keithly, J.H. *J. Food Sci.* **1996**, *61*, 560.
33. Miller, E.G.; Record, M.T.; Binnie, W.H.; Hasegawa, S. *Phytochemicals and Phytopharmaceuticals*; AOCS Press: Champaign, IL, **2000**; pp 95-105.

Chapter 7

Citrus Limonoid Bioavailability in Humans

Andrew P. Breksa III[1], Gary D. Manners[1], Robert A. Jacob[2], and Shin Hasegawa[1]

[1]**Western Regional Research Center, Agricultural Research Service, U.S. Department of Agriculture, Albany, CA 94710**
[2]**Western Human Research Center, Agricultural Research Center, U.S. Department of Agriculture, Davis, CA 95616**

The absorption, metabolism, and bioavailability of citrus limonoids in human subjects administered high doses of pure limonin glucoside has been reported (*1*). In this chapter, the results from this study are compared to the bioavailability results of other citrus secondary metabolites, and future research directions presented.

Citrus is recognized as one of the most healthful components of the human diet. Much of the contribution of citrus to human health and nutrition can be attributed to secondary metabolites present in citrus including antioxidants (ascorbic acid, flavanones, simple phenolics, carotenoids), folate, and pectin.

Limonoids, complex triterpenoid compounds, constitute another important class of secondary metabolites that occur in citrus in significant quantities. These compounds occur in all citrus tissues as limonoid aglycones, limonoid glucosides or limonoid A-ring lactones (Figure 1). Limonin glucoside is the most abundant limonoid glucoside found in citrus juices and is readily available from orange juice or citrus juice processing by-products. Like all of the limonoid glucosides, limonin glucoside is water soluble, tasteless, non-mutagenic (*2*) and has shown no significant toxic effects when fed to hamsters up to 0.5% of the animal diet (*3*). In contrast, limonoid aglycones, like limonin (Figure 1), occur in low levels in citrus juices. The aglycones are water insoluble and several of these compounds are responsible for the development of delayed bitterness in citrus juices at concentrations as low as 6 ppm (*4*). Limonoid A-ring lactones (limonoate A-ring lactone (Figure 1)) also occur in citrus as water soluble, tasteless metabolic precursors to limonoid aglycones and glucosides.

The limonoids have also been shown to possess biological activity indicative of their potential importance to human health and nutrition. Several *in vitro* cell line studies and *in vivo* studies in animals have shown that citrus limonoids possess anti-tumor activity (*2, 5, 6, 7, 8, 9, 10)* anti-HIV (*11*) and

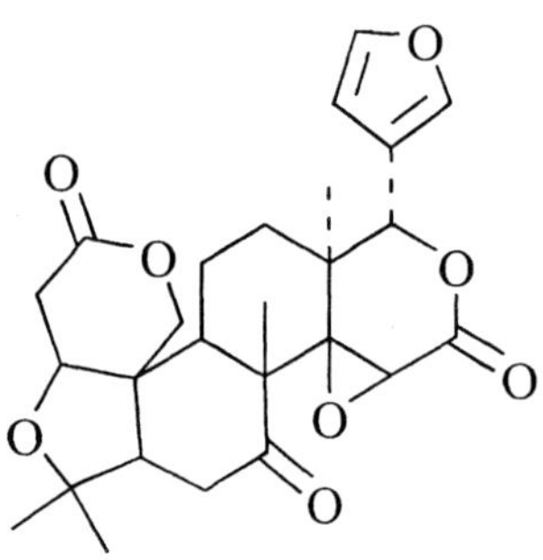

Limonin

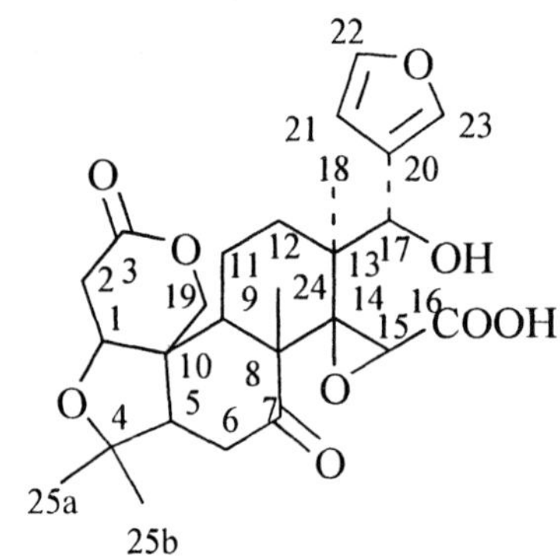

Limonoate A-ring lactone

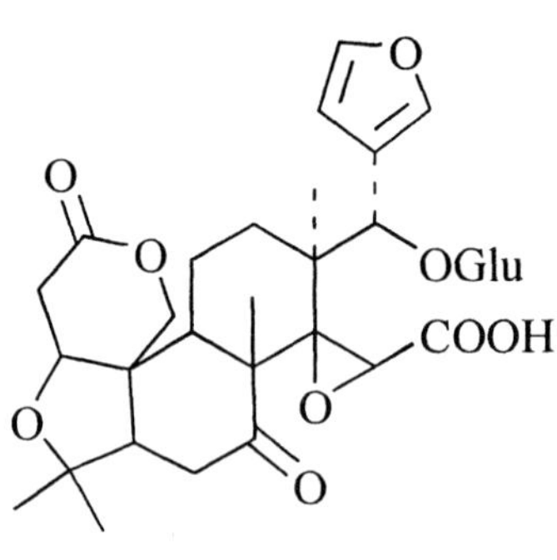

Limonin Glucoside

Figure 1. Structures of limonin, limonin glucoside, and limonoate A-ring lactone.

cholesterol lowering properties (*12, 13*). Similar studies have verified the biological activity, primarily antioxidant properties, of the flavonoids, anthocyanins and phenolic acids in citrus.

The observation of biological activity among secondary metabolites available to humans in fruits and vegetables as determined by *in vitro* and *in vivo* cell line and animal tests has become a common endorsement of the importance of these fruits or vegetables to human health and nutrition. The *in vitro* and *in vivo* animal test data are important indicators of the biological activities of naturally occurring chemicals compounds in fruits and vegetables, however, this data does not address the ability of these compounds to impart this activity after human consumption. In this sense, a biologically active compound must be available to act (be bioavailable) at the appropriate site (i.e. tumor formation site) in its active chemical form (bioassay test form). In the case of secondary metabolites from fruits and vegetables, the only proper assessment of these parameters can be accomplished through an analytically based human feeding study that establishes the presence of the biologically active secondary metabolites (bioavailability) in the body fluid associated with the target site in the human body.

Numerous studies have been undertaken to examine the bioavailability of biologically active polyphenolic secondary metabolites of fruits and vegetables. A review (*14*) of 97 bioavailability studies of anthocyanins, flavanols, flavanones, catechins, proanthocyanins, isoflavones, hydroxycinnamic acids and hydroxybenzoic acids provides extensive evidence of the absorption and bioavailability of these compounds after consumption by humans. In these studies the bioavailability of the polyphenols was primarily based upon the detection, in plasma and urine, of metabolic conjugates derived from polyphenol glycosides fed to the human subjects. Among all of the polyphenols studied, only a few specific catechins and isoflavones were shown to appear in plasma and urine in unconjugated forms. Some feeding studies provided evidence that polyphenol aglycones were not readily absorbed and metabolized by humans.

Human bioavailability studies of biologically active secondary metabolites in citrus have focused on flavonoids (*15, 16*), carotenoids and anthocyanins (*17*). Two independent groups assessed the bioavailability of flavone glucosides hesperidin and narirutin, by measuring plasma levels of the corresponding aglycones, hesperetin and naringenin, in subjects that consumed orange or grapefruit juices, and reported that the flavonoids were well absorbed with an apparent C_{max} of $\approx$ 5 h. In the first study, plasma samples were subjected to hydrolysis to generate the free aglycones prior to quantification and thus the exact identities of the bioavailable compounds were unknown. In the second study, a detailed analysis of the metabolites revealed that all of the metabolites of hesperetin were glucuronidated and that the aglycone was not present in plasma. In another recent study, researchers found that consumption of blood orange juice increased plasma concentrations of anthocyanin cyanidin 3-glucoside and carotenoids β-cryptoxanthin and zeaxanthin. Common themes across these reports include that secondary metabolites in citrus juices are bioavailable, that inter-individual variation in bioavailability is considerable and that there is a need to assess individual metabolites for biological activity to determine their potential in improving human health and nutrition.

In our limonoid bioavailability study, sixteen test subject were administered pure limonin glucoside (0.25, 0.5, 1.0, 2.0 g in 200 mL of buffered water) and their plasma analyzed by LC/MS for the presence of the aglycone of limonin glucoside, limonin, as a biomarker to establish limonoid absorption, metabolism and bioavailability of limonoids in humans (*1*). Limonin in low nmol/L amounts was detected in the plasma of all but one subject. Significant variation in the amount of bioavailable limonin was observed among subjects within each group. Similar variations have been observed in a study of the bioavailability of naringenin and hesperetin conjugates from orange juice (*15*). Fourteen of the sixteen subjects displayed the maximum concentration (C_{max}) of limonin at all limonin glucoside dose levels in plasma 6 h (T_{max}) post dose and all of the highest dosed subjects but one showed the presence of limonin in plasma prior to the 6 h post dose period. Two of the 0.5 g dose subjects and three of the eight 1.0 and 2.0 g dose subjects revealed the presence of limonin in plasma at 24 h post dose. The detection of limonin in five subjects 24 h post dose is contrary to studies with polyphenols that only have detectable amounts of polyphenol conjugates 10 to 12 h post dose (*15*). The lowest dose of limonin glucoside administered in this study is comparable to the amount a natural mixture of all limonoid glucosides in about four glasses of orange juice and is equivalent to the natural amount of limonin glucoside in about seven glasses of orange juice.

In the case of both polyphenolic aglycones and glycosides it is recognized that absorption and metabolism includes glycoside hydrolysis and subsequent conjugation to glucuronides or sulfates with or without methylation (*18, 19, 20*). In the course of this study, the presence or absence of limonin conjugates or limonin glucoside conjugates in subjects could not be confirmed since no conjugates of these compounds have been reported, and at present no standards or analytical methods exist for their detection or quantification.

While no derivatized conjugates of limonin were identified in this study, a second peak with a shorter retention time than limonin but with molecular ions and fragment ions from MS/MS experiments identical to those of limonin was detected in the plasma samples of subjects consuming the two highest dose levels of limonin glucoside. This substance was proposed to be a C-17 epimer of limonin due to the identical nature of this compound's MS/MS fragmentation pattern and chromatographic similarity to limonin. An alternative explanation for the observation of this limonin-like unknown (*m/z* 471.2) is offered by the recent reports of the *in-situ* conversion of limonoate A-ring lactone to limonin (*21, 22*) and the appearance of limonin as a fragmentation product of limonin glucoside (*23*) under MS ionization conditions. The fact that both limonoate A-ring lactone and limonin glucoside will elute prior to limonin when separated by C-18 reversed phase chromatography offers additional credence to this hypothesis.

While the chemical structure of the unknown compound cannot be conclusively related to limonin or an associated limonoid on the basis of the information available, its appearance in the plasma of the human subjects confirms that another compound with MS characteristics similar to limonin is bioavailable in humans administered high doses of limonin glucoside. Isolation and characterization of the unknown will be necessary if its identity is to be definitively established.

Future Work

Since the identity and activity of metabolic conjugates of citrus limonoids have not been established, the level of limonin detected may not reflect the potential therapeutic concentration of active limonoid glucoside metabolites. In light of the *in vivo* and *in vitro* validation of limonoids as effective anti-tumor agents, the significance of limonoid aglycones levels in plasma to human health will emerge from further studies that examine the detailed pharmacokinetics, and metabolic fate of the citrus limonoids in humans and the characterization and quantification of the most bioactive forms of these compounds.

Conclusion

Our results confirm that limonoids are absorbed and metabolized in humans, but does not provide significant evidence of the mode of the absorption and metabolism of these compounds. This documentation of the bioavailability of citrus limonoids in humans and the recognized biological activity of these compounds in mammalian systems is consistent with their prominent participation in the matrix of phytochemicals in citrus that contribute to improving human health and nutrition. The potential abundant supply of non-toxic, water-soluble limonoid glucosides from citrus processing industrial by-products endorses the reclamation of these compounds for use as nutraceuticals or as healthful fortifiers in functional foods.

Acknowledgement

The authors wish to acknowledge the financial support of this research supplied through a grant awarded by the Florida Department of Citrus. We also wish to acknowledge the technical assistance of Marlene Hidalgo (USDA/ARS/WRRC) and Giovanna Aiello (USDA/ARS/WHNRC) and biometric assistance from Mr. Bruce Mackey.

Literature Cited

1. Manners, G. D.; Jacob, R. A.; Breksa III, A. P.; Schoch, T. K.; Hasegawa, S. *J. Agric. Food Chem.* **2003**, 51, 4156-4161.
2. Lam, L. K. T.; Hasegawa, S.; Bergstrom, C.; Lam, S. H.; Kenney, P. In *Citrus Limonoids: Functional Chemicals in Agriculture and Foods;* Berhow, M. A., Hasegawa, S., Manners, G. D., Ed.; ACS Symposium Series 758; American Chemical Society, Washington, D.C., 2000, pp. 185-200.
3. Miller, E. G.; Record, M. T.; Binnie, W. H.; Hasegawa, S. In *Phytochemicals and Phytopharmaceuticals;* Shahidi, F., Ho, C-T., Ed.; American Oil Chemist's Society Press, Champaign, IL, 1999, pp 95-105.
4. Hasegawa, S.; Miyake, M.; Ozaki, Y.; Berhow, M. A. In *The Contribution of Low- and Non Volatile Materials to Flavor;* Pickenhagen, W., Ho, C., Spanier, A. M., Ed.; Allured, Carol Stream, IL, 1996, pp.137-145.
5. Lam, L. K. T.; Li, Y.; Hasegawa, S. *J. Agric. Food Chem.* **1989**, 37, 878-880.
6. Lam, L. K. T.; Hasegawa, S. *Nutrition and Cancer* **1989**, 12, 43-47.
7. Miller, E. G.; Gonzales-Sanders, A. P.; Couvillon, A. M.; Wright, J. M.; Hasegawa, S.; Lam, L. K. T. *Nutrition and Cancer* **1992**, 17, 1-7.
8. Lam, L. K. T.; Zhang, J.; Hasegawa, S.; Schut, H. A. J. In *Food Phytochemicals for Cancer Prevention I;* Huang, M. T.; Osawa, T. Ho, C.; Rosen, R. T., Ed.; ACS Symposium Series 546; American Chemical Society, Washington, D.C., 1994, pp 209-219.
9. Tanaka, T.; Kohno, H.; Kawabata, K.; Honjo, S.; Miyake, M.; Wada, K. In *Citrus Limonoids: Functional Chemicals in Agriculture and Foods;* Berhow, M. A., Hasegawa, S., Manners, G. D., Ed.; ACS Symposium Series 758; American Chemical Society, Washington, D.C., 2000, pp. 145-163.
10. Tanaka, T.; Maeda, M.; Kohno, H.; Murakami, M.; Kagami, S.; Miyake, M.; Wada, K. *Carcinogenesis* **2001,** 22, 193-198.
11. Battinelli, L.; Mengoni, F.; Lichtner, M.; Mazzanti, G.; Saija, A.; Mastroianni, C. M.; Vullo, V. *Planta Med.* **2003,** 69, 910-913.

12. Guthrie, N.; Chambers, A. F.; Carroll, K. K. *Proc. Am. Assoc. Cancer Res.* **1997,** 38, 113.
13. Guthrie, N.; Hasegawa, S.; Manners, G. D.; Carroll, K. K. In *Citrus Limonoids: Functional Chemicals in Agriculture and Foods;* Berhow, M. A., Hasegawa, S., Manners, G. D., Ed.; ACS Symposium Series 758; American Chemical Society, Washington, D.C., 2000, pp. 164-174.
14. Manach, C.; Williamson, G.; Morand, C.; Scalbert, A.; Remesy, C. *Am. J. Clin. Nutr.* **2005,** 81, 230S-242S.
15. Erlund, I.; Meririnne, E.; Alfthan, G.; Aro, A.; *J. Nutr.* **2001,** 131, 235-241.
16. Manach, C.; Morand, C.; Gil-Izquierdo, A.; Bouteloup-Demange, C.; Remesy, C. *Eur. J. Clin. Nutr.* **2003,** 57, 235-242
17. Riso, P.; Visioli, F.; Gardana, C.; Grande, S.; Brusamolino, A.; Galvano, F.; Galvano, G.; Porrini, M. *J. Agric. Food Chem.* **2005,** 53, 941-947.
18. Mizuma, T.; Awazu, S. *Biochim. Biophys. Acta* **1998,** *1425*, 398-404.
19. Shimoi, K.; Plada, H.; Furugori, M.; Goda, T.; Takase, S.; Sukuki, M.; Hara, Y.; Yamamoto, H.; Kinae, N. *FEBS Lett.* **1998,** *438*, 220-224.
20. Spencer, J. P. E.; Chowrimootoo, G.; Choudhury, R.; Debnam, E. S.; Srai, S. K.; Rice-Evans, C. *FEBS Lett.* **1999,** *458*, 224-230.
21. Zukas, A. A.; Breksa III, A. P.; Manners, G. D. *Phytochemistry* **2004,** 65, 2705-2709.
22. Breksa III, A. P.; Zukas, A. A.; Manners, G. D. *J. Chromatogr. A* **2005,** 1064, 187-173.
23. Tian, Q.; Schwartz, S. J. *Anal. Chem.* **2003,** 75, 5451-5460.

Health Properties of Bioactive Compounds in Citrus

Chapter 8

Citrus Flavonoid Nobiletin Suppresses Azoxymethane-Induced Rat Colon Tumorigenesis

Rikako Suzuki[1], Hiroyuki Kohno[1], Shigeyuki Sugie[1], Akira Murakami[2], Masamichi Yano[3], Hajime Ohigashi[2], and Takuji Tanaka[1]

[1]Department of Oncologic Pathology, Kanazawa Medical University, Ishikawa, Japan
[2]Division of Applied Life Science, Graduate School of Agriculture, Kyoto University, Kyoto, Japan
[3]National Institute of Fruit Tree Science, Shizuoka, Japan

We investigated the modulatory effect of citrus nobiletin on colon carcinogenesis initiated with azoxymethane (AOM) in rats. Starting one week after the initiation, rats received the diet mixed with 100 or 500 ppm nobiletin for 34 weeks. The inhibition rates of colonic adenocarcinoma in rats that received 100 or 500 ppm nobiletin after AOM exposure were 18% and 48%, respectively. Also, nobiletin feeding suppressed the prostaglandin E_2 levels and cell proliferation activity, and enhanced apoptosis in colonic adenocarcinomas. These results suggested that citrus nobiletin might be a possible chemopreventive agent against colon cancer development.

Introduction

In a recent literature review of citrus flavonoids, a broad spectrum of biological activities including anti-carcinogenic and anti-tumor activities were discussed (*1*). Epidemiological studies have revealed that flavonoid intake is correlated with a reduced risk of certain types of cancer (*2, 3*). Nobiletin (5,6,7,8,3',4'-hexamethoxyflavone, Figure 1) is a polymethoxy flavonoid and occurs exclusively in citrus fruits. We could ingest nobiletin from not only the citrus fruits, but also orange juice, since Valencia orange juice contains 46 ppm nobiletin (*4*). It is known that nobiletin possesses certain biological activities such as induction of apoptosis and reduction of proliferative activity in human colon cancer cells (*5*). This compound is reported to suppress the production of prostaglandin (PG) E_2 and promatrix metalloproteinase in human synovial cells (*6*). Previously, we found the inhibitory effect of nobiletin on phorbol ester-induced skin tumorigenesis in mice (*7*). Nobiletin also inhibited peritoneal dissemination of human gastric carcinoma cells in SCID mice (*8*). These observations encouraged us to examine the effect of nobiletin on chemically induced carcinogenesis in rodents.

Colorectal cancer, a common malignancy worldwide, is an important contributor to cancer morbidity and mortality, and to overall international cancer burden. This malignancy has increased in Asia owing to the changes in life style including dietary habit of increased meat consumption (*9, 10*). In Japan, colon cancer is one of the most important causes of death: the mortality rates were 16.32/100,000 for men and 9.74/100,000 for women in 2000 (*11*). In spite of several basic or clinical challenges to control colonic cancer death, no significant prolongation of survival has been obtained (*12*).

Although the content of nobiletin in citrus fruits is not abundant, this compound might have great potential as a cancer-preventing agent. Indeed, a variety of non-nutritive bioactive plant substances, such as flavonoids, fiber, coumarins, and limonoids are thought to have beneficial effects on human health including suppressing colonic malignancy (*13, 14*). We recently found that nobiletin inhibits azoxymethane (AOM)-induced colonic putative precursor lesions, aberrant crypt foci (ACF), of colonic adenocarcinoma in rats (*15*), suggesting that the compound might be effective in inhibiting colon carcinogenesis.

In the present study, we conducted an *in vivo* long-term experiment to investe the modifying effect of nobiletin on AOM-induced rat colon carcinogenesis. Since cell proliferation plays an essential role in carcinogenesis (*16*), we measured cell proliferation activity using biomarkers such as proliferating cell nuclear antigen (PCNA)-labeling index and polyamine level in colonic tumors and non-lesional colonic mucosa. To elucidate the mechanism of the modulating effect of nobiletin on colon carcinogenesis, apoptotic index was also assayed because certain chemopreventive agents exert their inhibitory action via induction of apoptosis (*14*). In addition, we measured PGE_2 levels in colonic adenocarcinomas and their surrounding colonic mucosa since close association between the high level of PGE_2 and colonic carcinogenesis has been suggested (*17*).

Materials & Methods

Animals, Chemicals, and Diets.

Four-week-old male F344 rats were obtained from SCL, Inc. (Shizuoka, Japan). They were maintained in the Kanazawa Medical University Animal Facility according to the Institutional Animal Care Guidelines. All animals were housed in plastic cages (3 or 4 rats/cage) with free access to drinking water and a basal diet, CE-2 (CLEA Inc., Tokyo, Japan), under controlled conditions of relative humidity (50±10%), lighting (12-h light/dark cycle), and temperature (23±2°C). AOM was purchased from Sigma Chemical Co. (St. Louis, MO, USA). Nobiletin (>99% purity) was isolated from *Citrus unshiu* (*7*). Experimental diets were prepared by mixing nobiletin into the basal diet at a dose of 100 or 500 ppm on a weekly basis.

Experimental Procedure.

Male F344 rats were divided into five groups, as shown in Figure 2. At 5 weeks of age, the rats in groups 1 through 3, designated for carcinogen treatment, were subcutaneously injected with AOM (20 mg/kg body weight) once a week for two weeks. Group 1 was fed the basal diet throughout the experiment. Groups 2 and 3 were fed the diets containing nobiletin at dose levels of 100 and 500 ppm, respectively, for 34 weeks, starting one week after the last injection of AOM. Group 4 was given 500 ppm nobiletin-containing diet alone, and group 5 served as an untreated control. The experiment was terminated at 36 weeks after the start.

All rats were provided with the experimental diets and tap water *ad libitum*, and weighed weekly. The food intake was also recorded weekly. At the termination of the study (week 36), all rats were sacrificed by an overdose of ether. At autopsy, all organs, especially the intestine, were carefully examined grossly, and then all abnormal lesions were examined histologically. Colons were fixed in 10% buffered formalin and processed for histopathological examination by routine methods. Intestinal neoplasms were diagnosed according to the criteria described by Pozharisski (*18*). The weighed liver and kidney were also submitted to histological examination for checking the toxicity of nobiletin.

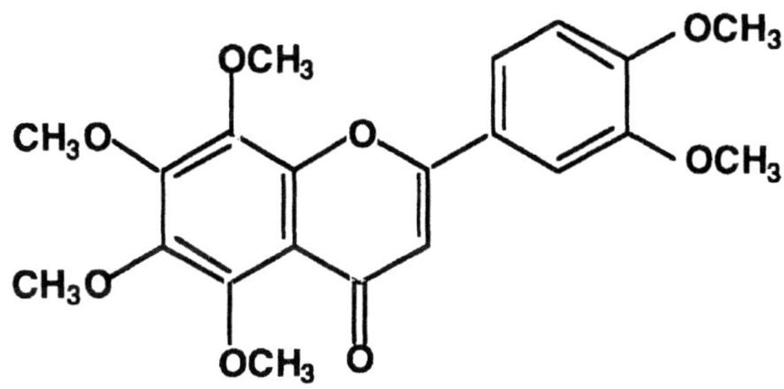

Figure 1. Chemical structure of nobiletin.

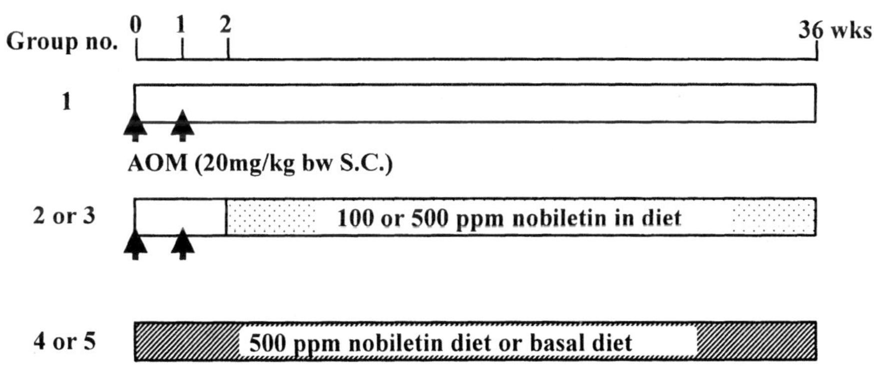

Figure 2. Experimental protocol.

Polyamine Level

Scraped colonic mucosa without tumors was stored at -70 °C until measured. Proteins were extracted from the mucosa, and then tissue polyamine levels in the extraction were determined by the method described by Koide *et al.* (*19*).

Measurement of PGE_2 Level

For PGE_2 determination, the scraped colonic mucosa of 5 rats each randomly selected and colonic adenocarcinomas from the experimental groups were homogenized in a 400 µL of PBS on ice. After centrifugation at 10,000 × g for 5 minutes, the supernatants obtained were diluted at the ratio of 1:9, and measured for PGE_2 concentration using a commercial kit (Cayman, Ann Arbor, MI, USA) according to the protocol of the manufacturer. Protein concentrations for tissue samples were determined using the Bradford method (*20*).

Measurement of PCNA and Apoptotic Indices in Colonic Neoplasms

PCNA-labeling and apoptotic indices were determined in all colonic tumors by immunohistochemistry. Tumor tissues fixed in 10% buffered formalin for 2 days were embedded in paraffin. Serial cross-sections of 3 µm were cut, and mounted onto gelatin-coated glass slides. A mouse monoclonal primary antibody against PCNA (1:50 dilution; PC10, DAKO Japan, Kyoto, Japan) and a rabbit polyclonal primary antibody against single stranded DNA (ssDNA, 1:300 dilution; DAKO Japan, Kyoto, Japan) were applied to the sections according to the manufacturer's protocol (DAKO LSAB 2 kit/HRP, DAKO Japan, Kyoto, Japan). All incubation steps were carried out for 15 min at 37°C. Negative controls were prepared by omitting the primary antibodies. All nuclei which densely immunoreacted with PCNA or ssDNA antibody were regarded as PCNA or ssDNA positive. The PCNA and apoptotic indices were determined by counting the number of positive cells among at least 200 cells in the tumor, and were indicated as percentages.

Statistical evaluation

Where applicable, data were analyzed using one-way ANOVA with Bonferroni correction or Fisher's exact probability test with $P<0.05$ as the criterion of significance.

Results

General Observation

Throughout the experiment, clinical signs of toxicity and poor condition were not observed in any rats. These observations were confirmed by histological examination of major organs (liver, kidney, heart, and lungs). Body and liver weights showed no significant differences among the groups (body and liver weights: group 1, 377±21 and 11.9±1.3; group 2, 376±19 and 11.7±1.7; group 3, 377±20 and 11.6±1.3; group 4, 392±14 and 12.9±1.0; and group 5, 387±14 and 12.8±0.9). Intakes of the diets with or without nobiletin in groups 1 through 5 were not significantly different (data not shown), suggesting that rats could tolerate the diets without experiencing adverse effects from consumption of 100 or 500 ppm nobiletin.

Incidence and Multiplicity of Intestinal Neoplasms

The incidence and multiplicity of colonic adenocarcinoma in the AOM alone group (group 1) were 67% and 1.33±1.28/rat, respectively (Figure 3). The incidence (33%, $P<0.05$) and multiplicity (0.40±0.58/rat, $P<0.01$) were significantly reduced by administration of 500 ppm of nobiletin (group 3) when compared to group 1. The differences on the incidences and multiplicities of colonic adenoma among groups 1-3 were not statistically significant. In groups 4 (500 ppm nobiletin alone) and 5 (no treatment), colonic tumors were not observed. Also, tumors were not found in any organs of animals in groups 4 and 5.

Polyamine Content and PGE_2 Level in Colonic Mucosa

The data on assays of polyamine content and PGE_2 level in the colonic mucosa determined at the end of the study are summarized in Figures 4A and 4B, respectively. As for the total polyamine content of colonic mucosa without tumors, significant difference was found between group 1 (16.8±1.2 nmol/mg protein, $P<0.001$) and group 5 (13.5±1.0 nmol/mg protein). The values of groups 2 (14.5±0.7 nmol/mg protein, $P<0.01$) and 3 (14.3±1.2 nmol/mg protein, $P<0.01$) for non-lesional colonic mucosa were significantly smaller than group 1. The PGE_2 content in colonic mucosa without tumors in group 1 (97.0±22.2 pg/mg protein, $P<0.05$) was significantly higher than group 5 (62.0±15.5 pg/mg protein). As for the colonic adenocarcinomas, the value of group 3 (77.6±20.2 pg/mg protein, $P<0.05$) was significantly lower than group 1 (111.1±35.3 pg/mg protein, $P<0.05$).

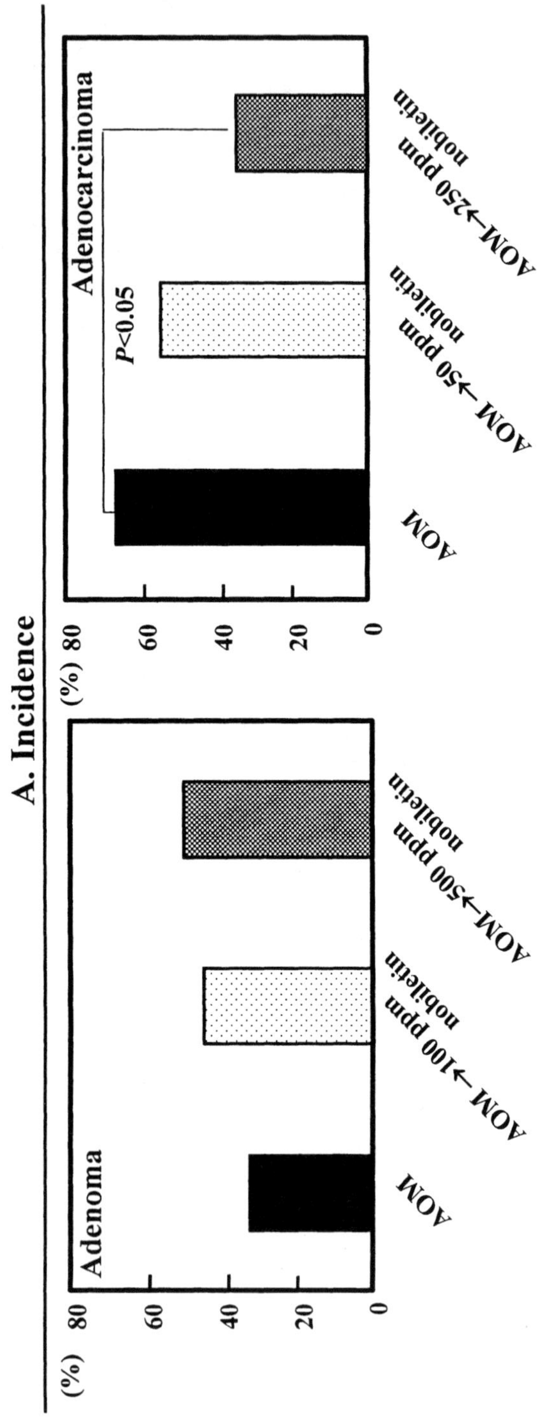
A. Incidence
Adenoma
(%)
80
60
40
20
0
AOM
AOM→100 ppm nobiletin
AOM→500 ppm nobiletin
Adenocarcinoma
P<0.05
AOM→50 ppm nobiletin
AOM→250 ppm nobiletin

B. Multiplicity

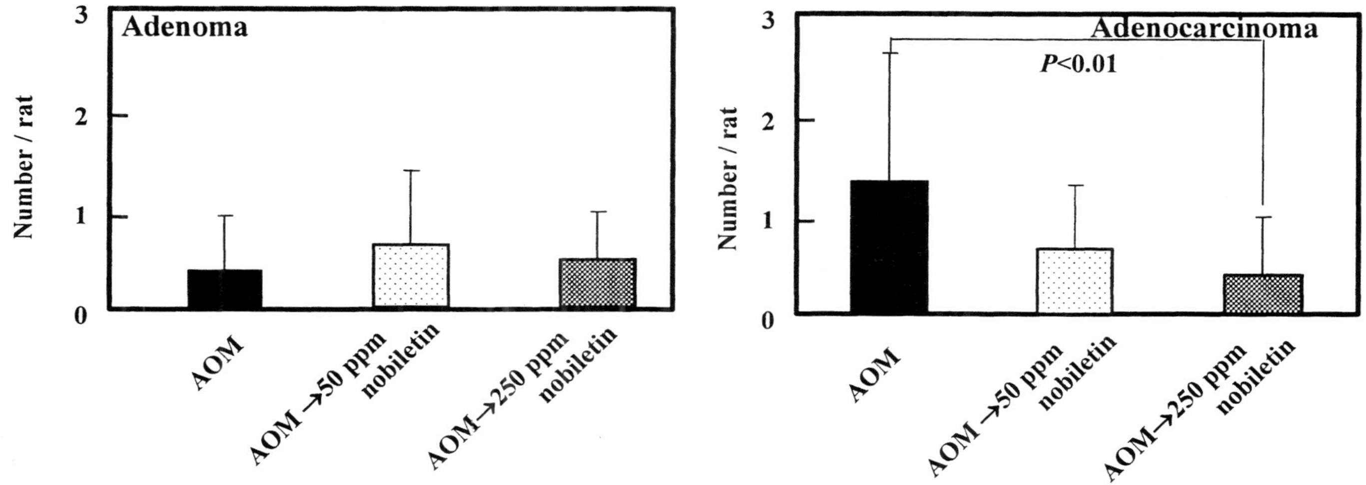

Figure 3. Incidence and multiplicity of large bowel tumors. "Modified from Biofactors, 22 (1-4), R Suzuki et al., Citrus nobiletin inhibits azoxymethane-induced large bowel carcinogenesis in rats, 111-114., Copyright (2004), with permission from IOS Press"

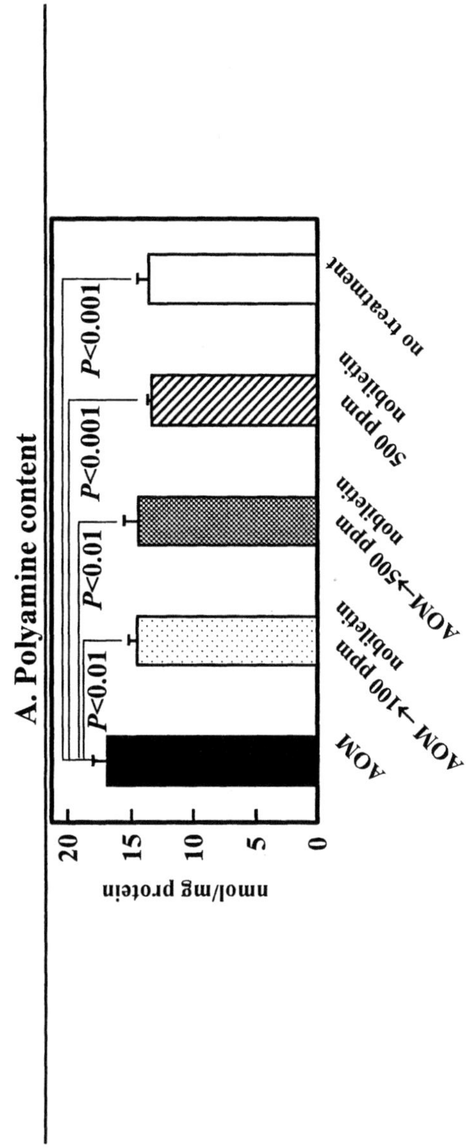
A. Polyamine content
nmol/mg protein
20
15
10
5
0
P<0.01
P<0.01
P<0.001
P<0.001
AOM
AOM→100 ppm nobiletin
AOM→500 ppm nobiletin
500 ppm nobiletin
no treatment

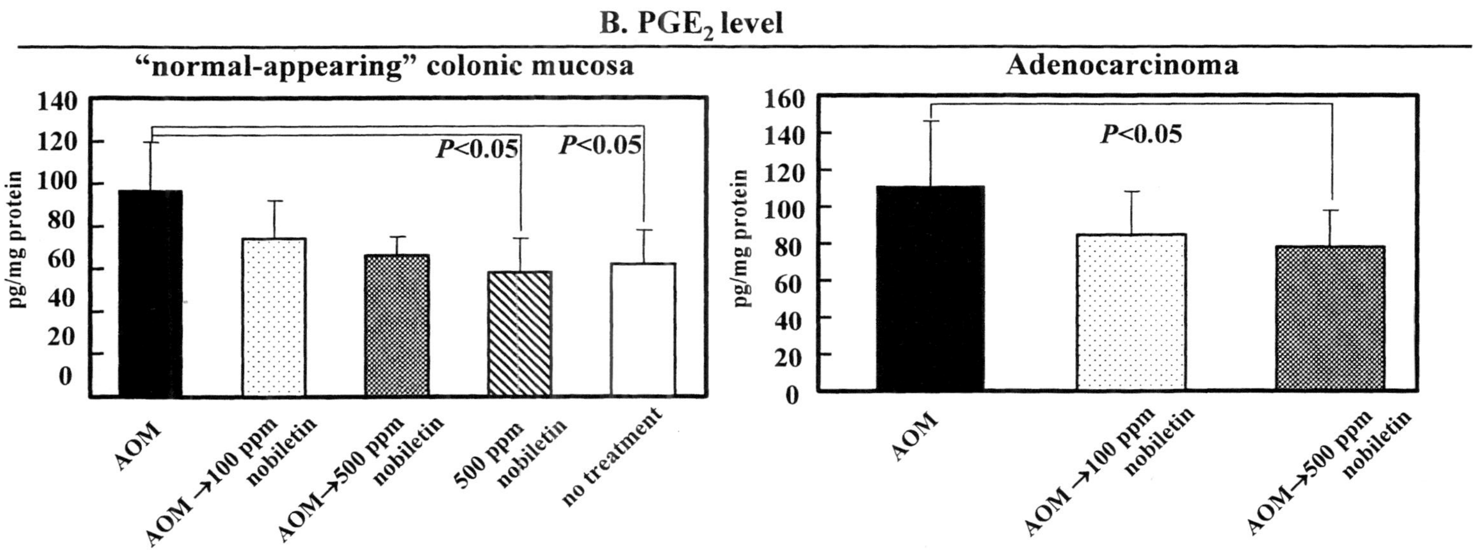

Figure 4. Colonic polyamine levels and PGE_2 contents of rats. "Modified from Biofactors, 22 (1-4), R Suzuki et al., Citrus nobiletin inhibits azoxymethane-induced large bowel carcinogenesis in rats, 111-114., Copyright (2004), with permission from IOS Press"

PCNA and Apoptotic Indices in Colonic Neoplasms

As shown in Figure 5A, the PCNA-positive index of adenoma developed in group 3 (25±4%, $P<0.01$) was statistically smaller than group 1 (31±4%). The indices of adenocarcinomas in groups 2 (44±6%, $P<0.001$) and 3 (44±5%, $P<0.01$) were also significantly lower than group 1 (54±6%). The apoptotic index in the colonic neoplasms is illustrated in Figure 5B. The index of adenocarcinomas in group 3 (5.08±0.44%, $P<0.05$) was significantly grater than group 1 (4.31±0.53%). Concerning the apoptotic indices of colonic adenomas, no statistical differences were found among the groups 1-3.

Discussion

The results described here indicate that dietary feeding of nobiletin suppresses the development of colonic adenocarcinomas induced by AOM. On the other hand, the incidence and multiplicity of colonic adenoma in rats receiving nobiletin at both doses were slightly higher than the AOM alone group. These results suggest that nobiletin predominantly may modulate the conversion of colonic adenomas to adenocarcinomas. In the current study, administration of 500 ppm nobiletin exerted an effective inhibitory ability in rat colon carcinogenesis when compared to the lower dose (100 ppm). This is in agreement with our previous findings that feeding with a higher dose (500 ppm) rather than a low dose (100 ppm) of nobiletin could inhibit ACF development in a short-term experiment (*15*). These results also suggested that nobiletin could inhibit chemically induced colonic carcinogenesis in a dose-dependent manner.

Cell proliferation is known to play an important role in carcinogenesis (*16*). Natural products possessing suppression effect on cell proliferation activity could be candidate chemopreventive agents (*14*). In the present study, dietary exposure to nobiletin at both doses significantly reduced cell proliferation. In our short-term assay of rat colonic ACF, the suppressive effect of nobiletin on the cell proliferation was noted (*15*). There are several reports demonstrating the inhibitory effect of nobiletin on cell proliferation in human cancer cell lines, such as hepatocellular (*21*), gastric (*22*), and colon (*5*). The expression of cell proliferation biomarkers documented in this experiment, PCNA-labeling index and polyamine level, were in accordance with these reports. Thus, it is likely that the prevention of AOM-induced colonic adenocarcinoma by dietary nobiletin is partly due to the alteration of cell proliferating activity in the colonic neoplasms and/or their surrounding mucosa.

Induction of apoptosis is one of the major contributing factors for anti-tumorigenesis properties of several natural compounds (*23*). Apoptosis might be one of the reliable biomarkers for detecting potential agents for cancer prevention (*24*). In human colon cancer cell lines, nobiletin strongly induces apoptosis (*5*). Our results suggest that the induction of apoptosis is one of the mechanisms for the chemopreventive action of nobiletin.

High levels of PGE_2 stimulates colon carcinogenesis (*17*). Cell proliferation and apoptosis are also modulated by PGE_2 production (*25*). In the current study, colonic mucosa without tumors of rat receiving AOM alone contained high amounts of PGE_2 when compared with the untreated group. Furthermore, the PGE_2 content of colonic adenocarcinoma in group 1 (AOM alone) was much higher than colonic mucosa without tumors. When rats were fed the diet containing nobiletin after AOM exposure, PGE_2 levels decreased in both colonic mucosa without tumors and colonic adenocarcinomas. Thus, the reduction of PGE_2 also may contribute to the chemopreventive activity of nobiletin. It is known that PGE_2 is produced from arachidonic acid by cyclooxygenase (COX) enzymes (*25*). COX-2, an inducible enzyme, plays a central role in the production of PGE_2 at inflammation sites (*26*), and is involved in colorectal cancer development (*27*). Although we did not determine the expression of COX-2, nobiletin is reported to reduce the COX-2 expression in several experimental conditions (*6, 7, 28*). The reduction of PGE_2 level in colonic mucosa or adenocarcinomas as described here might be contributed to the effect of nobiletin on COX-2 expression. Interestingly, nobiletin can interfere with the production of COX-2 but not with COX-1, a constitutively expressed enzyme, in human synovial cells (*6*). The potential roles of COX-2 inhibitors in the chemoprevention and treatment of colorectal tumors are well discussed (*29-31*). Nobiletin might exert a similarly effect with selective COX-2 inhibitors. Furthermore, nobiletin interferes with the gene expression of proinflammatory cytokines such as interleukin (IL)-1α, IL-1β and tumor necrosis factor-α, which are known to be inducers of PGE_2 (*6*). Such anti-inflammation effects of nobiletin also attenuate the production of PGE_2. Recently, nobiletin has been reported to suppress matrix metalloproteinases (MMP)-7 expression in human colorectal cancer cells (*32*). MMP-7 is known to be associated with the invasiveness (*33*) and metastasis (*34*) of cancer cells. MMP-7 also plays certain roles in the development and progression of colon cancer (*35*). Taken together, nobiletin may affect all processes of carcinogenesis and result in suppression of carcinogenesis.

The impotance of nobiletin as a chemopreventive agent is dependent on its absorption and biotransformation. Nobiletin preferentially accumulated in differentiated Caco-2 cell monolayers (*36*). As for the metabolites, nobiletin is extensively metabolized to demethylated derivatives (*36, 37*). To elucidate the mechanisms of the chemopreventive effect of nobiletin, further studies are warranted to determine the biological activities of these metabolites in carcinogenesis.

In conclusion, our investigation described here demonstrates for the first time that dietary administration of nobiletin suppresses the development of colonic adenocarcinomas induced by AOM. Potential mechanisms by which nobiletin inhibited AOM-induced colon carcinoigenesis include a reduction in

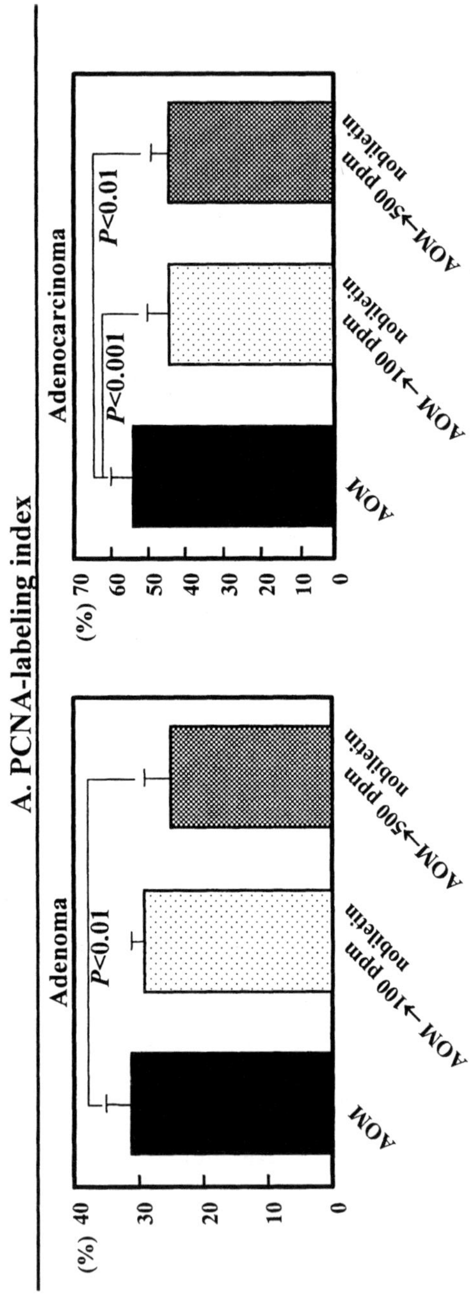
A. PCNA-labeling index
Adenoma
(%) 40
30
20
10
0
P<0.01
AOM
AOM→100 ppm nobiletin
AOM→500 ppm nobiletin
Adenocarcinoma
(%) 70
60
50
40
30
20
10
0
P<0.001
P<0.01
AOM
AOM→100 ppm nobiletin
AOM→500 ppm nobiletin

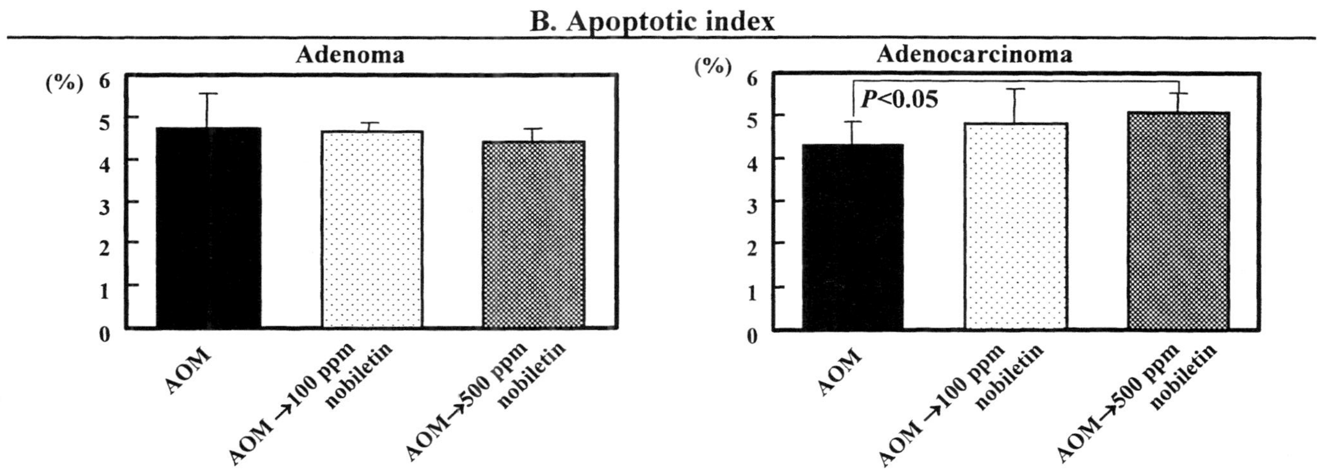

Figure 5. PCNA-labeling and apoptotic indices in the large bowel tumors in rats. "Modified from Biofactors, 22 (1-4), R Suzuki et al., Citrus nobiletin inhibits azoxymethane-induced large bowel carcinogenesis in rats, 111-114., Copyright (2004), with permission from IOS Press"

the amount of PGE_2 which might result in decreased cell proliferation, increased apoptosis, and finally suppression of AOM-induced colon carcinogenesis.

Acknowledgements

This work was supported in part by the Grant-in-Aid for Cancer Research, for the Third-Term Comprehensive 10-Year Strategy for Cancer Control from the Ministry of Health, Labour and Welfare of Japan; the Grants-in-Aid (nos. 15592007 and 15·2052) for Scientific Research from the Ministry of Education, Culture, Sports, Science and Technology of Japan; the grant (C2004-4) for the Collaborative Research from Kanazawa Medical University; and the grant (H2004-6) for the Project Research from the High-Technology Center of Kanazawa Medical University.

References

1. Manthey, J. A.; Grohmann, K.; Guthrie, N. *Curr. Med. Chem.* **2001**, *8*, 135-153.
2. Arts, I. C.; Hollman, P. C. *Am. J. Clin. Nutr.* **2005**, *81(1 Suppl.)*, 317S-325S.
3. Wattenberg, L. W. *Cancer Res.* **1985**, *45*, 1-8.
4. Kawaii, S.; Tomono, Y.; Katase, E.; Ogawa, K.; Yano, M. *J. Agric. Food Chem.* **1999**, *47*, 128-135.
5. Zheng, Q.; Hirose, Y.; Yoshimi, N.; Murakami, A.; Koshimizu, K.; Ohigashi, H.; Sakata, K.; Matsumoto, Y.; Sayama, Y.; Mori, H. *J. Cancer Res. Clin. Oncol.* **2002**, *128*, 539-546.
6. Lin, N.; Sato, T.; Takayama, Y.; Mimaki, Y.; Sashida, Y.; Yano, M.; Ito, A. *Biochem. Pharmacol.* **2003**, *65*, 2065-2071.
7. Murakami, A.; Nakamura, Y.; Torikai, K.; Tanaka, T.; Koshiba, T.; Koshimizu, K.; Kuwahara, S.; Takahashi, Y.; Ogawa, K.; Yano, M.; Tokuda, H.; Nishino, H.; Mimaki, Y.; Sashida, Y.; Kitanaka, S.; Ohigashi, H. *Cancer Res.* **2000**, *60*, 5059-5066.
8. Minagawa, A.; Otani, Y.; Kubota, T.; Wada, N.; Furukawa, T.; Kumai, K.; Kameyama, K.; Okada, Y.; Fujii, M.; Yano, M.; Sato, T.; Ito, A.; Kitajima, M. *Jpn. J. Cancer Res.* **2001**, *92*, 1322-1328.
9. Kono, S. *Eur. J. Cancer Prev.* **2004**, *13*, 127-132.
10. Jemal, A.; Tiwari, R. C.; Murray, T.; Ghafoor, A.; Samuels, A.; Ward, E.; Feuer, E. J.; Thun, M. J.; Society., A. C. *CA Cancer J. Clin.* **2004**, *54*, 8-29.
11. Bosetti, C.; Malvezzi, M.; Chatenoud, L.; Negri, E.; Levi, F.; La Vecchia, C. *Int. J. Cancer* **2005**, *113*, 339-341.
12. Bailar, J. C. r.; Gornik, H. L. *N. Engl. J. Med.* **1997**, *336*, 1569-1574.

13. Tanaka, T.; Kohno, H.; Mori, H. *Asian Pac. J. Cancer Prev.* **2001**, *2*, 165-177.
14. Tsuda, H.; Ohshima, Y.; Nomoto, H.; Fujita, K.; Matsuda, E.; Iigo, M.; Takasuka, N.; Moore, M. A. *Drug Metab. Pharmacokinet.* **2004**, *19*, 245-263.
15. Kohno, H.; Yoshitani, S.; Tsukio, Y.; Murakami, A.; Koshimizu, K.; Yano, M.; Tokuda, H.; Nishino, H.; Ohigashi, H.; Tanaka, T. *Life Sci.* **2001**, *69*, 901-913.
16. Mori, H.; Sugie, S.; Yoshimi, N.; Hara, A.; Tanaka, T. *Mutat. Res.* **1999**, *428*, 291-298.
17. Takahashi, M.; Wakabayashi, K. *Cancer Sci.* **2004**, *95*, 475-480.
18. Pozharisski, K. M. In *Pathology of Tumors in Laboratory Animals*; Turusov, V. S., Ed.; Tumours of the intestines; IARC Scientific Publications; Lyon, 1973; Vol. 1, pp. 119-140.
19. Koide, T.; Sakai, S.; Kawada, Y.; Hara, A.; Sawada, H. *Hinyokika Kiyo.* **1990**, *36*, 1103-1108.
20. Bradford, M. M. *Anal. Biochem.* **1976**, *72*, 248-254.
21. Ohnishi, H.; Asamoto, M.; Tujimura, K.; Hokaiwado, N.; Takahashi, S.; Ogawa, K.; Kuribayashi, M.; Ogiso, T.; Okuyama, H.; Shirai, T. *Cancer Sci.* **2004**, *95*, 936-942.
22. Yoshimizu, N.; Otani, Y.; Saikawa, Y.; Kubota, T.; Yoshida, M.; Furukawa, T.; Kumai, K.; Kameyama, K.; Fujii, M.; Yano, M.; Sato, T.; Ito, A.; Kitajima, M. *Aliment. Pharmacol. Ther.* **2004**, *20 Suppl 1*, 95-101.
23. Johnson, I. T. *Food Chem Toxicol.* **2002**, *40*, 1171-1178.
24. Sun, S. Y.; Hail, N. J.; Lotan, R. *J. Natl. Cancer Inst.* **2004**, *96*, 662-672.
25. Trifan, O. C.; Hla, T. *J. Cell Mol. Med.* **2003**, *7*, 207-222.
26. Geng, Y.; Blanco, F. J.; Cornelisson, M.; Lotz, M. *J. Immunol.* **1995**, *155*, 796-801.
27. Wendum, D.; Masliah, J.; Trugnan, G.; Flejou, J. F. *Virchows Arch.* **2004**, *445*, 327-333.
28. Tanaka, S.; Sato, T.; Akimoto, N.; Yano, M.; Ito, A. *Biochem. Pharmacol.* **2004**, *68*, 433-439.
29. Reddy, B. S. *Environ. Mol. Mutagen.* **2004**, *44*, 26-35.
30. Reddy, B. S.; Rao, C. V. *J. Environ. Pathol. Toxicol. Oncol.* **2002**, *21*, 155-164.
31. Subongkot, S.; Frame, D.; Leslie, W.; Drajer, D. *Pharmacotherapy* **2003**, *23*, 9-28.
32. Kawabata, K.; Murakami, A.; Ohigashi, H. *Biosci. Biotechnol. Biochem.* **2005**, *69*, 307-314.
33. Adachi, Y.; Itoh, F.; Yamamoto, H.; Iku, S.; Matsuno, K.; Arimura, Y.; Imai, K. *Tumour Biol.* **2001**, *22*, 247-253.
34. Kioi, M.; Yamamoto, K.; Higashi, S.; Koshikawa, N.; Fujita, K.; Miyazaki, K. *Oncogene* **2003**, *22*, 8662-8670.

35. Heslin, M. J.; Yan, J.; Johnson, M. R.; Weiss, H.; Diasio, R. B.; Urist, M. M. *Ann. Surg.* **2001**, *233*, 786-792.
36. Murakami, A.; Kuwahara, S.; Takahashi, Y.; Ito, C.; Furukawa, H.; Ju-Ichi, M.; Koshimizu, K. *Biosci. Biotechnol. Biochem.* **2001**, *65*, 194-197.
37. Yasuda, T.; Yoshimura, Y.; Yabuki, H.; Nakazawa, T.; Ohsawa, K.; Mimaki, Y.; Sashida, Y. *Chem. Pharm. Bull. (Tokyo)* **2003**, *51*, 1426-1428.

Chapter 9

Comparison of the Chemoprotection Conferred by Grapefruit and Isolated Bioactive Compounds against Colon Cancer

Nancy D. Turner[1,2], Jairam Vanamala[1–3], Tety Leonardi[1], Bhimanagouda S. Patil[2,3], Mary E. Murphy[4], Yingxue C. Liu[4], Naisyin Wang[4], Leonard M. Pike[2,3], Robert S. Chapkin[1], and Joanne R. Lupton[1]

[1]Faculty of Nutrition, [2]Vegetable and Fruit Improvement Center, [3]Department of Horticultural Sciences, and [4]Department of Statistics, Texas A&M University, College Station, TX 77843

Grapefruit, and isolated bioactive citrus compounds, are suggested to protect against some cancers. The ability of grapefruit pulp powder (irradiated or non-irradiated) and isolated compounds (apigenin, hesperidin, limonin, naringin, naringenin, nobiletin) to protect against colon cancer development were compared in Sprague Dawley rats. Rats were injected with saline or a colon carcinogen (azoxymethane, AOM, 15 mg/kg body weight, 2x, weeks 3 and 4) after starting the diets. All test diets, except hesperidin and nobiletin, reduced ($P < 0.04$) preneoplastic lesions (aberrant crypt foci, ACF) and increased ($P < 0.05$) apoptosis. Hesperidin, nobiletin and apigenin were the only diets that did not decrease ($P < 0.04$) proliferation of colonocytes. Untreated grapefruit pulp powder, limonin and naringenin prevented ($P < 0.05$) proliferative zone expansion in AOM-injected rats. The data indicate untreated grapefruit pulp powder, and certain isolated compounds, reduce ACF formation through changes in colonocyte proliferation and apoptosis. Because irradiated grapefruit pulp powder was not as effective as untreated grapefruit pulp powder in controlling proliferative zone expansion, it may not be as effective as untreated grapefruit pulp powder in colon cancer prevention.

Introduction

Based on epidemiological results, colon cancer incidence could be lowered by consumption of an appropriate diet and implementation of beneficial lifestyles (*1*). However experiments conducted to determine the benefit derived from specific diet inputs have met with conflicting results (*2-4*). Much of the difficulty in ascribing beneficial effects to particular dietary components is the inability to isolate the effect of that food or nutrient, compared to the other changes that occur in the diet. Vitamin C, a significant portion of which is derived mostly from citrus, has long been considered a beneficial compound in addition to meeting nutritional requirements. Using experimental models of colon cancer, various investigators have started to identify protective compounds in a variety of citrus foods (*5-8*). Yet few of these studies have attempted to directly compare the effectiveness of isolated compounds to the intact citrus fruit in an attempt to establish their relative positive or negative contributions toward the overall effect of the intact fruit.

Many horticulturalists would like to increase the levels of the protective compounds through breeding or production practices. However, until we know the relative contributions to the protection against colon cancer or whether some compounds may either not be protective or be promotive of the disease, it will not be possible to make sound recommendations. Therefore, it is important to establish the relative effectiveness of various different isolated bioactive compounds, as compared to the intact fruit and to determine whether post harvest production practices influence the benefit derived from the fruit.

The goal of this work was to compare the ability of a variety of citrus-derived flavonoids and liminoids to protect against the promotion stage of colon cancer in comparison to the effect obtained with the intact fruit pulp. In addition, we wanted to know whether a proposed postharvest irradiation treatment to control fruit flies would alter the protective ability of the fruit. The measurements included the number and multiplicity of aberrant crypt foci (ACF, a preneoplastic lesion of colon cancer), the proportion of proliferating colonocytes and the expansion of the proliferative zone, as well as the incidence of apoptosis in the colons of male Sprague-Dawley rats.

Materials and Methods

Experiment I

Weanling, male Sprague-Dawley rats were adapted to wire-mesh cages for 5-7 days prior to starting the experimental diets. The diets were based on the AIN-76 formulation, and met all of the National Research Council (NRC) nutritional requirements for the rat. In this experiment we compared the effect of whole grapefruit pulp (either control or irradiated) to isolated compounds (naringin or limonin) and a control treatment, using a 2X5 factorial design. Fruit was irradiated (300 Gy, ^{137}Cs) and pulp devoid of seeds and peel was collected (*9*). The whole pulp was added at the expense of dextrose and pectin so that the total fiber content and energy density of the diets were the same as the control diet (Table I). The isolated compounds were included at the expense of dextrose. The level of whole pulp provided 200 mg/kg of naringin, so the isolated naringin was also provided at 200 mg/kg of the diet in order to determine the relative contribution of this level of naringin to the overall protection provided by the intact pulp. For a comparison of the relative effectiveness of naringin and limonin, we included both the isolated compounds in the diet at the same level.

Table I. Experimental Diet Composition[a]

Diet Ingredients	*Control Diet*	*Untreated Grapefruit*	*Irradiated Grapefruit*	*Naringin*	*Limonin*
			g/100 g		
Dextrose	51.06	49.87	49.87	51.04	51.04
Casein	22.35	22.35	22.35	22.35	22.35
Pectin	6.00	5.82	5.82	6.00	6.00
Mineral mix	3.91	3.91	3.91	3.91	3.91
Vitamin mix	1.12	1.12	1.12	1.12	1.12
D,L-methionine	0.34	0.34	0.34	0.34	0.34
Choline bitartrate	0.22	0.22	0.22	0.22	0.22
Corn oil	15.00	15.00	15.00	15.00	15.00
Treatments	0.00	1.37	1.37	0.02	0.02

[a] Dextrose, casein, mineral mix, and D,L-methionine were purchased from Bio-Serv, Frenchtown, NJ. Pectin was purchased from Danisco Cultor, New Century, KS. The vitamin mix and choline bitartrate were purchased from Harlan, Indianapolis, IN. Corn oil was provided as a gift from Traco Labs, Champaign, IL.

Experiment II

Weanling, male Sprague-Dawley rats were adapted to wire mesh cages for 5-7 days prior to consuming the experimental diets. The diets were based on the AIN-76 diet and contained the same ingredients listed in Table I. In this experiment, we compared the effect of four flavonoids isolated from citrus fruits (100 g of diet contained either 0.1 g apigenin, 0.1 g hesperidin, 0.02 g naringenin, 0.01 g nobiletin) and a control diet, in a randomized design. All the compounds were added to the diet at the expense of dextrose and the levels used were based on existing studies in the literature indicating that these levels were effective in protecting against cancers for a variety of tissues and animal models.

Experimental Timelines and Carcinogen Treatment

In both experiments, 10 rats were randomly assigned to each experimental treatment group. Prior to receiving the experimental diets all rats received a commercially available pelleted diet. Experimental diets were provided for 3 weeks prior to the first injection of azoxymethane (15 mg/kg body weight) or saline (Experiment I only). A second injection was given 7 days later. Rats continued to consume the experimental diets for another 6 weeks before sample collection.

Aberrant Crypt Foci, Proliferation and Apoptosis

Six weeks after the last carcinogen injection, samples were collected from the resected colons in order to determine the number and multiplicity of aberrant crypt foci (ACF), and colonocyte proliferation and apoptosis. Half of the colon was fixed in 70% ethanol for 24 h before the aberrant crypts were documented after methylene blue staining (*10*). A 1 cm section of the distal colon was split and fixed in 4% paraformaldehyde or an ethanol gradient. Proliferation was determined in sections prepared from ethanol fixed tissues using a PCNA antibody (*11*). Apoptosis was documented in the paraformaldehyde fixed tissues using the TUNEL assay (*12*). Proliferative or apoptotic indices represent the proportion of labeled cells within each crypt column. Proliferative zone was calculated as the position of the highest labeled cell divided by the total number of cells within a crypt column.

Statistics

Data were analyzed using both exploratory and inferential statistical methods. Graphical displays in exploratory data analysis suggested that measurements in the different subgroups had different variances. In order to perform pairwise multiple comparisons among the treatment groups under these conditions, adjusted p-values (*13*), which controlled family-wise type I error rates were calculated. All results are reported as a percent of the response observed for the control diet.

Results

Experiment I

None of the experimental diets altered the food intake or body weight gain of the rats indicating that this level of dietary consumption had no deleterious effects on the rats (data not shown). However, all of the experimental diets provided a significant level of protection against the formation of high multiplicity aberrant crypt foci, compared to the control diet (Table II). Similarly all of the experimental diets resulted in a lower proliferative index in comparison to the control diet. However, when the proliferative zone was evaluated, only the untreated grapefruit and limonin diets caused a significant reduction, compared to the control diet (Table II). All the experimental diets caused a greater proportion of apoptotic cells in the colon crypts, when compared to the control diet. Yet the greatest increase was observed in the rats consuming the untreated grapefruit and limonin diets (Table II).

Table II. Physiological Responses to Dietary Treatments Expressed as a Percent of the Control Diet (%) in Experiment I

Variable	*Untreated Grapefruit*	*Irradiated Grapefruit*	*Naringin*	*Limonin*
HMACF	41.0 ^{*a}	48.2 ^{*a}	48.2 ^{a}	345 ^{*a}
Proliferative index	494 ^{*a}	66.5 ^{*a}	57.1 ^{a}	44.1 ^{*a}
Proliferative zone	68.8 ^{*a}	76.9 ^{a}	73.3 ^{a}	66.5 ^{*a}
Apoptotic index	287 ^{*a}	179 ^{*b}	180 ^{*b}	262 ^{*a}

NOTE: HMACF = high multiplicity aberrant crypt foci (contain 4 or more aberrant crypts).

* Different from control diet ($P < 0.05$).

^{a,b} Means within a row without a common superscript letter differ ($P < 0.05$).

Experiment II

There was no effect of dietary treatment on average food intake or body weight gain in Experiment II, indicating the treatments did not have a negative impact on the rats over this period of time. Only the apigenin and naringenin diets inhibited the formation of high multiplicity ACF, relative to the number found in rats consuming the control diet (Table III), even though there was a tendency for hesperidin and nobiletin to reduce the lesion incidence. Part of the protection provided by naringenin may have been the result of this compound's ability to reduce the proportion of proliferating cells and suppress expansion of the proliferative zone, as compared to the control diet. Both apigenin and naringenin caused a greater proportion of cells to undergo apoptosis relative to the proportion in the rats consuming the control diet (Table III). There were no significant differences between the rats consuming the control diet and the rats consuming either the hesperidin or nobiletin diet.

Table III. Physiological Responses to Dietary Treatments Expressed as a Percent of the Control Diet (%) in Experiment II

Variable	*Apigenin*	*Hesperidin*	*Naringenin*	*Nobiletin*
HMACF	42.9 ^{*a}	59.1 ^{a}	49.2 ^{*a}	70.1 ^{a}
Proliferative index	72.2 ^{a}	86.8 ^{a}	67.6 ^{*b}	76.4 ^{a}
Proliferative zone	85.4 ^{a}	91.6 ^{a}	81.6 ^{*a}	86.3 ^{a}
Apoptotic index	178 ^{*ab}	135 ^{a}	197 ^{*b}	129 ^{a}

NOTES: HMACF = high multiplicity aberrant crypt foci (contain 4 or more aberrant crypts); Apoptotic index was measured on the luminal surface.
* Different from control diet ($P < 0.05$).
^{a,b} Means within a row without a common superscript letter differ ($P < 0.05$).

Discussion

Our goal was to compare the effectiveness of a variety of isolated compounds with the whole fruit pulp in an attempt to ascribe levels of activity to the various compounds. We found the untreated grapefruit pulp and isolated limonin provided the greatest level of protection against this early stage of colon cancer development, effected through changes in the regulation of proliferation and apoptosis in Experiment I. The level of isolated limonin included in the diet was the same as for isolated naringin. but this level of limonin was 10-fold that found in the intact grapefruit pulp. Thus, the protection derived from the grapefruit pulp was a combination of effects generated by the multitude of compounds found in the intact food.

In addition to the potential contribution of limonin in the intact food, at this early stage of colon carcinogenesis, elevated doses of isolated limonin may prove protective against the disease process. Inhibition of high multiplicity ACF in this experiment is comparable to the results obtained when 0.02 g/100 g or 0.05 g/100 g of limonin were included in the diet of male Fisher 344 rats prior to injection with AOM (*14*). Tanaka et al. (*14*) noted no difference in the formation of aberrant crypt foci between the two doses. Results from our study and that of Tanaka et al. (*14*) would suggest that the maximal benefit derived from supplemental limonin was achieved with the 0.02 g/100 g of diet level.

Isolated naringin, at the level found in the untreated grapefruit pulp, provided a level of protection against the formation of preneoplastic lesions of colon cancer that was not too dissimilar from the intact food source. It was only when we determined effectiveness in controlling cell proliferation and apoptosis was a difference in the whole food and the isolated compound identified. This would suggest that in its pure form, naringin would help protect against this early stage of the disease. Yet, the fact that it was less effective in controlling proliferation and stimulating apoptosis either means that the isolated compound is operating through other mechanisms than changes in cell cycle activity or may not be as effective during the later stages of cancer development.

Although the untreated and irradiated grapefruit pulp resulted in similar levels of lesions being formed, the irradiated grapefruit was less effective in controlling colonocyte proliferation and inducing apoptosis. Similar to the results with naringin, these observations suggest the possibility that irradiated grapefruit may not be as effective at controlling the later stages of colon cancer development. Therefore, changes in the chemical profile of the irradiated grapefruit had a net negative impact on the fruit's chemoprotective capacity. Some of the possible chemical changes in the irradiated fruit have been reported (*9*). However, considering the number of compounds that may have changed as a result of irradiation, it is not possible at this time to delineate the exact cause of the loss of chemoprotective ability.

Because of its ability to improve all of the variables measured, naringenin was considered the most protective of all the compounds tested in Experiment II. Even though it was less effective, apigenin was also able to reduce high multiplicity ACF formation and increase apoptosis, relative to the control diet. The lack of effect on proliferation from apigenin ingestion by rats in this experiment is in contrast to cell culture experiments in which apigenin caused G2/M cell cycle arrest (*15*). Hesperidin was included in the diet at the same level as apigenin, but none of the observations for hesperidin were different from the control diet. However, within the experimental diets there were no differences noted, except for the reduction in proliferative index and apoptosis noted for naringenin. Together, the data from Experiment II indicate that there were important differences in potency of these compounds.

In comparing the responses from Experiment I and Experiment II we find that there were similar levels of protection, compared to the control diets, in lesion formation from untreated and irradiated grapefruit, naringin, limonin, apigenin and naringenin. Even though there were beneficial effects on proliferation and apoptosis with these compounds, the degree of positive changes was the greatest for untreated grapefruit and limonin. We also find that not all of the effective compounds were operating through similar mechanisms since they had variable abilities to mediate colonocyte proliferation and apoptosis. In a direct comparison between naringenin (aglycone) and naringin (glucoside), we found little numerical differences in the ability of these flavanones to protect against colon cancer. However, within the individual experiments, naringenin provided a significant change from the results obtained with the control diet for all of the variables measured. The long-term implications of these small changes would likely only become apparent with a study in which tumor formation was determined.

One of the most likely explanations for the difference in responses observed with the isolated compounds and the intact untreated grapefruit is that the compound present in the whole fruit could have a greater probability of arriving in the colon, compared to the free, isolated compounds. Bioactive compounds can be susceptible to hydrolysis and/or metabolism/conjugation in the small intestine, which may limit systemic availability (*16-18*). Intact pulp containing bioactive compounds would have a higher probability of allowing the compounds to pass through the small intestine into the colon before they are released from within the cell walls as a result of microbial fermentation. However, without a mechanism of delivering the intact, isolated compound to the colon, it will be impossible to distinguish whether the diminished responses were due to metabolism and hydrolysis of the molecules that reduce their bioactivity or whether the compounds in fact have only small individual effects. Therefore, at this time the best recommendation for consumers is to include citrus fruits as part of an otherwise healthy diet that includes a variety of fruits and vegetables if their goal is to reduce their risk of colon cancer.

Acknowledgments

This work was supported by funding from the USDA (2001-52102-11257), the Texas Higher Education Coordinating Board (ATP 003658-0359c-2001, ATP 010366-0194-2001), and the National Institute of Environmental Health Sciences (P30-ES09106).

References

1. Tomeo, C. A.; Colditz, G. A.; Willett, W. C.; Giovannucci, E.; Platz, E.; Rockhill, B.; Dart, H.; Hunter, D. J. *Cancer Causes Control* **1999**, *10*, 167-180.
2. Michels, K. B.; Giovannucci, E.; Joshipura, K. J.; Rosner, B. A.; Stampfer, M. J.; Fuchs, C. S.; Colditz, G. A.; Speizer, F. E.; Willett, W. C. *J. Natl. Cancer Inst.* **2000**, *92*, 1740-1752.
3. Voorrips, L. E.; Goldbohm, R. A.; van Poppel, G.; Sturmans, F.; Hermus, R. J. J.; van den Brandt, P. A. *Am. J Epidemiol.* **2000**, *152*, 1081-1092.
4. Bingham, S.A.; Day, N.E.; Luben, R.; Ferrari, P.; Slimani, N.; Norat, T.; Clavel-Chapelon, F.; Keese, E.; Nieters, A.; Boeing, H.; Tjonneland, A.; Overvad, K.; Martinez, C.; Dorronsoro, M.; Gonzalez, C.A.; Key, T.J.; Trichopoulou, A.; Naska, A.; Vineis, P.; Tumino, R.; Krogh, V.; Bueno-de-Mesquita, H.B.; Peeters, P.H.; Berglund, G.; Hallmans, G.; Lund, E.; Skeie, G.; Kaaks, R.; Riboli, E. *Lancet* **2003**, *361*, 1496-1501.
5. Miyagi, Y.; Om, A. S.; Chee, K. M.; Bennink, M. R. *Nutr. Cancer* **2000**, *36*, 224-229.
6. Kossoy, G.; Ben-Hur, H.; Stark, A.; Zusman, I.; Madar, Z. *Oncol. Rep.* **2001**, *8*, 1387-1391.
7. Frydoonfar, H. R.; McGrath, D. R.; Spigelman, A. D. *Colorectal Dis.* 2002, *5*, 149-152.

8. Tanaka, T.; Makita, H.; Kawabata, K.; Mori, H.; Kakumoto, M.; Satoh, K.; Hara, A.; Sumida, T.; Tanaka, T.; Ogawa, H. *Carcinogenesis* **1997**, *18*, 957-965.
9. Vanamala, J.; Cobb, G.; Turner, N.D.; Lupton, J.R.; Yoo, K.S.; Pike, L.M.; Patil, B.S. *J. Agric. Food Chem.* **2005**, *53*, 3980-3985.
10. Bird, R.P. *Cancer Res.* **1987**, *48*, 6187-6192.
11. Warren, C.A.; Lupton, J.R.; Popovic, N.; Hong, M.Y.; Taddeo, S.S.; Murphy, M.E.; Chapkin, R.S.; Turner, N.D. *FASEB J.* **2003**, *17,* A1202.
12. Hong, M. Y.; Chapkin, R. S.; Wild, C. P.; Morris, J. S.; Wang, N.; Carroll, R. J.; Turner, N. D.; Lupton, J. R. *Cell Growth Djff* **1999**, *10*, 749-758.
13. Westfall, P.H. *J. Amer. Stat. Assoc.* 1997, *92*, 299-306.
14. Tanaka, T.; Maeda, M.; Kohno, H.; Murakami, M.; Kagami, S.; Miyake, M.; Wada, K. *Eur. J. Cancer Prev.* **2001**, *12*, 195-200.
15. Wang, W.; VanAlstyne, P.C.; Irons, K.A.; Chen, S.; Stewart, J.W.; Birt, D.F. *Nutr. Cancer* **2004**, *48*, 106-114.
16. Liu, Y.; Liu, Y.; Dai, Y.; Xun, L.; Hu., M. *J. Alt. Compl. Med.* **2003**, *9*, 631-640.
17. Rechner, A.R.; Kuhnle, G.; Bremner, P.; Hubbard, G.P.; Moore, K.P.; Rice-Evans, C.A. *Free Rad. Biol. Med.* 2002, *33*, 220-235.
18. Choudhury, R.; Chowrimootoo, G.; Srai, K.; Debnam, E.; Rice-Evans, C.A. *Biochem. Biophys. Res. Comm.* **1999**, *265*, 410-415.

Chapter 10

Citrus Limonoids and Flavonoids: Enhancement of Phase II Detoxification Enzymes and Their Potential in Chemoprevention

Hassan Ahmad[1,2], Jiaxing Li[2], Maria Polson[1], Kimberly Mackie[1], Walter Quiroga[1], and Bhimanagouda S. Patil[2]

[1]Department of Chemistry, University of Texas–Pan American, 1201 West University Drive, Edinburg, TX 78539
[2]Vegetable and Fruit Improvement Center, Department of Horticultural Sciences, Mail Code 2119, Texas A&M University, College Station, TX 77843

Enhancement of the detoxification pathway for the elimination of toxic electrophiles by the Phase-II enzymes (Glutathione S-transferase, GST; and NAD(P)H:quinine reductase, QR) is one means of cellular protection that may be anticarcinogenic. Effects of citrus limonoids (nomilin, limonin, aglycone mixtures) and flavonoids (hesperidin, naringin, and crude flavonoids mixture) were investigated in various tissues of mice. Three doses of 20 mg of citrus limonoids and flavonoids were given to 10-week-old female A/JOlaHsd mice over a period of one week. Limonoid aglycones were more effective inducers of GST activity than their respective glucosides. Nomilin and an aglycone mixture were the most potent inducers of GST. Citrus flavonoids showed the most significant induction of GST and QR in the stomach. The GST and QR induction by the limonoids and flavonoids appeared to be tissue-specific and related to the structures of the compounds. The enhanced level of phase-II enzymes by citrus flavonoids suggests their importance in chemoprevention.

Introduction

For over a quarter century, a consensus supported by a growing number of epidemiologic studies suggests that consumption of diets rich in fruits and vegetables is associated with lower risks of developing various types of malignant cancers (1-6). Multiple mechanisms are undoubtedly involved in the protective effects of diets rich in fruits and vegetables. It is difficult to identify the specific, individual contributions from various components of the diet to overall cancer risk reduction, and the issue is only confounded by the potential synergism between the constituents. Nonetheless, there is much evidence that specific compounds from fruits and vegetables such as flavonoids, carotenoids and limonoids among others protect against chemical carcinogenesis. A compelling body of evidence now indicates that substantial protection against chemical carcinogenesis can be achieved by non-nutrient components of vegetables and fruits capable of inducing enzymes that are involved in carcinogen metabolism. Although the anticarcinogenic effects of many nonnutrient phytochemicals are not entirely understood, an enhanced detoxification of carcinogenic electrophiles by Phase-II detoxification enzymes, such as glutathione S-transferase (GST) and NAD(P)H:quinone reductase (QR), appears to be the single most important component of the mechanisms responsible for their anticarcinogenic activity (7-9). Both of these phase II enzymes are highly inducible in mammals (10,11). Thus, induction of Phase II enzymes by naturally occurring or synthetic agents represents a promising strategy for cancer prevention.

GSTs are ubiquitous enzymes that protect cells by detoxification of carcinogens by catalytic and non-catalytic binding mechanisms. GSTs catalyze the conjugation of tripeptide glutathione (GSH) to a wide variety of endogenous and exogenous chemicals with electrophilic functional groups. These include the products of oxidative stress, pollutants and carcinogens, which upon conjugation with GSH yield water soluble thioesters (12-15). A multitude of GST isoenzymes belonging to various gene families are reported to be present in mammalian tissues (16-18). The most abundant cytosolic mammalian GST isoenzymes are grouped into four major classes, α, μ, π, and θ (18-20). This classification is based on substrate specificity, primary structure, kinetics, and immunological properties of the isoenzymes (18-20). A large number of carcinogens are known to be metabolized by GST (16,21,22). Numerous studies strongly implicate the induction of GST with enhanced detoxification of carcinogens. For example, 1,2-dithiol-3-thione has an anticarcinogenic effect against aflatoxin B_1-induced hepatocarcinogenesis in rats. This is believed to be due to induction of GSTs which exhibit a 4 to 6-fold increase in the specific activity of "aflatoxin-GSH conjugation" (23). More recent studies, which focus on the search for biomarkers of cancer risk and prevention, strongly suggest that individuals deficient in protection rendered by Phase-II detoxification enzymes, especially GSTs, are at an increased risk of cancer (24-28).

Quinonides are formed as intermediates during Phase-I metabolism of various carcinogens. QR mediates the two-electron reduction of quinones leading to the formation of relatively stable hydroquinones, through redox-cycling. This shields against their ability to generate oxidative stress. Induction of QR, therefore, is considered important in diminishing the toxicity of quinone metabolites. The hydroquinone intermediates that are produced by QR are susceptible to conjugation with glucuronic acid by UDP-glucuronosyl transferases to produce water soluble glucoronyl conjugates (29,30). It is, therefore, believed that the induction of NAD(P)H:quinone reductase is also an important component in the overall mechanisms by which various Phase-II enzyme-inducing agents protect from chemical carcinogenesis, especially those mediated by quinonide (31-34).

Phase I enzymes catalyze reactions largely through oxidation and reduction. Phase II enzymes promote conjugation of toxic Phase I enzyme-products with endogenous ligands such as GSH, amino and glucuronic acids. This sequence of reactions usually leads to more soluble and easily excretable products. Monofunctional inducers are, therefore, more desirable and preferred as the agents for achieving chemoprevention (24,31,32). Chemoprotection can be achieved by preferentially raising the levels of Phase II enzymes, and many inducers of this type are already present in the human diet. Numerous studies have shown that administration of phenolic antioxidants, e.g. flavonoids, produce marked elevations of GSTs and other Phase II enzymes in many tissues and cell lines (35-39).

Limonoids are a group of triterpenoids. Their general structure contains a furan ring attached to C1, oxygen-containing functional groups, a 14,15 epoxide group and an oxymethylene at C19 (See Figure 1). In citrus, limonin and nomilin are the most prevalent limonoids. Citrus limonoids are known to possess anticarcinogenic activity in various organs such as the forestomach (40), lung (41), colon (42), oral cavity (43-45), skin (46) and breast cancer cell lines in vitro (47). Our recent studies have demonstrated the differential inhibition of the proliferation of human cancer cells by citrus limonoids (48). In another recent investigation, limonoid glucosides at micromolar concentrations are lethal to neuroblastoma cells in culture (49). In another study, we have demonstrated that citrus flavonoids have stronger antioxidant activity compared to limonoids (50). Since citrus is one of the major fruits of the human diet, evaluating the potential of phytochemicals in chemoprevention from citrus fruits is of particular interest. Here, we report the effect of citrus flavonoids and limonoids on the induction of phase II enzymes (Fig. 1).

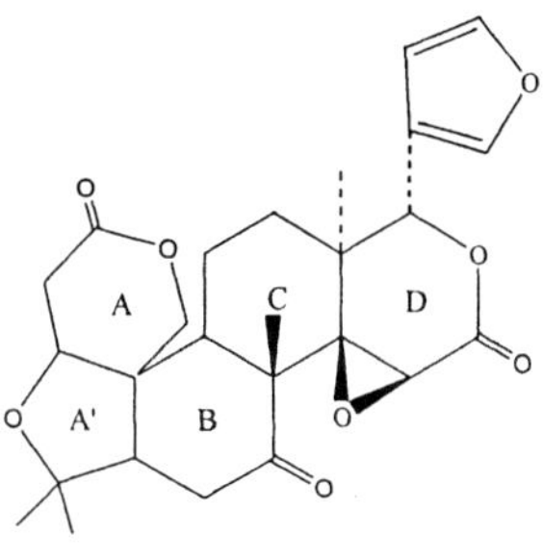

A

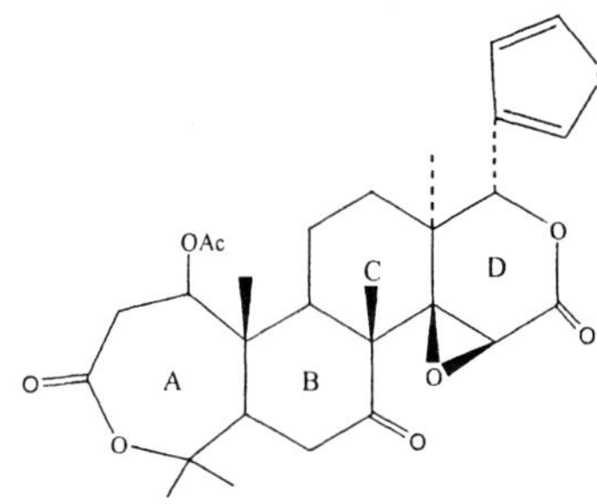

B

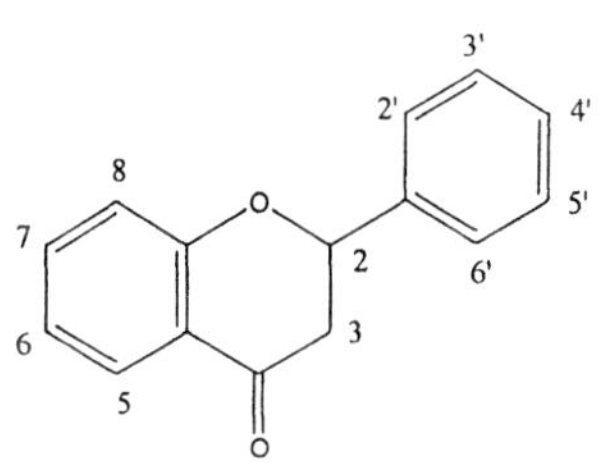

C

Figure 1. Structures of two citrus limonoids: (a) limonin (b) nomilin and (c) a general flavanone: Hesperidin 3'=OH, Naringin 3'=H; Hesperidin 4'=OMe, Naringin 4'=OH.

Materials and Methods

Most of the reagents used in this study were obtained from Sigma Chemicals Co. St. Louis, MO. The citrus flavonoids and limonoids were isolated by using established procedures (51-53). The structures of the purified compounds were analyzed and verified with HPLC-ESI/MS.

Treatment of Animals

Female Albino A/JOlaHsd mice, 5-6 weeks old, were purchased from Harlan Sprague Dawley, Inc., Indianapolis, IN. Guidelines approved by the Institutional Review Committee for animal use and care were followed. The animals were acclimatized at our animal care facility for two weeks prior to start of the experiments. The animals were housed under controlled lightning conditions (12 hours light and 12 hours dark cycle) and were fed semi-purified diet (AIN-76, ICN Laboratories, Cleveland, OH) and water *ad libitum*. The control and experimental groups, each containing five mice, were formed. The experimental groups received three doses of citrus flavonoids, limonoids, or mixtures in corn oil, administered by gavage every other day, while the control mice received only appropriate amounts of corn oil. Each dose consisted of 20 mg of flavonoid, limonoid or mixtures dissolved in 0.25 mL of corn oil. The animals were sacrificed by cervical dislocation forty-eight hours after the last dose. The organs were harvested and rinsed with cold phosphate-buffered saline. A small amount of excised tissue from each group was used for enzyme activity assays, while the remaining tissues were frozen at -20°C until used. Details of these procedures are published elsewhere (54).

Sample preparation and Enzyme Activity

Organ homogenates (10% (w/v)) were prepared from each group in 10 mM phosphate buffer, pH 7.0, containing 1.4 mM β-mercaptoethanol. The homogenization was carried out with a Potter-Elvehjem type homogenizer. The homogenates were centrifuged at 22,000 x g for 45 min in a Beckman T30 Avanti centrifuge.

GST activity against 1-chloro-2,4-dinitrobenzene (CDNB) was determined as described by Habig *et al.* (55) and QR activity against 2,6-dichlorophenolindophenol (DCPIP) was determined as described by Benson *et al.* (56). The Beckman-DU640 UV/Visible spectrophotometer equipped with enzyme kinetics software was programmed to calculate the enzyme units. One unit of enzyme activity is defined as the amount of enzyme that used 1 μmole of substrate per minute at 25°C. Protein concentration was determined by the dye binding method of Bradford (57) using bovine serum albumin as a standard. Resutls are presented as means ± S.D. of n=4-5 per group and the student's t-test was used to assess the significance of the data.

Results and Discussion

Effect of Flavonoids on GST Activity

GST activity was significantly ($p < 0.01$) induced in the liver by 4-bromoflavone while no significant effect on GST activity was observed in mice treated with citrus-derived flavonoids (Fig 2). In the intestine, GST activities were increased ($p < 0.1$) by 4-bromoflavone, a synthetic flavonoid that has been shown to considerably induce the phase II detoxification enzyme activities of GST and QR with *in vivo* and *in vitro* models (58). Hesperidin and naringin showed a slight decrease in GST activity in the intestine, although not significantly, while the mixture had no significant effect (Fig. 2).

GST activity in the stomach, with CDNB as substrate, was increased ($p < 0.1$) by 4-bromoflavone and to a lesser extent by the crude mixture of flavonoids ($p < 0.15$). Hesperidin and naringin (nearly the same as the mixture – I wouldn't separate their relative changes) only slightly increased this activity (Fig. 2). GST activities were also increased by the 4-bromoflovone ($p < 0.1$) in the lung. While naringin and the mixture of flavonoids had no effect, the GST activity was slightly decresed with hesperidin treatment.

Effect of Flavonoids on QR Activity

The levels of QR activity were low but naringin significantly increased ($p < 0.01$) the QR activity in the liver by 1.6 fold to the control, and it was also induced ($p < 0.1$) by hesperidin but to a lesser extent (Fig. 3). In intestine, the QR activity was significantly induced by 4-bromoflavone (3.6 fold to the control) and hesperidin (1.7 fold to the control). On the other hand, naringin and the flavonoid mixture had no affect on QR in the intestine (Fig. 3). Stomach showed maximum induction of QR activity by the synthetic and various citrus flavonoids. The greatest induction occurred with 4-bromoflavone in the intestine. The induction by the natural compounds was greatest with the mixture in the stomach. The enzyme activity was increased differentially by 4- bromoflavone, hesperidin, and naringin, 1.6, 1.2, and 1.4 fold to the control, respectively, while naringin had no significant effect (Fig. 3).

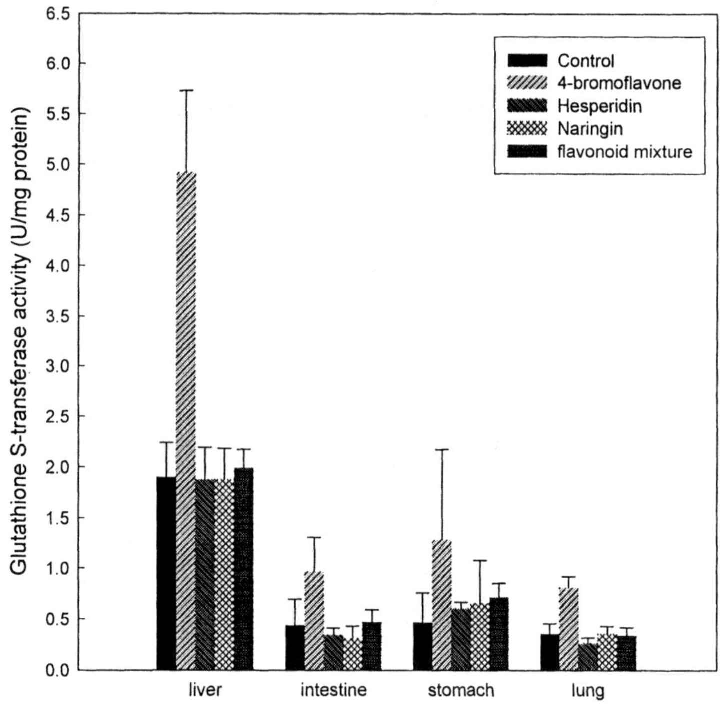

Figure 2. Effects of citrus flavonoids on glutathione S-transferase activities in mouse tissues. Experimental groups received hesperidin, naringin and crude flavonoid mixture (20 mg/dose) and the control animals received only corn oil. Details are given in the text.

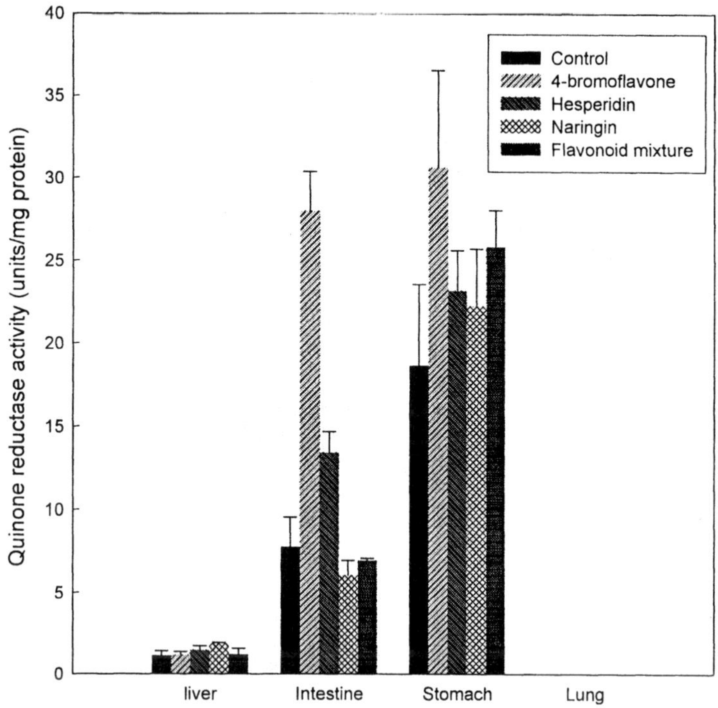

Figure 3. Effects of citrus flavonoids on quinone reductase activities in mouse tissues. Experimental groups received hesperidin, naringin and crude flavonoid mixture (20mg/dose) and the control animals received only corn oil. Details are given in the text.

Although enzyme activity data for GST and QR do not show an overall induction of activities throughout the various tissues studied, they do suggest a differential induction based on organ type. The results of the citrus-derived flavonoids in the stomach suggest that these particular flavonoids may be specific inducers of Phase II enzymes in the stomach. Since phase II enzyme inducers are known to differentially induce various isoenzymes of GST (54), it is essential to carry out detailed studies before full potential of flavonoids could be recognized. The results of hesperidin and naringin (Fig 3) suggest the likelihood of these compounds being QR-specific inducers in the intestine and liver.

Although a number of studies report the protective role of flavonoids in male F344 rats (59, 60), they lack an elucidating mechanism of action for these flavonoids. To our knowledge no studies have been performed to demonstrate whether the flavonoid structures are important in inducing phase-II enzymes. A number of reports suggest that antioxidant structures are important in determining their antioxidant, antiproliferative and enzyme inhibition activities

(61, 62). The two flavonoids used in this study belong to the flavanone group. Since they do not have the C2-C3 double bond their structures are not planar. However they differ in the hydroxylation of the 3',4'-catechol moiety (Fig. 1). These variations in flavonoid structures are known to affect cellular activities. Therefore, further investigation into structural differences and the pattern of induction of enzyme isoforms is needed. Additionally, new studies regarding the absorption and bioavailability of these flavonoids are needed to elucidate their metabolic fate *in vivo* as well as possible mechanisms of action.

Effect of Limonoids on GST Activity

Limonoid aglycones appear to have better GST inducing capabilities (Fig. 4) compared to the limonoid glucosides (data not presented). The highest increase in GST activity was observed in the stomach of mice treated with nomilin (2.96 fold to the control). The stomach was the only organ in which all three limonoids caused significant induction of GST activity. In liver, only nomilin increased ($p < 0.01$) the levels GST activity. None of the limonoids caused any significant changes in the GST activity levels in either intestine or lung.

Nomilin and the aglycone mixture actually significantly decreased the GST activity in the lung. Despite only slight overall changes in the enzyme levels in various tissues, it appears that nomilin is the most potent GST inducer of all the compounds tested. The induction of GST activity due to nomilin was markedly higher in the stomach, followed by liver and intestine. These data are consistent with the earlier report by Lam and Hasegawa, who demonstrated that the nomilin is effective inducer of GST and protected the stomach against chemical carcinogenesis (40). The aglycone mixture-induced GST activity was found to be higher in the stomach, followed by intestine. Limonin, however, effectively induced GST only in the stomach. The effectiveness of limonin on GST induction in other tissues, if any, was marginal (Fig. 4). Similar levels of GST induction were also reported by Lam and Hasegawa for limonin (63). Furtermore, it has been suggested that natural products possessing a furan moiety are inducers of the GST enzymes (63). In our study, both limonoids showed marginal to significant levels GST induction (Fig. 4) despite both having a furan ring (Fig 1). Further studies are thus needed to establish the role of furan ring in the regulation of the phase II enzymes induction. It also appears that stomach showed maximum induction of enzyme activities by the flavonoids and limonoids. Additionally, protection against chemical carcinogenesis by the limonoids is particularly effective in stomach (40). Possibly the localized effects on stomach could be due to the maximum exposure of the inducer in this tissue due to poor solubility of the limonoids. In light of these findings, it is important to investigate bioavailability of the inducers in target tissues over a period of time in order to accurately judge the potential of these compounds in various tissues.

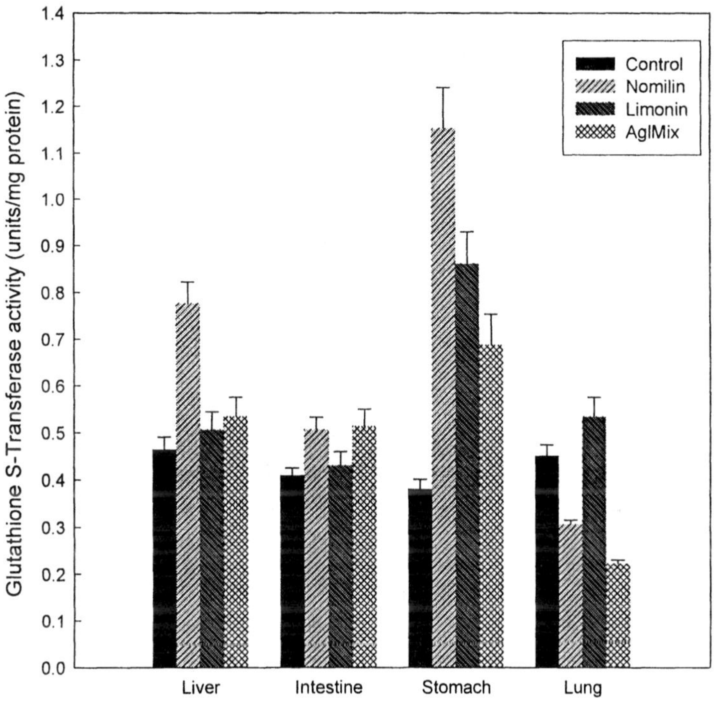

Figure 4. Effects of citrus limonoids on glutathione S-transferase activities in mouse tissues. Experimental groups received limonin, nomilin and aglycone mixture (AglMix) (10 mg/dose) and the control animals received only corn oil. Details are given in the text.

Conclusions

Induction of phase II detoxification enzymes GST and QR in particular is considered as a significant mechanism of cancer chemoprevention. In this study we have investigated the ability of citrus flavonoids and limonoids to induce GST and QR. Our data suggest that citrus flavonoids exhibited slightly more inductive effects on phase II enzymes compared to the limonids in general. Both inducers were more effective in inducing the Phase II enzymes in stomach compared to other tissues. However more studies are needed to establish whether the selective induction of phase II enzymes in the stomach is due to the more effective exposure of the inducers to this tissue compared to others.

Acknowledgements

The study was supported in part by the NIH grants GM08038 and GM50080 to HA, USDA-IFAFS 2001-52102-11257, USDA-CRIS/HATCH H-08802 and THECO/ATP grant 003658-0359-2001 to BSP.

References

1. Wattenberg, L. W. *Cancer Res.* **1983** *43,* 2448-2452.
2. Bueno de Mesquita, H. B., Maisonneuve, P., Runia, S. and Moerman, C. H. *Intl. J. Cancer*, **1991,** *48*, 540-549.
3. Temple N.J. *J. National Cancer Institute,* **1999,** *91*, 1164.
4. Williams G.M., Wynder, E.L *in Nutrition and Cancer Prevention* Watson, R. R. and Mufti, S. I. Eds.. CRC Press, Inc., Boca Raton, FL 1996 p. 1.
5. Terry, P., Giovannucci, E., Michels, K.B., Bergkvist, L., Hansen, H., Holmberg, L., Wolk, A. *Journal of the National Cancer Institute,* **2001,** *93*, 525-533.
6. Schulze, M.B., Hoffmann, K., Kroke, A., Boeing, H., *British Journal of Nutrition,* **2001,** *85*, 363-373.
7. Kensler, T.W. *Environ. Health Prospect.* **1997**, *105*, Suppl 4, 965-970.
8. Beglieter, A., Leith, M.K., Curphey, T.J., Doherty, G.P., *Oncol. Res.* **1997**, *9*, 371-382.
9. Talalay, P. *Biofactors*, **2000**, *12*, 5-11.
10. Talalay, P., Fahey, J.W., Holtzclaw, W.D., Prestera, T., Zhang, Y. *Toxicol. Lett.* **1995**, *82/83,* 173-179.
11. Sreerama, L., Hedge, M.W., Sladek, N.E. *Clin Cancer Res.* **1995**, *1*, 1153-1163.
12. Jakoby, W.B. *Adv. Enzymol. Relat. Areas Mol. Biol.*, **1978,** *40*, 383-414.

13. Booth, J., Boyland, E., and Sims, P. *Biochem. J.* **1960,** *74,* 117-122
14. Habig, W.H., Pabst, M.J., and Jakoby, W.B. *J. Biol. Chem.,* **1974,** *249,* 7130-7139.
15. Morgenstern, R. and DePierre, J. W. *Eur. J. Biochem*, **1983**, *134*, 591-597.
16. Hayes, J. D. and Pulford, D. J. *Critical Reviews in Biochemistry and Molecular Biology* **1995**, *30*, 445-600.
17. Mannervik, B. and Danielson, U.H. *CRC Crit. Rev. Biochem.* **1988**, *23,*283-337.
18. Tsuchida, S. and Sato, K *Crit. Rev of Biochem. and Mol. Biol.* **1992**, *27,*337-384.
19. Awasthi, Y.C., Sharma, R., and Singhal, S.S. (1994) *Int. J. Biochem.*, **26**:295-308.
20. Landi, S. (2000) *Mutation Research* **463**:247-283.
21. Singh, S.V., Srivastava, S.K., and Awasthi, Y.C. *FEBS Lett.* **1985**, *179,*111-114.
22. Singh, S.V., Creadon, G., Das, M., Mukhtar, H., and Awasthi, Y.C. *Biochem. J.*, **1987,** *243*, 351-358.
23. Cabral, J.R.P. and Neal, G.E. *Cancer Lett.* **1983**, *19*,125-132.
24. Clapper, M and Szarka, C.E. *Chemico-Biological Interaction.* **1998,** *11-12,*377-388.
25. Inoue, H., Kiyohara, C., Shinomiya, S., Marugame, T., Tsuji, E., Handa, K., Hayabuchi, H., Eguchi, H., Fukushima, Y., Kono, S. *Cancer Letters,* **2001,** *163*, 201-206.
26. Gsur, A., Haidinger, G., Hinteregger, S., Bernhofer, G., Schatzl, G., Madersbacher, S., Marberger, M., Vutuc, C., Micksche, M. *International Journal of Cancer*, **2001,** *95*,152-155.
27. Spurdle, A.B., Webb, P.M., Purdie, D.M., Chen, X., Green, A., Chenevix-Trench, G. *Carcinogenesis*, **2001,** *22*, 67-72.
28. Parl, F.F. *Cancer Lett.* **2005,** *221*, 123-129.
29. Lind, C., Vadi, H., and Ernster L. *Arch. Biochem. Biophys.* **1978,** *190,* 97.
30. Lind, C. *Biochem. Pharmacol.*, **1985,** *34*, 895-897.
31. Talalay, P. (1992) in "Cancer Chemoprevention" Wattenberg, L., M. Lipkin, M., Boone, C. W., and Kelloff, G. J. Eds., CRC Press, Boca Raton, FL, p. 469.
32. Talalay, P., De Long. M. J., and Prochaska H. J. *Proc Natl. Acad Sci. USA* **1988,** *85,* 8261-8265.
33. Talalay, P. *Adv. Enzyme Reg.* **1989,** *28*: 237-250.
34. Benson, A.M., Hunkeler, M.J., and Talalay, P. *Proc. Natl. Acad. Sci. U.S.A.,* **1980**, *77,* 5216-5220.
35. Galati G, O'brien, P.J. *Free Radical Biology & Medicine*, **2004**, *37*, 287-303.
36. Steele, V. E.; Kelloff, G.J.; Balentine, D.; Boone, C. W.; Mehta,R.; Baheri, D.; Sigman, C.C.; Zhu, S.; Sharma, S. *Carcinogenesis* **2000**, *21*, 63-67.

37. Weisburger, J. M. *Proc. Soc. Exp. Biol. Med.* **1999,** *220*, 271-275.
38. Middleton, E., Kandaswami, C., in The flavonoids; Advances in Research Science. 1986, Harborne Ed., Chapman and Hall, London, p619.
39. Zhao, J., Agarwal, R. *Carcinogenesis*, **1999**, *20*, 2101-2108.
40. Lam, L. K. T., and Hasegawa, S. *Nutr Cancer* **1989,** *12*, 43-47.
41. Lam, L. K. T., Zhang, J., Hasegawa, S., and Schut, H. A. J. In: *Food Phytochemicals for Cancer Prevention I. Fruit and Vegetables* Huang, M. T., Osawa, T., Ho, C. T., Rose, R. T. Eds. Amer. Chem. Soc., Washington, DC, 1994. p. 209.
42. Tanaka, T, Maeda, Kohno M. H., Murakami, M,. Kagami, S., Miyake, M., and Wada, K. *Carcinogenesis* **2000,** *22*, 193-198.
43. Miller, E. G., Gonzales-Sanders, A. P., Couvillon, A. M., Binnie, W. H., Hasegawa, S. and Lam, L. K. T. *Food Technol* **1994,** *48*, 110-114.
44. Miller, E. G., Gonzales-Sanders, A. P., Couvillon, A. M., Wrigh, J. M., Hasegawa, S., Lam, L. K. T., and Sunahara, G. I. In *Food Phytochemicals for Cancer Prevention I. Fruit and Vegetables.* Huang, M. T, Osawa, T., Ho, C. T., Rosen, R. T. Eds. Amer. Chem. Soc., Washington, DC, 1994, p. 220
45. Wright, J. L., Miller, E. G., Binnie, W. H., Guo, I. Y., and Hasegawa, S. *J Dent Res* **1996,** *75,* 436.
46. Lam, L. K. T., Zhang, J., Hasegawa, S. *Food Tech* **1994,***48*, 104-108.
47. Guthrie, N., Morley, K., Hasegawa, S., Manners, G. D., Vandenberg, T. In *Citrus Limonoids-Functional Chemicals in Agriculture and Foods.* Berhow, M. A, Hasegawa, S., Manners, G. D. Eds. Amer. Chem. Soc., Washington, DC, 2000. p. 164.
48. Tian, Q., Miller, E. G., Ahmad, H., Tang, L., Patil, B. S. *Nutr. Cancer* **2001,** *40*, 180-184.
49. Poulose, S. M., Harris, E. D., Patil, B. S. *J. Nutrition* **2005**, 135, 870-877.
50. Yu, J., Wang, L., Walzem, R. W., Miller, E. G., Pike, L. M., Patil, B. S. *Journal of Agriculture and Food Chemistry* **2005**, 53, 2009-2014.
51. Raman, G. R., Cho, M., Brodbelt, J., Patil, B. S. *Phytochemical Analysis* **2005** *(In Press).*
52. Raman, G. R., Jayaprakasha, G. K., Cho, M., Brodbelt, J., Patil, B. S. *Separation and Purification Technology* **2005**, (*In Press*).
53. Raman, G., Jayaprakasha, G. K., Cho, M., Brodbelt, J. S., Patil, B. S. *Analytical Letters* **2004** 37, 3005-3016.
54. Ahmad, H., Tijerina, M. T. and Tobola, A. S. *Biochem. Biophys. Res. Commun.,* **1997,** *236*, 825-828.
55. Habig, W. H., Pabst, M. J., and Jakoby, W.B. *J. Biol. Chem.* **1974,** *249*, 7130-7139.
56. Benson, A. M., Hunkeler, M. J., and Talalay, P. *Proc. Natl. Acad. Sci. U.S.A.* **1980,** *77*, 5216-5220.

57. Bradford, M. M. *Anal. Biochem.* **1976,** *72*, 248-254.
58. Song, L, L., Kosmeder II, J, W., Lee, S. K., Gerhauser, C., Lantvit, D., Moon, R. C., Moriarty, R. M., Pezzuto, J. M. Cancer Res., **1999**, *59*, 578–585.
59. Tanaka T ; Makita H ; Kawabata K ; Mori H ; Kakumoto M ; Satoh K ; Hara A ; Sumida T ; Tanaka T ; Ogawa H *Carcinogenesis* **1997**, *18*, 957-965.
60. Tanaka T ; Makita H ; Ohnishi M ; Mori H ; Satoh K ; Hara A ; Sumida T ; Fukutani K ; Tanaka T ; Ogawa H *Cancer Res* **1997,** *57*, 246-252.
61. Rice-Evans, C. A., Miller, N. J., Paganga, G. *Free Rad. Biol. & Med.* **1996**, *20*, 933-956.
62. Depeint, F., Gee, J, M., Williamson, G., Johnson, I. T. *Proc. Nutr. Soc.* **2002,** *61,* 97-103.
63. Lam, L. K. T, Zheng, B. L. *Nutr Cancer* **1992,** *17*, 19-26,

Chapter 11

Prevention of Drug-Induced Programmed and Unprogrammed Cell Death by Citrus Flavonoids

Sidhartha D. Ray[1,2], Daniel Zinkovsky[1], Ellida Bulku[1], and Bhimanagouda S. Patil[2]

[1]Molecular Toxicology Laboratories, Division of Pharmaceutical Sciences, Arnold and Marie Schawrtz College of Pharmacy and Health Sciences, Long Island University, Brooklyn, NY 11201
[2]Vegetable and Fruit Improvement Center, Department of Horticultural Sciences, Mail Code 2119, Texas A&M University, College Station, TX 77843

Cell life and cell death in vivo are delicately balanced and linked processes dependent upon several "death" or "survival" signals from inside and outside the cell. These signals are regulated by several vital intracellular events associated with DNA, RNA, caspases, proteins, and ions. Drugs and other chemicals are known to threaten the stability of such key intracellular molecules by causing ion deregulation, oxidative stress, DNA fragmentation and activation of caspases. Citrus flavonoids, such as hesperidin (HES) and rutin (RUT), are known to specifically interfere with such deleterious pathways, minimize macromolecular perturbations, and exhibit their prolific antitoxic properties. This study was designed to investigate whether HES and RUT pre-exposures (1.25g/kg orally for 14 days) have the ability to counteract hepatotoxicity and nephrotoxicity induced by toxic doses of acetaminophen (APAP, 500 mg/kg, ip) and diclofenac (DCLF, 200 mg/kg, po) respectively *in vivo*. Additional objectives were to determine whether exposure to these flavonoids protect the liver and kidneys from oxidative stress and genomic DNA fragmentation, the prime players responsible for turning on various forms of cell death. Results indicate that HES and RUT pre-exposures showed dramatic prevention of hepato-

and nephrotoxicity by minimizing toxicant-induced oxidative stress and genomic DNA fragmentation which are instrumental in orchestrating apoptotic (programmed) and necrotic (unprogrammed) cell deaths in these organs *in vivo.*

Introduction

ROS (reactive oxygen species) and RNS (reactive nitrogen species) are formed during a variety of biochemical and pathological reactions. The steady-state formation of pro-oxidants (free radicals) is normally balanced by a similar rate of consumption of antioxidants. Oxidative stress results from an imbalance between formation and neutralization of pro-oxidants. Various metabolic and pathologic processes disrupt this balance by increasing the formation of free radicals in proportion to the available antioxidants (thus, oxidative stress). Examples of increased free radical formation are immune cell activation, inflammation, ischemia, microbial infection, cancer and CYP450 mediated drug metabolism. Metabolism of xenobiotics usually leads to the formation of biological reactive intermediates (BRIs). Free radical formation and the effect of these reactive molecules on cell function are collectively called "oxidative stress." These free radicals are highly reactive, unstable molecules that have an unpaired electron in their outer shell, and they have the intrinsic ability to interact and destroy cellular micro and macromolecules, such as DNA, RNA, proteins, lipids and carbonyls [1, 2]. These reactions between cellular components and free radicals can ultimately result in genomic instability (DNA fragmentation), mitochondrial dysfunction (cytochrome c release and disruption of electron transport chain), cell membrane damage (lipid peroxidation) and eventually cell death (apoptosis, necrosis or both). Sophisticated in vitro and in vivo experiments have now shown that a number of citrus flavonoids have the ability to interrupt specialized biochemical and molecular pathways and modulate apoptogenic and necrogenic responses of a wide variety of drugs and chemicals [3 – 9].

Medicinal plants and a range of phytochemicals have been used for centuries to inhibit hepatic and nephrotic dysfunctions emanating from infectous agents, intentional or accidental exposure to toxic substances and a multitude of physiological disturbances. Although the vast majority of information concerning their use was considered anecdotal, a recent upsurge in credible mechanistic research using phytochemicals as tools has changed the notion dramatically. Well-designed in vivo and in vitro studies have lent credence to the concept that some phytochemicals may delay, prevent, or at least, ameliorate hepatic and nephrotic dysfunctions arising from drug-induced toxicity. The present study focused on the potential for some of the key citrus flavonoids, HES and RUT, to favorably influence the course of acute liver and kidney injuries induced in mice by the well-known analgesic acetaminophen and a non-steroidal anti-inflammatory drug (NSAID), diclofenac. This study employed reliable and sensitive serum markers for the determination of hepatotoxicity (alanine aminotransferase activity) and nephrotoxicity (blood urea nitrogen). Tissue histopathology was used to assess organ injuries, the extent of their protection and involvement of various forms of cell deaths (apoptosis, necrosis and apocrosis). Toxicant-induced cell injury and cell death were indirectly evaluated by the levels of oxidative stress (lipid peroxidation) and changes (both quantitative and qualitative) in the integrity of the genomic DNA. Overall, results showed that oral ingestion of HES or RUT (1.25g/kg) are extremely effective in lessening drug-induced hepato- and nephrotoxicity produced by APAP and DCLF in an animal model.

Materials & Methods

Animals, Chemicals, and Diets.

Male ICR mice (25–35 g) were obtained from Harlan Sprague-Dawley, Inc., Indianapolis, IN, USA. Animals were housed in an environment of controlled temperature, humidity, 12h light/dark cycle and given free access to lab chow. APAP, DCLF, HES and RUT were purchased from Sigma Chemical Co. (St. Louis, MO, USA). All chemicals were analytical/ACS grade or higher and used without purification. All animal procedures received prior approval by the Institutional Animal Care and Use Committee and met or exceeded current local, state, and federal regulations.

Experimental Procedure.

Acetaminophen (ip), diclofenac (po), HES (po) and RUT (po) were dissolved in normal saline (isotonic, pH adjusted to 7.4) and were administered at the doses of 500, 200, 1250, and 1250 mg/kg body weight, respectively. Flavonoids were administered (orally gavaged; in a total volume of 0.5 ml) daily for 14 days prior to drug exposures. On day-14 two hours after the flavonoid exposure, toxicants were administered. All the animals were sacrificed 24 h later and the blood and the tissues (kidneys and liver) were collected for biochemical and morphological analyses. For histopathology, portions of fresh livers and kidneys, with discernable visible damage, were sectioned and preserved in 10% phosphate-buffered formalin. The remaining portions of the tissues were collected in liquid N_2 and preserved at -70°C until analysis for other parameters. For oxidative stress [10] and DNA damage [11], portions of frozen tissues were homogenized and used for the assays.

Determination of Hepatotoxicity and Nephrotoxicity

The extent of hepatotoxicity was inferred from the increases in serum alanine aminotransferase [EC 2.6.1.2] activity (ALT:U/L) and histopathology. The final concentrations of toxicants and flavonoids employed in this investigation were based on several prior pilot experiments. Also, it was an important goal to employ non-hepatotoxic and nephrotoxic doses of flavonoid modulators, and severely hepato- and nephrotoxic doses of acetaminophen and diclofenac, which would produce appreciable organ injury in the absence of total organ failure. Serum ALT activity was determined using a sigma kit (# 59-UV) based on the method of Wroblewski and LaDue [12], and BUN (blood urea nitrogen) levels were determined using a sigma kit (#67-UV) based on the methods of Talke and Schubert [13].

Estimation of lipid peroxidation

The lipid peroxidation (induced by oxidative stress) was monitored by measuring thiobarbituric acid reactive substances using malondialdehyde (MDA) as standard. The extent of drug-induced lipid peroxidation in the liver and kidneys was inferred from the increase in MDA production based on the methods of Ray and Fariss [14] and Ray et al. [10]. Variously treated tissue homogenates were used to determine concentrations of MDA. The values are expressed as nmol MDA/g liver and presented in the graphs as % control changes.

Quantitative Apoptotic DNA fragmentation assay

Portions of variously treated tissues were taken (evidence of damage) and DNA damage was quantified in each sample individually [1; 15]. To measure tissue DNA fragmentation by spectrophotometry, a portion of the frozen tissue was homogenized in chilled lysis buffer (pH 8.0). Homogenates were then centrifuged at 27,000xg for 20 min to separate intact chromatin in the pellet from fragmented/damaged DNA in the supernatant. Pellets and supernatants were treated with perchloric acid, and boiled at 90°C for 15 min, and centrifuged at 1500xg for 10 min to coprecipitate protein along with other debris. Resulting supernatants were then treated with Burton's diphenylamine reagent for 16–20 h at room temperature in the dark [16]. DNA fragmentation in samples [(fragmented DNA in supernatant)/(fragmented DNA in supernatant + intact DNA in pellet)] were expressed as a percentage of total DNA appearing in the supernatant fraction. DNA fragmentation in samples were expressed as percentage of total DNA appearing in the supernatant fraction. Control tissues produced 4-8% fragmented DNA (which was treated as 100%).

Agarose gel-electrophoresis to probe caspase-activated DNA fragmentation

Liver and kidney samples collected in liquid N_2, and stored at -70°C were used in this assay. DNA was extracted from the tissues to assess Ca^{2+}-activated, endonuclease (or caspase-activated DNAse)-dependent, ladderlike DNA fragmentation based on the modified method of Ray et al.,[17]. DNA (10 μg/lane) laddering was determined by constant voltage mode electrophoresis (60 V, Large Submarine from Hoeffer Instruments, San Francisco, CA, USA) on a 1.2% agarose gel containing 0.4 μg/ml ethidium bromide. A λDNA BstE II-digest served as a molecular weight size standard. Gels were illuminated with 300 nm UV light and a photographic record was made with instant Polaroid film (#667).

Data analysis and statistics

Results are presented as mean $\pm$ SEM (standard error of means) unless otherwise indicated. Data were compared by ANOVA followed by Schiffs' 'F' test.

Results

Prevention of APAP-induced hepatotoxicity and DCLF-induced nephrotoxicity by HES and RUT pre-exposures

Serum ALT and BUN were used as indexes of the degree of liver and kidney injuries (Figs. 1 & 2). Figure 1 shows the effects of APAP, HES and RUT alone, and combinations of APAP with HES and RUT on serum ALT 24 h following exposure. Flavonoids alone failed to produce liver injury to any extent. The degree of liver injury by a 500 mg/kg dose of APAP alone was reflected as a sharp increase in serum ALT activity that exceeded the control (20±4 U/l) by greater than 879-fold. Exposure to the flavonoids prior to APAP considerably reduced the liver injury and there was a near complete protection as reflected in ALT levels (HES+APAP: 180 U/L and RUT+APAP: 220 U/L). Grossly, centrilobular areas were most severely affected by a 500 mg/kg dose of APAP and both the flavonoids significantly reduced the impact of the drug in all the areas of the liver. Likewise, DCLF caused severe nephrotoxicity, which was very effectively prevented by both HES and RUT pre-exposures (Figure 2). DCLF-alone caused a 7-fold increase in BUN which was reduced to less than 3-fold due to flavonoid pre-exposure.

Modulation of APAP and DCLF-induced liver and kidney lipid peroxidation and its reversal by HES and RUT

To gain further insight into the mechanism of action of these flavonoids, lipid peroxidation, which is predominantly a marker of oxidative stress was evaluated in both these organs. APAP and DCLF both are well known ROS producers, and ROS in turn produces MDA accumulation via lipid peroxidation. These effects are presented in Fig. 3 and 4. Lipid peroxidation was also used as an indirect marker of organ injury. APAP and DCLF, when administered individually caused massive oxidative stress resulting in appreciable lipid peroxidation (accumulation of TBARS). A powerful inhibition in lipoperoxidative effects, essentially nullifying the drug-induced increase in lipid peroxidation and minimizing MDA accumulation in both tissues was found when APAP and DCLF were administered to HES and RUT treated animals. The values of MDA levels in organs exposed to HES in combination with either APAP or DCLF, and RUT in combination with APAP and DCLF, were nearly identical to vehicle or flavonoid-alone-exposed organs.

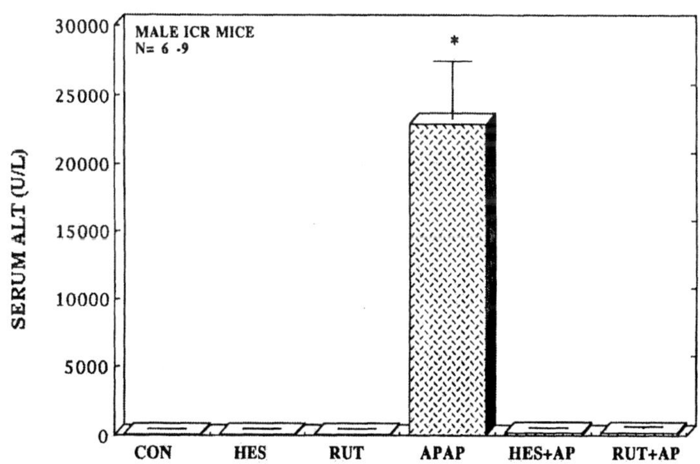

Figure 1. Protection of acetaminophen-induced liver injury by HES and RUT pre-exposures.

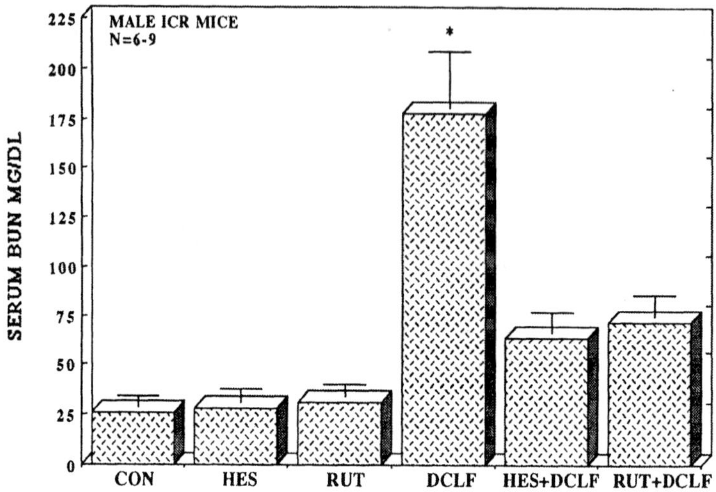

Figure 2. Protection of diclofenac-induced kidney injury by HES and RUT pre-exposures.

Reversal of APAP and DCLF-induced depletion of total glutathione levels in the liver and kidneys by HES and RUT

Besides lipid peroxidation, antioxidative properties of citrus flavonoids were also scrutinized by monitoring changes in the total glutathione level in these organs. Organotoxic doses of APAP (Figure 5) and DCLF (Figure 6) markedly decreased the levels of total glutathione (oxidized plus reduced) in both the liver and kidneys demonstrating massive oxidative stress. HES and RUT exposures for 14 days did not produce any change in the levels of total glutathione either in the liver or kidneys (Control: 8.1 μmol/g liver). The decrease in glutathione was more pronounced in the liver (46% lower than control) due to APAP exposure compared to DCLF-induced decrease in kidneys (only 26% lower than control). Exposure to HES or RUT prior to the toxicant exposure significantly ameliorated drug-induced depletion of total GSH in both liver and kidneys which may suggest neutralization of ROS and/or BRIs produced during drug metabolism. Both HES and RUT were equally effective in counteracting oxidative effects produced by these drugs.

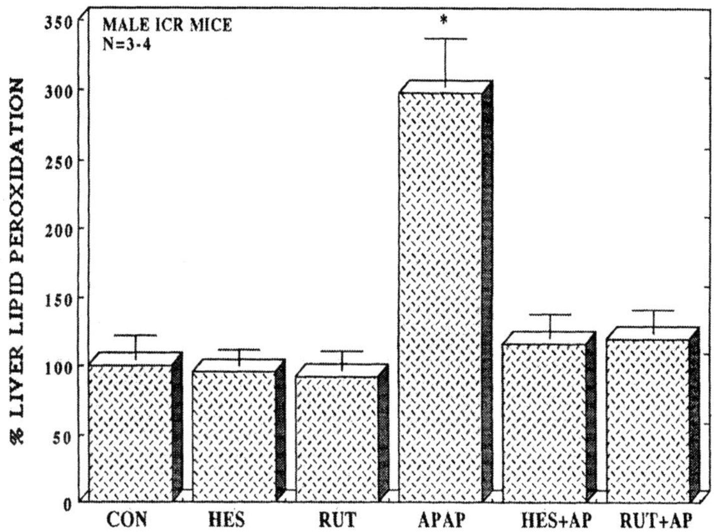

Figure 3. Prevention of acetaminophen-induced oxidative stress in the liver by HES and RUT pre-exposures.

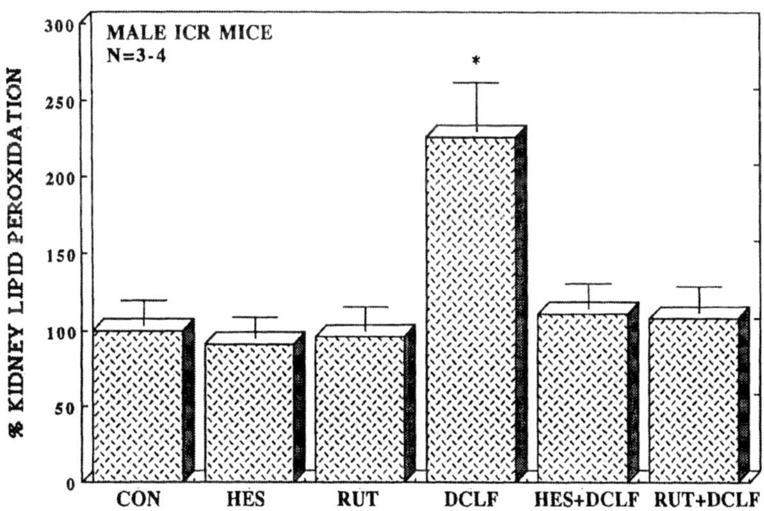

Figure 4. Prevention of diclofenac-induced oxidative stress in the kidney by HES and RUT pre-exposures.

HES and RUT mediated protection of genomic integrity and prevention of DNA fragmentation culminated by APAP and DCLF-induced organ injury

Quantitative changes in the integrity of the genomic DNA during exposure to organotoxic doses of APAP and DCLF are shown in Figures 7 and 8. Quantitative evaluation of chromatin damage in the form of DNA fragmentation based on a density-dependent sedimentation assay is presented in these figures. Orderly fragmentation of DNA in the form of a ladder due to endonucleolytic attack is reportedly considered as an apoptosis-related event, whereas the quantitative assay reliably predicts the extent of fragmented and intact DNA. DNA fragmentation is considered one of the later steps in apoptotic program, which involves caspase-activated DNAse-dependent degradation of higher order chromatin structure into 50 to 300 kb and subsequently into 200 bp length. Both the toxicants caused massive DNA fragmentation at 24 h (APAP: 298% and DCLF: 238%), whereas both HES and RUT when administered alone failed to alter the genomic structure to any extent. Interestingly, however, DNA fragmentation levels were near normal levels in the HES+APAP/DCLF and RUT+APAP/DCLF exposed animals. Overall, the pattern of quantitative spectrophotometric DNA fragmentation mirrored the hepatotoxicity and nephrotoxicity profiles discussed in Figures 1 and 2 and patterns of oxidative stress described in Figures 3-6.

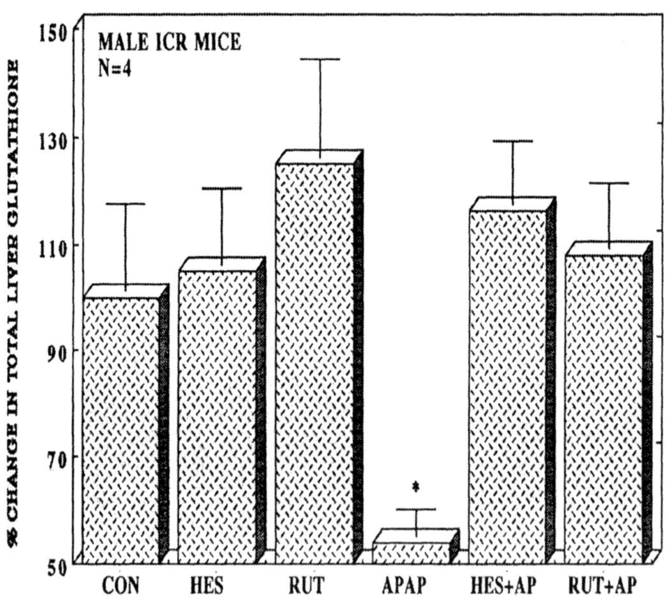

Figure 5. Acetaminophen-induced oxidative stress in the liver as determined indirectly by total tissue glutathione concentrations.

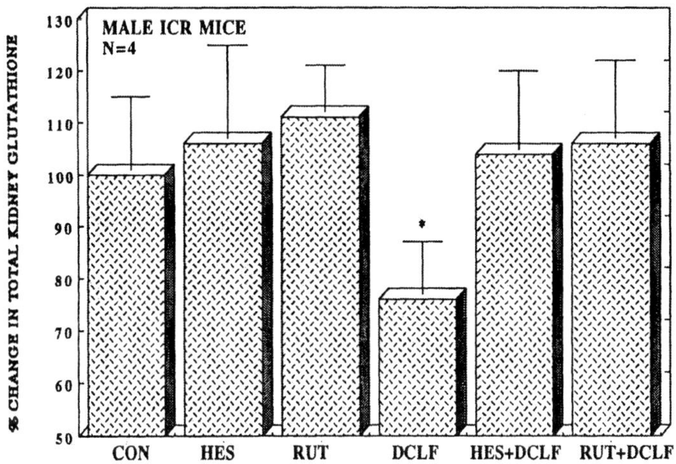

Figure 6. Diclofenac-induced oxidative stress in the kidney as determined indirectly by total tissue glutathione concentration.

Inhibition of caspase-activated-DNAse activity (endonuclease activation) and prevention of genomic destruction in the liver and kidneys by HES and RUT during hepatotoxicity induced by APAP and nephrotoxicity induced by DCLF

Apoptotic-type DNA laddering which is predominantly dependent on caspase-activated-DNAse (Ca^{2+}-Mg^{2+}-endonuclease) activity was evaluated by agarose gel electrophoresis. The data from these experiments examining qualitative DNA damage are shown in Fig. 9 (A and B). Similar to the spectrophotometric assay, the electrophoretogram generated by gel electrophoresis shows that APAP and DCLF overdose culminated a dramatic orderly degradation of liver and kidney DNA and a typical ladder of DNA fragments consisting of multiple repetitive bands diagnostic of caspase-activated-DNAse activity (see lane 5 in both panels A and B). DNA isolated from the control, HES and RUT alone groups (lanes 1 through 3) remained totally intact and devoid of any fragmentation. All the DNA remained confined in the well. Using the 1-kb DNA ladder as a marker size (lane 4), the fragmentation pattern observed in APAP and DCLF alone exposed tissues presumably represents 200-bp multiples of DNA. The toxicant-induced loss of large molecular weight DNA (see fluorescence intensities in the lane 5 in both panels) were readily apparent on the gels. The lanes 6 and 7 in both panels show the degree of prevention by the flavonoids. As is evident on the gels, both HES and RUT were superbly effective in inhibiting CAD-activity and preventing the genomic disintegration. In fact, lanes 1 to 3 are nearly identical to lanes 6 and 7 mirroring the intactness of the DNA. The overall pattern of DNA fragmentation and a clear-cut ladder suggested presumable involvement of massive cell death via apoptosis, and the absence of a ladder in HES+APAP/DCLF and RUT+APAP/DCLF tissues indicated minimization of cell death.

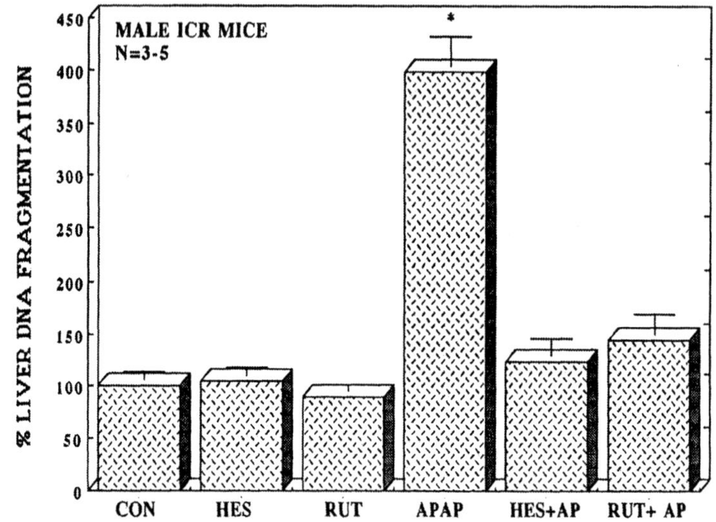

Figure 7. Effects of citrus flavonoids on acetaminophen-induced genomic DNA fragmentation in the liver.

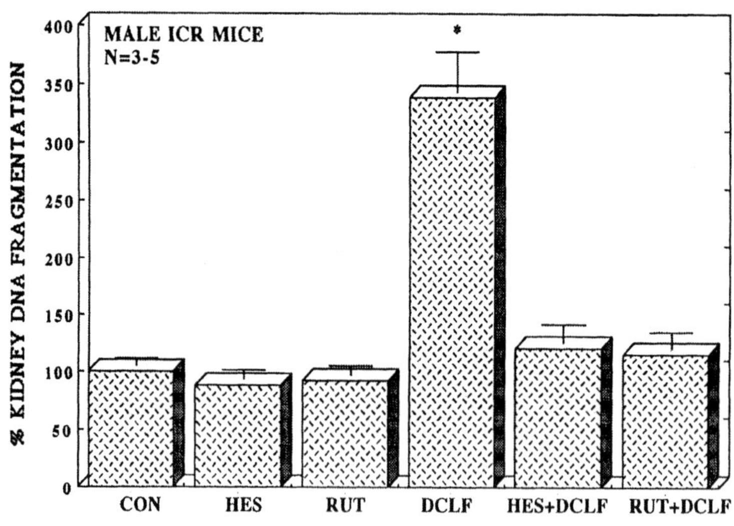

Figure 8. Effects of citrus flavonoids on diclofenac-induced genomic DNA fragmentation in the kidney.

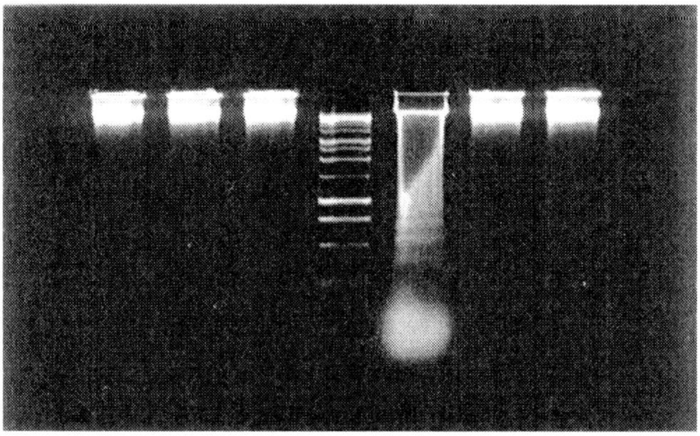

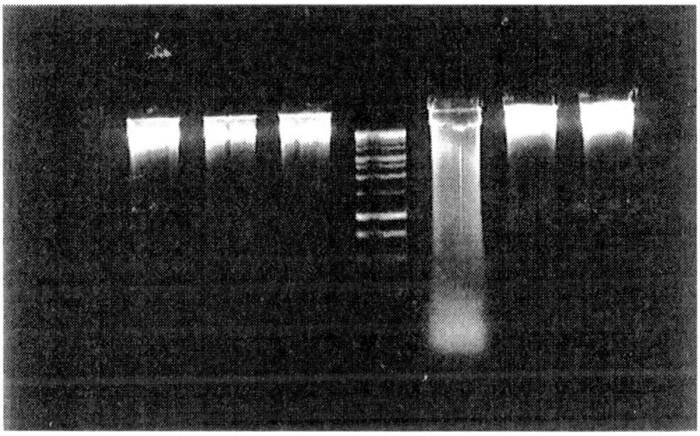

Figure 9A (Top). Effects of citrus flavonoids on acetaminophen-induced endonuclease-mediated genomic DNA fragmentation in the liver. Figure 9B (Bottom). Effects of citrus flavonoids on diclofenac-induced endonuclease-mediated genomic DNA fragmentation in the kidney (see legends for details).

Discussion

Polyphenols are among the most abundant phytochemicals in human food items and of these, flavonoids are probably the most studied. Although the last decade has generated a plethora of research papers in the field of phytochemicals, the mechanisms of actions of flavonoids in cellular processes remain unclear. Most scientists agree that vitamins C and E, beta-carotene, and selenium play a role in the prevention of various degenerative diseases, yet new research indicates that there may be many other antioxidants that are also important for maintaining good health. Interestingly, antioxidants can either function independently or in a concerted fashion. In a series of previous publications, we have shown that relatively low concentrations of flavonoids have the ability to counteract cytotoxic properties of a variety of xenobiotics. For example, an admixture of grape seed proanthocyanidins has the ability to counteract hepatotoxic properties of acetaminophen [1], nephrotoxic properties of $CdCl_2$ [18], splenotoxic properties of dimethylnitrosamine [19], pneumotoxic properties of amiodarone, and cardiotoxic properties of doxorubicin [19]. Additionally, in a long-term exposure study, we have recently shown that continuous grape seed proanthocyanidin exposure considerably reduces hepatocarcinogenic properties of dimethylnitrosamine [20]. These diverse antitoxic and anticarcinogenic properties may have been due to a variety of reasons: (i) minimizing the effects of pro-oxidants by acting as potent antioxidants, (ii) increasing the synthesis of glutathione via activation of glutathione synthase, (iii) reducing drug metabolism by influencing specific CYP450 isozymes, (iv) reducing the CAD activity by specifically interfering with CAD-ICAD complex and caspase-3 processing, (v) promoting DNA repair by turning on PARP activity, (vi) upregulating expression of antiapoptotic genes and down -regulating pro-apoptotic genes and finally, (vii) by maintaining mitochondrial vitality (electron transport chain activity, optimal ATP production and minimizing cytochrome c release). Therefore, it is difficult to pinpoint the exact loci of interactions between HES and RUT with APAP and DCLF. Several investigations have already shown antoxidative and anti-DNA damaging properties of these two flavonoids [5, 7, 21, 22, 23].

Following exposure to toxic doses, hepatocytes metabolize APAP to its reactive BRI, N-acetyl-p-benzoquinoneimine (NAPQI). When NAPQI accumulation overwhelms the glutathione, antioxidants drop and protective mechanisms falter in the cells, excess NAPQI interacts with vital intracellular macromolecules such as cell membrane lipids, essential cytosolic enzymes and DNA, leading to oxidative damage. In this study, liver enzyme leakage, accumulation of MDA, depletion of glutathione and DNA fragmentation signify APAP-induced lipid peroxidation, oxidative stress and DNA damage, respectively. Each of these effects can lead to cell death. Both the flavonoids, HES and RUT, considerably attenuate all the deleterious effects induced by APAP-and minimized cell death (Figures 1, 3, 5, 7, 9A). Whether HES and RUT dealt with these events independently or in a concerted manner is not known.

Similarly, DCLF (Voltaren) is a well-known prescription NSAID, which includes seven others, etodolac (Lodine), indomethacin (Indocin), ketorolac (Toradol), nabumetone (Relafen), sulindac (Clinoril), and tolmetin (Tolectin). DCLF is the most common NSAID used to reduce inflammation and pain associated with arthritis and other conditions, such as osteoarthritis, rheumatoid arthritis, and ankylosing spondylitis. DCLF is known to bind exclusively to plasma albumin. There is considerable interest in the toxicity of DCLF because of its clinical use and for the study of the mechanisms of nephrotoxicity. Most common toxic effects of DCLF are usually gastrointestinal complications, hematotoxicity, renal dysfunction, and hypersensitivity reactions. Bioactivation of DCLF can cause a rare but potentially severe liver injury, which may be due to the formation of reactive metabolites. CYP450-mediated metabolism of DCLF leads to the formation of 5′-hydroxydiclofenac and 4′-hydroxydiclofenac. In humans, cytochrome P450s, 2C9, and 3A4 all metabolize DCLF, although only P450 2C9 is capable of producing benzoquinoneimine. The *p*-benzoquinoneimine derivative of 5′-hydroxydiclofenac has been a prime suspect in causing cell injury due to its ability to covalently bind to macromolecules in situations where intracellular levels of NADH, NADPH, GSH, and other reducing agents are very low. Although the true scenario behind initiation of liver injury remains unknown, many clinical studies reveal that a variety of immune and nonimmune mechanisms contribute towards development of toxicity. Covalently bound protein adducts of DCLF have been detected in hepatic tissues of mice and rats, as well as human hepatocytes, and DCLF is eliminated following conjugation by sulfate and glucuronic acid. Excretion of conjugates and accumulation of conjugates have been correlated to renal function and end-stage renal disease, respectively. Usually after detoxification pathways are impaired, and if metabolite(s) is/are formed in excessive amounts, they can cause cell injury leading to cell death. Although concrete evidence is lacking, it is quite possible that cytochrome P450-mediated DCLF metabolism involves production of both ROS and RNS. This study also investigated the potential involvement of these free radicals and their after-effects during DCLF-induced nephrotoxicity in vivo. DCLF-induced kidney lipid peroxidation and a reduction in total glutathione strongly suggested participation of massive oxidative stress (Figures 4 & 6). Lack of clearance of serum urea nitrogen supported the foregoing observations.

Under oxidative conditions, the superoxide anion is the first ROS formed, which if not scavenged, ultimately leads to a highly reactive species, the hydroxyl radical, which attacks nucleic acid, protein and lipid-rich membranes causing severe cell damage. APAP's and DCLF's potential to generate this ROS is well documented. In this regard, the most studied markers of oxidative damage are lipid peroxidation [malondialdehyde (MDA) formation] and DNA damage [2, 15]. The efficacy of HES and RUT to thwart APAP- and DCLF-induced lipid peroxidation were nearly identical in this investigation. This effect may have unraveled several important properties of HES and RUT: (i) ability of these flavonoids to percolate and discern an appreciable effect in both tissues (liver and kidney) despite their tremendous size difference, (ii) ability to scavenge a variety of BRIs (NAPQI, 4'OH-DCLF and 5'OH-DCLF), (iii) ability to interfere with different drug metabolizing enzymes (2E1, 3A4, 2C9) and lastly, (iv) the capacity to communicate with every intracellular compartment despite their remarkable structural differences. These observations were fascinating.

The DNA fragmentation or DNA-laddering observed in this study is a qualitative picture of both mitochondrial (which is only 4%) and nuclear DNA fragmentation combined. The presence of a ladder instead of a smear in APAP (Figure 9A) and DCLF (Figure 9B) treated tissues is suggestive of massive induction of apoptotic death. The absence or abolition of a genomic ladder is also a clear-cut indication of absence of various forms of cell death, particularly apopotic type. In this experimental set up, HES and RUT both very effectively protected the genomic integrity in the liver and kidneys after the drug exposure. Nagata and his collaborators [24], in an elegant series of investigations, have shown that the endonuclease, which is responsible for inducing DNA ladder, is a caspase-activated DNAse (CAD). This enzyme pre-exists in living cells as an inactive complex with an inhibitory subunit, dubbed ICAD. Activation of CAD occurs by means of caspase-3-mediated cleavage of the inhibitory subunit, resulting in the release and activation of the catalytic subunit. Although, final activation of CAD may be or may not be Ca^{2+}-dependent, experiments are in progress in our laboratories to unravel APAP's and DCLF's intervening role at such critical regulatory steps. Masking the activation of CAD-ICAD complex by switching the redox balance of the cell (and/or inhibiting caspase-3) may have been another novel pathway by which HES and RUT prevented attack on the genomic DNA. This observation is consistent with some of our earlier findings [1], where a strong antiendonucelolytic property of a polyphenolic flavonoid was demonstrated [1].

The most important endogenous antioxidant defense systems are composed of the thiol-containing tripeptide glutathione and small thiol-containing proteins such as thioredoxin, glutaredoxin, and peroxiredoxin. Of these, glutathione is found at millimolar concentrations in most cells and it is the major contributor to the redox state of the cell. Glutathione exists in cells in both a reduced form (GSH) and an oxidized form (GSSG); it may also be covalently bound to proteins through a process called glutathionylation. The ratio of GSH to GSSG is determined by the overall redox state of the cell. Glutathione is synthesized enzymatically by γ-glutamylcysteine synthetase (γGCS) and glutathione synthetase, with the former being the rate-limiting enzyme. One important task for cellular glutathione is to scavenge free radicals and peroxides produced during normal cellular respiration, which would otherwise oxidize proteins, lipids, and nucleic acids. Mechanisms operating to counteract oxidative damage involve transactivation of genes encoding enzymes that participate in glutathione metabolism and synthesis. Typically, these enzymes belong to the phase I and II families of detoxification genes. Possible involvement of HES and RUT in these events can not be ruled out. Substantial depletion of glutathione by the drugs and an absence of its depletion in HES and RUT treated tissues suggested profound protective ability of these flavonoids. The antioxidant activity of the flavonoids varies considerably among the different backbone structures and functional groups. Some of the flavonoids have even proven to be more potent than α-tocopherol/ascorbic acid in scavenging ROS. The difference in ROS scavenging between the flavonoids can be accounted for by the variation in the number and kind of functional groups present. This study did not reveal any such difference between HES and RUT in minimizing oxidative stress or events linked to oxidative stress.

Collectively, these data suggest that citrus flavonoids, HES and RUT possess potent antioxidative and antitoxic properties. Both these flavonoids have the ability to protect the integrity of the genome against diverse molecular entities. By vitue of these properties, HES and RUT prevent all forms of cell death.

References

1. Ray, S. D.; Kumar, M. A.; Bagchi, D. *Arch Biochem Biophys.* **1999,** *369*, 42-58.
2. Ray, S. D.; Lam, T. S.; Rotollo, J. A.; Phadke, S.; Patel, C.; Dontabhaktuni, A. et al. *Biofactors* **2004,** *21(1-)4,* 223-232.
3. Yang, K.; Lamprecht, S. A.; Liu, Y.; Shinozaki, H,; Fan, K.; Leung, D.; Newmark, H.; Steele, V. E,; Kelloff, G. J.; Lipkin, M. *Carcinogenesis.* **2000,** *21(9),* 1655-1660.
4. Chen, Y.C.; Shen, S.C.; Lin, H.Y. *Biochem. Pharmacol.* **2003**, *66*, 1139-1150.
5. Choi, Y. J.; Kang, J. S.; Park, J. H.; Lee, Y. J.; Choi, J. S.; Kang, Y. H.; *J Nutr.* **2003,** *133(4),* 985-991.
6. Kwon, Y. K.; Jun, J. M.; Shin, S. W.; Cho, J.W.; Suh, S. I.; *Int J Oncol* .**2005,** *26(6)*, 1597-1603.
7. Tirkey, N.; Pilkhwal, S.; Kuhad, A.; Chopra, K.; *BMC Pharmacol.* **2005,** *5(1)*, 2-8.
8. Miller, N. J.; Rice-Evans, C. A. *Food Chem.* **1997,** *60,* 331–337, 1997.
9. Volate, S. R.; Davenport, D. M.; Muga, S. J.; Wargovich, M. J. *Carcinogenesis*. **2005**, *26(8)*, 1450-6.
10. Ray, S.D.; Balasubramanian, G.; Bagchi, D.; Reddy, C.S. *Free Radic. Biol. Med.* **2001**, *31*, 277-291.
11. Ray, S. D.; Kamendulis, L. M.; Gurule, M. W.; Yorkin, R. D.; Corcoran, G. B. *FASEB J.* **1993,** *7(5)*, 453-463.
12. Wroblewski, F. Ladue, J. S. *Proc Soc Exp Biol Med.* **1956,** *91(4)*, 569-571.
13. Talke, H.; Schubert, G. E. *Klin Wochenschr*. **1965,** *43*, 174-175.
14. Ray, S. D.; Fariss, M. W. *Arch Biochem Biophys.* **1994,** *311(1)*, 180-190.
15. Hickey, E. J.; Raje, R. R.; Reid, V. E.; Gross, S. M.; Ray, S. D. *Free Radic Biol Med.* **2001,** *31(2)*, 139-152.
16. Burton, K. *Biochem J.* **1956,** *62(2)*, 315-323.
17. Ray, S. D.; Mumaw, V. R.; Raje, R. R.; Fariss, M. W. *J Pharmacol Exp Ther*. **1996,** *279(3)*, 1470-1483.
18. Ray, S. D.; Patel, D.; Wong, V.; Bagchi, D. *Res Commun Mol Pathol Pharmacol.* **2000,** *107(1-2)*, 137-166.

19. Ray, S. D.; Wong, V.; Rinkovsky, A.; Bagchi, M.; Raje, R. R.; Bagchi, D. *Res Commun Mol Pathol Pharmacol.* **2000,** *107(1-2)*, 105-128.
20. Ray, S. D.; Parikh, H.; Bagchi, D. *Mutation Res.* **2005,** (In Press).
21. Webster, R. P.; Gawde, M. D.; Bhattacharya, R. K. *Cancer Lett.* **1996,** *109(1-2)*, 185-191.
22. Yoshikawa, Y.; Suzuki, M.; Yamada, N.; Yoshikawa, K. *FEBS Lett.* **2004,** *566(1-3)*, 39-42.
23. Matsuda, H.; Wang, T.; Managi, H.; Yoshikawa, M. *Bioorg Med Chem.* **2003,** *11(24)*, 5317-5323.
24. Sakahira, H.; Enari, M.; Nagata, S. *Nature.* **1998** 391(6662), **96-99**.

Chapter 12

Antioxidant Effects of Citrus Flavonoid Consumption

John R. Burgess and Juan E. Andrade

Department of Foods and Nutrition, Purdue University, West Lafayette, IN 47907–2059

Grapefruit juice is a rich source of nutrients and citrus flavonoids which are proposed to provide important health benefits. Many flavonoids are good antioxidants *in vitro* and this property is one that is hypothesized to mediate their biological effects *in vivo*. In two studies we tested the effects of citrus flavanones and grapefruit juice on lipid oxidation and the antioxidant defense system *in vivo*. The first tested the dose-response effect of naringenin consumption in rats adequate or deficient in vitamin E and selenium on growth and multiple measures of antioxidant defense, lipid oxidation and oxidative stress. The second was a human intervention trial of three months in duration testing the effects of regular consumption of grapefruit juice on antioxidant nutrient status and oxidative stress in young adult women. No evidence of antioxidant or pro-oxidant activity was observed, however, in rats inhibition of adipose accumulation was observed.

Our work has focused on understanding adaptations to oxidative stress involving the endogenous antioxidant defense system and the potential role of non-nutrient phytochemicals in modulating this system. The results of two studies testing the effect of citrus phytochemicals on this system will be presented. This chapter will include: i) a brief summary of the multifaceted antioxidant defense system with a focus on the enzyme and antioxidants of interest to our lab, ii) a discussion of the evidence that flavonoids are good antioxidants *in vitro,* iii) a reminder of the extensive metabolism of phytochemicals in small intestine and liver, iv) a summary of the results of our rat feeding study, v) followed by a discussion of the results of the intervention study that we conducted with grapefruit juice in humans. The chapter will conclude with thoughts on lessons learned for future research.

The multifaceted endogenous antioxidant defense system in mammals includes primary antioxidants that help break the chain reaction initiated with the formation of reactive oxygen species (ROS) (*1*). These include both dietary antioxidants as well as endogenously synthesized compounds. Secondary antioxidants include enzymes which detoxify ROS and those that help support the function of the primary antioxidants. The defense system also includes enzyme systems that repair the damage caused by excessive ROS such as lipases like phospholipase (PL) A_2 which catalyzes the removal of oxidized lipids from the membrane, as well as regenerating systems that form replacement molecules. Finally, a robust antioxidant defense system which is found in healthy organisms exhibits the ability to adapt, up-regulate key components of its system to protect itself in the face of greater oxidative stress.

Figure 1 illustrates the multifaceted nature of the antioxidant defense system in the plasma membrane. The interaction of a ROS with polyunsaturated fatty acids (PUFA) in the membrance can lead to the initiation of lipid peroxidation forming a lipid peroxyl radical esterified in the membrane (LOO·). If not removed this chemical species can propagate the chain reaction, but alternatively it can be reduced by an electron supplied by tocopherol or ubiquinol. Regeneration of these fat-soluble antioxidants can take place via the action of quinone reductases (QR) or ascorbate (ASC). The resulting lipid hydroperoxide can be released from the phosholipid membrane via PLA_2, and after diffusing to the soluble portion of the cell be reduced by peroxidases utilizing reducing equivalents supplied by glutathione (GSH). Coupled interactions with GSH-reductase and glucose-6-P dehydrogenase (G6PDH) help maintain a constant supply of electrons from NADPH to fully support the system (*2,3*).

We use a dietary deficiency of vitamin E and selenium in rats as a model to study the components of this system which will upregulate to defend the cells of the animals from oxidative stress. In this model we have seen significant enhancements in QR, G6PDH, PLA_2 as well as ASC and GSH synthesis (*3-5*).

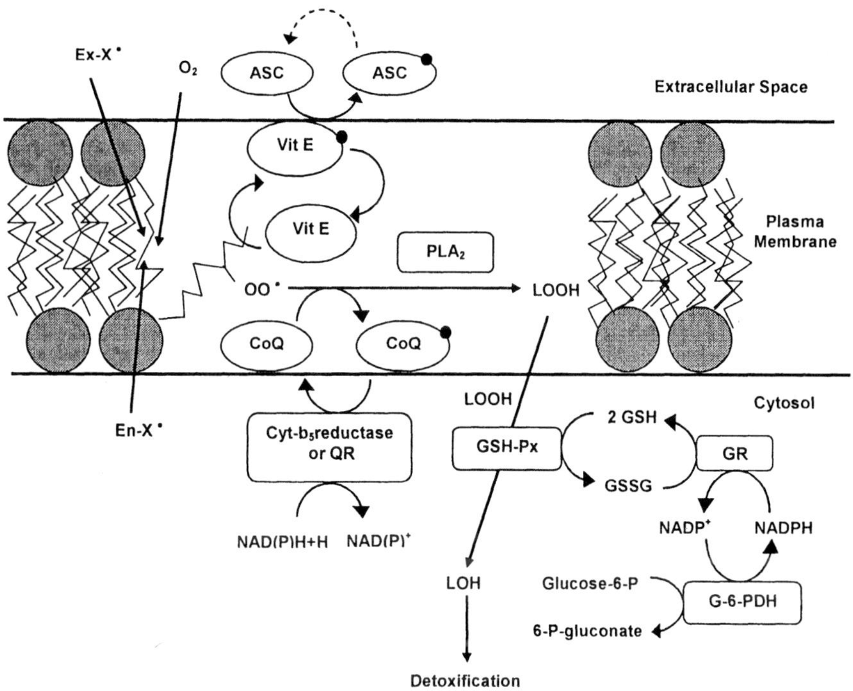

Figure 1. The multifaceted endogenous antioxidant defense system. Abbreviations: radical form (•), endogenous free radical (En-X•), exogenous free radical (Ex-X•), ascorbate (ASC), vitamin E (vit E), coenzyme Q (CoQ), phospholipases A_2 (PLA_2), fatty acid hydroperoxide (LOOH), cytochrome b_5 reductase (Cyt b_5 reductase) quinone reductase (QR), glutathione peroxidase (GSH-Px), fatty acid alcohol (LOH), glutathione (GSH), glutathione disulfide (GSSG), glutathione reductase (GR), glucose-6-phosphate dehydrogenase (G-6-PDH), 6-phospho-gluconate (6-P-gluconate), glucose-6-phosphate (Glucose-6-P), nicotinamide adenine dinucleotide (NAD), nicotinamide adenine dinucleotide phosphate (NADP).

A key question for understanding the potential health benefits of non-nutrients substances in foods is what effects do they have on the multifaceted endogenous antioxidant defense system? We know that fruit and vegetable intake is associated with lower incidence of chronic disease, that the essential nutrients in these fruit and vegetables can't account for all of the benefits observed, that flavonoids are proposed to contribute to these beneficial effects (*6*), and that these natural compounds in plants are good antioxidants in the test tube. The proposed antioxidant mechanisms for flavonoids are: peroxyl radical scavenging, chelation of transition metals, and enhancements of the endogenous antioxidant defense system (*7*). The first two mechanisms have been shown to occur *in vitro* and are hypothesized to occur *in vivo*. The third mechanism is proposed to occur *in vivo* (*8*).

As outlined by Williams et al. (*9*), and using quercetin, the most abundant flavonoid in foods, as a model, the structural characteristics that confer the strongest antioxidant properties for flavonoids *in vitro* are: viscinal diol on the B-ring, 2,3-unsaturation on the C ring, as well as the 4-oxo group (Figure 2). To illustrate this point Table 1 shows the results of a total peroxyl radical antioxidant potential (TRAP) assay represented in lag time in which equimolar concentrations of a variety of flavonoids were evaluated *in vitro*. The assay utilizes the azo-dye initiator AAPH and the chemical dye dichloroflourescein diacetate as the visualization agent (*10*). Note Trolox, a water-soluble form of vitamin E used as a standard in these types of assays- illustrates a lag time of about 500 seconds. Epigallocatechin gallate (EGCG) which contains an additional hydroxyl group on the B-ring as well as a gallic acid moiety is a stronger antioxidant than quercetin, but the citrus flavanones which have fewer functional hydroxyl groups on the B ring and lack the 2,3 unsaturation on the C ring are less strong.

Although many flavonoids are good antioxidants *in vitro* whether this property mediates their health benefits *in vivo* is debated because of their known extensive metabolism. Overall absorption of flavonoids is estimated to vary considerably based on the amounts excreted in the urine (*11*). Contributing to this variation is the well-documented metabolism of the flavonoid structure which can occur via first-pass metabolism, by the colonic bacteria, and via the liver (*12,13*). These modifications include: removal of the sugar (most naturally occurring forms are glycosylated); conjugation of hydroxyl groups with glucuronic acid, sulfate, or glycine; O-methylation; and ring opening via colonic bacteria. Thus, for most flavonoids very little of the parent compound is found intact in blood or tissues.

So the question that we wanted to address was whether flavonoids act through enhancing the endogenous antioxidant defense system. We used the established model of vitamin E and Se deficiency that shows strong adaptive properties. We also had previously shown that a synthetic antioxidant (tBHQ at

Table 1. Total Peroxyl Radical Antioxidant Potential (TRAP) *In vitro* Determination of Dietary Flavonoids and t-BHQ

Treatment	*N*	*Lag Time (s)*	*SE*
Trolox	24	498 [c]	45
EGGC	4	973 [a]	39
Quercetin	4	679 [b]	19
(-)Epicatechin	4	403 [d]	35
t-BHQ	4	380 [d]	12
Naringenin	4	321 [e]	23
Hesperetin	4	268 [e]	6

NOTE: Results are expressed as mean lag times (s, seconds) and standard errors (SE). Means with different (a, b, c, d, e) superscript letters are significantly different after One-way ANOVA and post-hoc testing with Tukey ($P<0.05$).

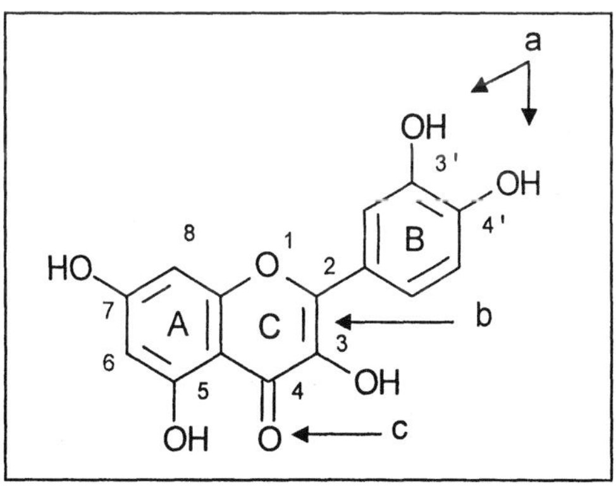

Figure 2. Flavonoids structural requirements for antioxidant activity, example, quercetin: orthodihydroxy substitution in B ring (a); 2, 3 unsaturation in C ring (b); and 4 carbonyl (oxo) substitution (c) (7,9).

100 mg/kg diet) which was well absorbed and distributed could prevent deficiency if included in the diet (*14*). We chose a test compound that was not as strong an antioxidant *in vitro* as other choices in the hopes of avoiding the complication of the chemical exhibiting primary antioxidant properties in the animal. And we supported this choice with a rationale based on previous studies in rats that naringenin, at 30 mg/kg diet, appeared to influence liver coenzyme Q amounts and total aldehydes (*15*). Also it had been reported in the literature that the citrus flavanones influence cell signaling cascades (*16*).

Effects of Naringenin Consumption on Oxidative Stress in Rats

The details of this experiment will be published elsewhere, but briefly, weaned Long-Evans hooded rats were randomized into 8 experimental diet groups for 6 weeks (*17*). The basal diet was Torula-yeast based to control Se and the oils were tocopherol-stripped to control vitamin E. A low oxidative stress diet (LOX) was supplemented with tocopheryl acetate (30 mg/kg) and sodium selenite (0.5 mg/kg) and a high oxidative stress diet (HOX) was deficient in both antioxidant nutrients. Naringenin was added to these diets to reflect intakes at 0 30, 60 & 120 mg per kg diet to reflect levels indicative of typical intake from citrus food sources. The major outcome measures that are reported here reflect oxidative stress effects on growth, liver lipid peroxidation and the endogenous antioxidant defense system. Rats consuming a diet without vitamin E and selenium show severely depleted levels by three weeks, but continue to grow at the same rate as control rats for up to five weeks at which point their rate of growth declines. This observation along with increases in liver to body weight ratio are taken as physiological effects of the oxidative stress caused by the antioxidant nutrient deficiency (*18*). In these experiments rats consuming the HOX diet exhibited growth decline at six weeks as expected, but this was not prevented by naringenin consumption (Table 2). No difference in food intake was observed with any of the treatments.

We measured the activity of the QR, also known as NAD(P)H quinone oxidoreductase (*19*), in liver homogenates as a key marker of oxidative stress adaptation (Figure 3) and observed, as previously shown, that the HOX was associated with a 2-3 fold increase in activity. NAR consumption showed no effect in the LOX, but in the HOX groups consumption of NAR at increasing amounts was associated with greater QR activity with the 120 mg/kg diet group exhibiting significantly greater (about 1/3 greater) activity than 0 NAR group.

The concentration of total aldehydes as a marker of oxidative stress/lipid peroxidation was measured in liver homogenates and, as expected, found to be significantly greater in the HOX vs LOX group (Figure 4). However, no effect of

Table 2. Effects of Naringenin Consumption and Oxidative Stress on Total Weight, Weight Gain, Parametrial Fat Mass and Food Intake at the 6th Week of the Study

		Treatment (mg/kg diet)			
Variable	*Oxidative Condition*	*0*	*30*	*60*	*120*
Total weight (g)	LOX ^{x}	246 ± 25	227 ± 16	244 ± 31	235 ± 23
	HOX ^{y}	236 ± 16	236 ± 17	227 ± 23	211 ± 16
Weight gain (g)	LOX ^{x}	27.6 ± 3.2	26.3 ± 2.0	29.8 ± 5.1	29.7 ± 2.9
	HOX ^{y}	23.5 ± 5.9	24.6 ± 4.1	24.1 ± 6.2	23.7 ± 2.5
Liver Index (g/100g BW)	LOX ^{x}	3.00 ± 0.23	2.78 ± 0.31	2.88 ± 0.12	2.91 ± 0.21
	HOX ^{y}	3.33 ± 0.17	3.47 ± 0.46	3.38 ± 0.21	3.42 ± 0.30
Parametrial fat (g/100g BW)	LOX ^{x}	1.14 ± 0.25 ^{a}	0.93 ± 0.07 ^{a,b}	0.93 ± 0.18 ^{a,b}	0.70 ± 0.11 ^{b}
	HOX ^{y}	0.77 ± 0.22	0.71 ± 0.17	0.76 ± 0.16	0.79 ± 0.21
Food intake (g/day/rat)	LOX	13.9 ± 1.9	12.9 ± 1.7	14.5 ± 1.9	13.5 ± 1.6
	HOX	13.8 ± 2.2	14.0 ± 1.7	13.3 ± 1.2	13.2 ± 1.5

NOTE: Results are expressed as means ± standard deviations (SD). Factor statistical differences among oxidative conditions are represented by x,y superscripts after Two-way ANOVA (P<0.05). Naringenin treatment effects are represented by a,b superscripts after post-hoc testing with Tukey (P<0.05).

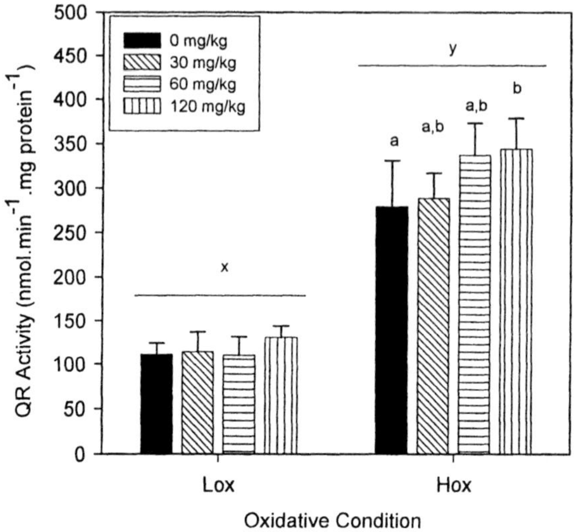

Figure 3. The effect of naringenin (NAR) consumption and high oxidative stress (HOX) versus low oxidative stress (LOX) on rat liver homogenate quinone reductase activity. Bar values are means ± SD. Factor statistical differences among oxidative conditions are represented by x,y superscripts after Two-way ANOVA (P<0.05). Naringenin treatment effects are represented by a,b superscripts after post-hoc testing with Tukey (P<0.05).

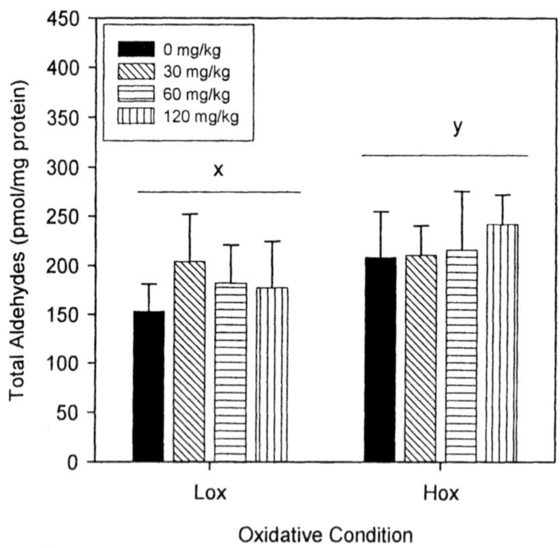

Figure 4. The effect of naringenin (NAR) consumption and high oxidative stress (HOX) versus low oxidative stress (LOX) on rat liver homogenate total aldehydes. Factor statistical differences among oxidative conditions are represented by x,y superscripts after Two-way ANOVA (P<0.05).

NAR consumption was observed within each group. Thus NAR intake did not prevent the increase in oxidative stress markers resulting from the HOX diet, deficient in vitamin E and Se. Thus, naringenin showed no antioxidant effect *in vivo* in rats.

Because extracts of flavonoid-rich plants are sold as supplements to different population groups with various disease conditions, any relevant information of toxic effects of flavonoid mediated via oxidative damage is of interest (*20*). Several reports have identified flavonoids with multiple hydroxylations in the B-ring to have stronger prooxidant activities. However, these activities are mostly present in conditions of high concentration of transition metals such iron and copper (*20,21*). Higher iron and copper concentrations under physiological conditions are not likely due to their selective chelation by specialized storage proteins (*1*). Therefore, the role of flavonoids as prooxidant *in vivo* is uncertain. In these studies no evidence of a prooxidant effect was observed with NAR consumption in either the LOX or HOX condition.

Effects of Narigenin Consumption on Lipid Oxidation in Rats

The results were not entirely negative for a potential positive health benefit of NAR. In collaboration with colleagues at Purdue we measured the amount of visceral fat associated with the rat parametrial fat pad and found a NAR effect in LOX state (Table 2). In ongoing studies spearheaded by our colleagues and published elsewhere (*22*), we have observed NAR effects on lowering adipose and blood triglyceride levels. This effect may be mediated through transcription factors as we have observed upregulation of $PPAR_{\alpha}$ and $PPAR_{\alpha}$-regulated genes. More about the potential beneficial effects of citrus flavonoids on blood lipids and adiposity will be discussed in chapters by Drs. Manthey and Fujioka.

Antioxidant Effects of Grapefruit Juice Consumption in Humans

Here we will report some of the results of a randomized intervention trial in humans of three months in duration. The primary objective was to test the effect of regular grapefruit juice consumption on mineral and antioxidant nutrient status, factors that can reduce disease risk in healthy people. We also looked at satiety and satiation. The collaborators on this project were Dr. Connie Weaver, who conducted the mineral status studies, and Dr. Rick Mattes, who performed the satiety and satiation work. Here the antioxidant nutrient status effects will be presented in part.

College women (18 – 30 y) were recruited to participate in a three-month intervention trial. Participants were randomized after screening into two treatment groups which involved balancing for blood ferritin concentrations and oral contraceptive use. Participants in the first treatment group were asked to consume two servings of grapefruit juice each day, and the second group served as the control and participants were asked to consume a calorie-matched fruit-flavored beverage. The juices were generously supplied by Tropicana as ruby red grapefruit juice (RRGJ) and Capri Sun Surfer Cooler as the placebo. The juice was provided in 64 oz. unmarked refrigerated cartons and subjects picked up their supply on a weekly basis. Compliance with juice consumption was monitored by the subjects filling out a juice consumption verification form and by measuring the amount of juice in returned cartons. Subjects were required to provide blood samples and 3-day diet records at monthly intervals during the study. They were also required to provide a urine sample at the end of the intervention period. The project was approved by the Purdue University Committee on the Use of Human Research Subjects.

Ninety two women completed the study in two phases (n=46 per each group). The effect of RRGJ consumption on the status of fat- and water-soluble antioxidants, total antioxidant potential in the serum, and blood lipids are summarized in the Table 3. Statistical analyses were conducted using the data from completers of the protocol. The effect of juice consumption on the outcome measures was tested by repeated measures ANOVA using the GLM procedure with the SAS program (Cary, S.C.). Also, an ANCOVA was conducted using baseline values as the covariate. Consumption of RRGJ led to a 45% increase in plasma ascorbate concentrations and this was statistically greater than the 16% increase observed with the consumption of the placebo, and similar to that reported for orange juice (*23*). This result was expected because the RRGJ contained vitamin C (30+ mg/serving) whereas the Capri Sun Surfer Cooler did not. Evaluation of the naringenin concentration in the plasma was conducted by first treating the blood samples with a non-specific esterase to convert esterified forms to free flavanone. The values obtained were quite variable for those consuming RRGJ, ranging from 0.0 to 2,612 nM, with a mean of 333.8 nM similar to a previous report (*24*). Other than in two samples, no naringenin was found in the blood samples from participants consuming the placebo drink. The mean concentrations of the fat-soluble antioxidants α-tocopherol and coenzyme Q10 increased in the plasma with time of intervention, however there was not a statistically significant treatment effect. Similarly, the total radical absorbance potential (TRAP) increased with time of intervention with no significant effect of RRGJ. Blood lipids such as total cholesterol (Total-CHL) and high density

Table 3. The Effect of Consuming RRGJ on Plasma Concentrations of Fat- and Water-soluble Antioxidants, Serum TRAP, and Blood Lipids

	Baseline		*3 Months*	
Variable	*RRGJ*	*Placebo*	*RRGJ*	*Placebo*
α-tocopherol (μM)	17.2 ± 5.2	16.8 ± 6.3	18.9 ± 5.0 [a]	18.1 ± 5.1 [a]
γ-tocopherol (μM)	3.8 ± 1.2	4.1 ± 1.2	4.2 ± 1.4	4.5 ± 1.3
Coenzyme Q10 (μM)	0.36 ± 0.18	0.33 ± 0.18	0.40 ± 0.10 [a]	0.42 ± 0.12 [a]
β-carotene (μM)	0.44 ± 0.31	0.41 ± 0.28	0.38 ± 0.29	0.32 ± 0.22
TRAP (mmol/L)	1.11 ± 0.10	1.10 ± 0.10	1.31 ± 0.09 [a]	1.29 ± 0.10 [a]
Triglycerides (mg/dL)	90.5 ± 50.0	84.2 ± 41.6	91.7 ± 53.1	97.6 ± 50.3
Total-CHL (mg/dL)	184 ± 41	170 ± 28	191 ± 44 [a]	181 ± 31 [a]
HDL-CHL (mg/dL)	51.0 ± 9.6	50.8 ± 12.3	52.0 ± 10.6 [a]	52.6 ± 11.7 [a]
Naringenin (nM)	nd	nd	334 ± 488	12 ± 62 [x]
Ascorbate (μM)	49.5 ± 16.8	44.8 ± 18.6	71.7 ± 23.6 [a]	52.1 ± 26.0 [a,y]

NOTE: Values are means ± SD, n=45-46 participants per group. [a] Statistically different from baseline (time effect; $P<0.05$). [x] Statistical differences between groups at three months ($P<0.001$). [y] Statistical differences between groups and time interaction ($P<0.05$). Total cholesterol (Total-CHL), high density lipoprotein cholesterol (HDL-CHL), not determined (nd).

lipoprotein cholesterol (HDL-CHL) increased with time intervention as well, but without significant effect of RRGJ.

Oxidative stress was evaluated using urinary 8-epi-prostaglandin $F_{2\alpha}$ (8-isoprostane) which is a non-enzymatic eicosanoid-like compound formed from lipid peroxidation (*25*). The results are presented in Figure 5. Although the amount of 8-isoprostane excreted in the urine decreased over time, no statistically significant differences were observed between the two groups.

In summary, consumption of ruby red grapefruit juice significantly improved vitamin C status in this population of college-age women. The naringin found in RRGJ was variably absorbed and resulted in average blood naringenin concentrations that were sub-micromolar. Measures of oxidative stress decreased in the urine and antioxidant protection increased in the blood over time with intervention but no statistically significant effect of RRGJ consumption was observed. This population was chosen based on the rationale for low mineral status and thus would not be considered a high oxidative stess model. Consistent results with humans considered to be under high oxidative stress is not always observed (*26*), thus populations under low oxidative stress are unlikely to reveal an additional antioxidant benefit. Future studies examining the antioxidant health benefits of citrus and other phytochemicals should be conducted in study populations exhibiting documented high oxidative stress. Moreover, the statistical power can be improved by incorporating a crossover design.

Summary and Overall Conclusions

The reported study results tested the hypothesis that the citrus flavonoid naringenin, either in pure form in the diet or as a component of grapefruit juice, would act as an antioxidant *in vivo*, either directly or through enhancing key components of the endogenous antioxidant defense system. No evidence of significant antioxidant effect was found, but in rats naringenin consumption was associated with higher activity of quinone reductase, a key antioxidant defense enzyme, but only in rats under the oxidative stress due to vitamin E and selenium deficiency. In humans, consumption of ruby red grapefruit juice led to increased concentrations of the water-soluble antioxidant vitamin C, for which the juice is a good dietary source. However, no statistically significant improvement in other biological antioxidants, antioxidant capacity or markers of oxidative stress were observed. This result was most likely due to the study population being healthy young college-age women not suffering from an elevated oxidative stress state. No evidence of a prooxidant effect for narigenin was observed in either *in vivo* study.

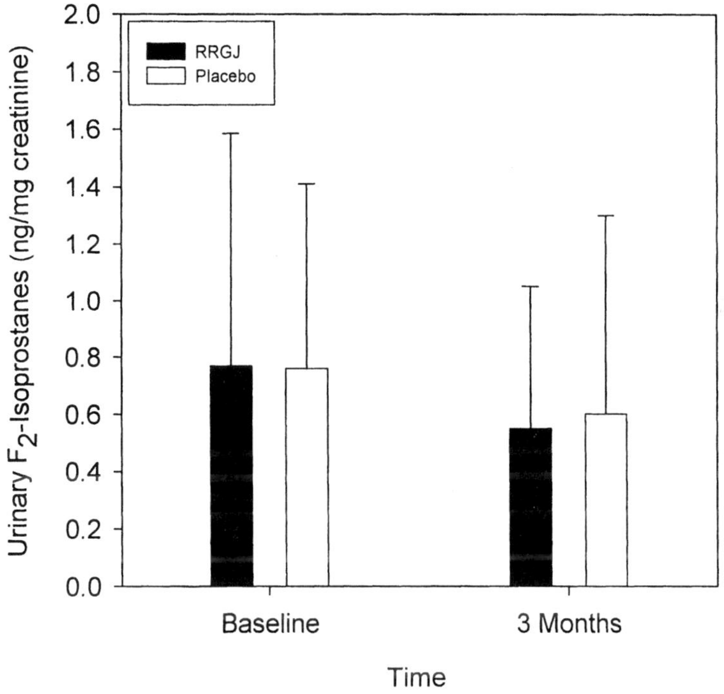

Figure 5. The effect of ruby red grapefruit juice (RRGJ) consumption for 3 months in duration versus a placebo beverage on urinary excretion of 8-epi-prostaglandin $F_{2\alpha}$ (8-isoprostane) in college age women. No significant differences were observed.

Literature Cited

1. Halliwell, B. *Annu Rev Nutr* **1996**, *16*, 33-50.
2. Villalba, J. M.; Navarro, F.; Gomez-Diaz, C.; Arroyo, A.; Bello, R. I.; Navas, P. *Mol Aspects Med* **1997**, *18*, S7-13.
3. Navarro, F.; Navas, P.; Burgess, J. R.; Bello, R. I.; De Cabo, R.; Arroyo, A.; Villalba, J. M. *Faseb J* **1998**, *12*, 1665-73.
4. Kuo, C. F.; Cheng, S.; Burgess, J. R. *Journal of Nutrition* **1995**, *125*, 1419-29.
5. De Cabo, R. Ph.D. thesis, Purdue University, West Lafayette, IN, 2000.
6. Hertog, M. G.; Feskens, E. J.; Hollman, P. C.; Katan, M. B.; Kromhout, D. *Lancet* **1993**, *342*, 1007-11.
7. Pietta, P. G. *J Nat Prod* **2000**, *63*, 1035-42.
8. Myhrstad, M. C.; Carlsen, H.; Nordstrom, O.; Blomhoff, R.; Moskaug, J. J. *Free Radic Biol Med* **2002**, *32*, 386-93.
9. Williams, R. J.; Spencer, J. P.; Rice-Evans, C. *Free Radic Biol Med* **2004**, *36*, 838-49.
10. Valkonen, M.; Kuusi, T. *J Lipid Res* **1997**, *38*, 823-33.
11. Hollman, P. C. H.; Katan, M. B. In *Flavonoids in health and disease*; Rice Evans, C. A., Packer, L., Eds.; Antioxidant in health and disease; Marcel Dekker, Inc.: New York, 1988, pp 483-522.
12. Hollman, P. C.; Katan, M. B. *Biomed Pharmacother* **1997**, *51*, 305-10.
13. Ross, J. A.; Kasum, C. M. *Annu Rev Nutr* **2002**, *22*, 19-34.
14. Burgess, J. R.; Gao, F. In *Food Phytates*; Reddy, N. R., Sathe, S. K., Eds.; CRC Press: Boca Raton, 2002, pp 189-197.
15. Andrade, J. E.; Burgess, J. R. *Faseb J* **2002**, *16*, A1009.
16. Virgili, F.; Acconcia, F.; Ambra, R.; Rinna, A.; Totta, P.; Marino, M. *IUBMB Life* **2004**, *56*, 145-51.
17. Andrade, J. E.; Burgess, J. R. *Faseb J* **2005**, *19*, A1158.
18. Burgess, J. R.; Kuo, C. F. *J Nutr Biochem* **1996**, *7*, 366-374.
19. Jaiswal, A. K. *J Biol Chem* **1994**, *269*, 14502-8.
20. Cao, G.; Sofic, E.; Prior, R. L. *Free Radic Biol Med* **1997**, *22*, 749-60.
21. Hanasaki, Y.; Ogawa, S.; Fukui, S. *Free Radic Biol Med* **1994**, *16*, 845-50.
22. Cho, K. W.; Andrade, J. E.; Burgess, J. R.; Kim, Y. C. *Faseb J* **2005**, *19*, A1154.
23. Sanchez-Moreno, C.; Cano, M. P.; de Ancos, B.; Plaza, L.; Olmedilla, B.; Granado, F.; Martin, A. *Am J Clin Nutr* **2003**, *78*, 454-60.
24. Erlund, I.; Meririnne, E.; Alfthan, G.; Aro, A. *J Nutr* **2001**, *131*, 235-41.
25. Morrow, J. D.; Roberts, L. J. *Prog Lipid Res* **1997**, *36*, 1-21.
26. Moller, P.; Vogel, U.; Pedersen, A.; Dragsted, L. O.; Sandstrom, B.; Loft, S. *Cancer Epidemiol Biomarkers Prev* **2003**, *12*, 1016-22.

Chapter 13

Citrus sp.: A Source of Flavonoids of Pharmaceutical Interest

Ana Ortuño[1], Pedro Gómez[1], Ana Báidez[1], Víctor Frías[2], and José A. Del Río[1]

[1]Department of Plant Biology, Faculty of Biology, University of Murcia, Campus Espinardo, Murcia 30100, Spain
[2]Department of Research and Development, Agrométodos S. A., Álamos 1, Urb. Monteclaro, Pozuelo de Alarcón, Madrid 28223, Spain
*Corresponding author: aortuno@um.es

Flavonoids in *Citrus* sp. are a widely distributed group of polyphenolic compounds characterized by a common benzo-γ-pyrone structure. Flavonoids are present in a large variety of edible plants, especially in *Citrus* species. All flavonoids described in *Citrus* sp. to date can be classified into four clearly differentiated groups: flavones, flavonols, flavanones and their corresponding glycosides with these two possible types of of glycoside substitution: β-neohesperidosides (2-O-α-L-rhamnopyranosyl-β-D-glucopyranose) or β-rutinoside (6-O-α-L-rhamnopyranosyl-β-D-glucopyranose) (*1*).

Depending on the particular citrus species, the biosynthetic pathways result in the synthesis of: naringin, the 7-β-neohesperidoside of naringenin (4′,5,7-trihydroxyflavone), which is the major flavonoid in *Citrus paradisi*; neohesperidin, the 7-β-neohesperidoside of hesperetin (3′,5,7-trihydroxy-4′-methoxy flavanone), which is the principal flavonoid in *Citrus aurantium*; or hesperidin, the 7-β-rutinoside of hesperetin, which is the principal flavonoid in *Citrus sinensis* and *Citrus limon* (Figure 1).

The flavanone glycosides are accumulated in the greatest quantity, although the concentration of these compounds depends on the age of the plant. The highest concentration occur in young tissues showing pronounced cell divisions, in which they may represent 40-45% of the dry weight (*2-8*). However, less is known about other structural groups of *Citrus* flavonoids, the flavones and flavonols, although they have been studied in greater depth in other plant families (*9*).

The flavones in *Citrus* are found in both glycosylated and aglycon states, the latter showing a greater variety of compounds with their structure frequently multi-substituted by hydroxyl and/or methoxyl groups (see Figure 1). Among these polymethoxyflavones are sinensetin (5,6,7,3′,4′-pentamethoxyflavone), tangeretin (5,6,7,8,4′-pentamethoxyflavone), quercetogetin (3,5,6,7,3′,4′-hexamethoxyflavone), nobiletin (5,6,7,8,3′,4′-hexamethoxyflavone), and 3,5,6,7,8,3′,4′-heptamethoxyflavone (*10-12*).

Flavonoids	*R8*	*R7*	*R6*	*R5*	*R3*	*R4'*	*R3'*	*Name*
		Ram-Glu						
Flavanones	-	α1-6		OH	-	OCH_3	OH	**Hesperidin**
	-	α1-2		OH	-	OCH_3	OH	**Neohesperidin**
	-	α1-2		OH	-	OH	-	**Naringin**
Polymetho-xyflavones	-	OCH_3	OCH_3	OCH_3	-	OCH_3	OCH_3	**Sinensetin**
	OCH_3	OCH_3	OCH_3	OCH_3	-	OCH_3	-	**Tangeretin**
	OCH_3	OCH_3	OCH_3	OCH_3	-	OCH_3	OCH_3	**Nobiletin**
	OCH_3	OCH_3	OCH_3	OCH_3	OCH_3	OCH_3	OCH_3	**Heptamethox.**
	-	OCH_3	OCH_3	OCH_3	OCH_3	OCH_3	OCH_3	**Quercetogetin**

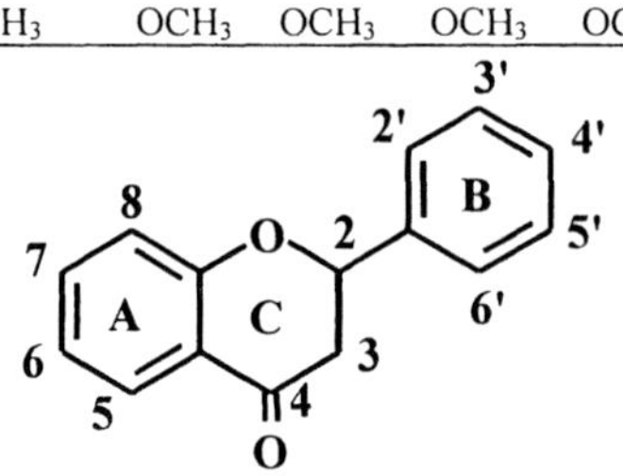

Figure 1. Chemical structures of the flavanones, naringin, neohesperidin and hesperidin, and the polymethoxyflavones, sinensetin, tangeretin, nobiletin, heptamethoxyflavone, quercetogetin.

These compounds not only play an important physiological and ecological role but are also of comercial interest because of their multitude of applications in the food and pharmaceutical industries. For example, naringin can act as antioxidant (*13*), protecting against lipid peroxidation (*14, 15*), and as an antimutagenic (*16*). Furthermore, naringin can be used as an alternative to caffeine or quinine in tonic beverages and other non-alcoholic drinks and produces a distinctly bitter taste at low concentration (*17*). Hesperidin influences vascular permeability, increases capillary resistance and has both analgesic and anti-inflammatory properties (*18, 19*). It is also an effective antioxidant due to its ability to quench the oxygen free radicals which are involved in cancer (*20-22*). Naringin and neohesperidin also have another important industrial application in that they can be chemically converted into their corresponding intensely sweet dihydrochalcones (*23-26*). Diosmin possesses antihemorroidal, antioxidant and anti-lipid peroxidation properties and protects against free radicals (*18, 27*).

Polymethoxyflavones are also of interest for their pharmacological potential (*28-30*), the most important of which are their anticarcinogenic properties (*31*) due to their ability to absorb UV light (*32*). They also have antimutagenic and antiproliferative effect against tumours (*33-35*), anti-inflammatory activities (*36-37*), and anti-allergic and analgesic properties (*38*).

In addition, the taxonomic interest of these compounds is widely known and they have been used in an industrial context to detect the adulteration of citric juices.

Biosynthesis of Flavonoids in *Citrus*

The distribution of flavonoids in 51 species of *Citrus* (39, *40*) shows that the principal flavonoids in *Citrus* are 7-O-glycosylated flavanones, determined by HPLC method. Thirty-one percent of the species studied express flavonoids with a neohesperidoside type glycosylated structure and 63% with a rutinoside type; six percent exhibit both structures in similar proportions.

Substitution of the B ring of the flavonoid skeleton constitutes a fundamental factor in the taxonomic state of the different species of *Citrus*. Eighty percent of species yield a 3'-hydroxy-4'-methoxyflavanone substitution model in their most abundant flavonoids, with only 10% being exclusively 4'-hydroxy and 10% with both substitution types

In the case of those *Citrus* species containing rutinosides, 97% have hesperidin as the principal flavonoid. The *Citrus* species which contain neohesperidosides, 97% have neohesperidin (3' hydro-4'methoxy) and naringin (4'-OH) as the principal flavonoids. Approximately, 3% of species express neohesperidoside type flavanones, with substitution at the 4' position (-OH or -OMe).

Seventy-five percent of the flavones of the citrus species are the rutinoside type. Among the most important compounds are diosmin (3'-hydroxy-4'methoxy) and isorohifolin (4'-hydroxy) in the form of rutinoside-type glycosides, and rohifolin (4'-hydroxy) and neodiosmin (3'-hydroxy-4'-methoxy) in the form of neohesperidoside-type glycosides.

The highest concentrations of flavanones-glycosides in *Citrus* occur in leaves, flowers and fruits, their presence being hardly noticeable in roots (*41*). The relative levels of flavonoids are highly characteristic of a given organ (leaves, flowers and fruits) and are markedly affected by the age of the developing organ. The biosynthesis of flavonoids is associated with the process of growth and development of leaves, flowers and fruit (*2*). The highest levels of polymethoxyflavones are associated with young developing states in fruits and they are only located in the peel.

In mature fruit, the highest levels of naringin are produced by Marsh and Red Blush grapefruit (around 3 g/100 g dry weight (DW). In *Citrus aurantium*, the highest levels of neohesperidin are produced by cv. Bouquet de Fleurs (around 4 g/100 g DW). The mature fruit of the pigmented orange variety, cv. Sanguinelli, showed the highest expression of hesperidin (around 4 g/100 g DW) (Figure 2) at levels similar to those found in tangelo Nova, a mandarin hybrid (*Citrus reticulata* B) x tangelo orlando (*Citrus reticulata* x *Citrus paradisi* Macf.). The highest levels of diosmin are detected in *Citrus limon* cv. Fino-49 (around 0.4 g/100 g DW).

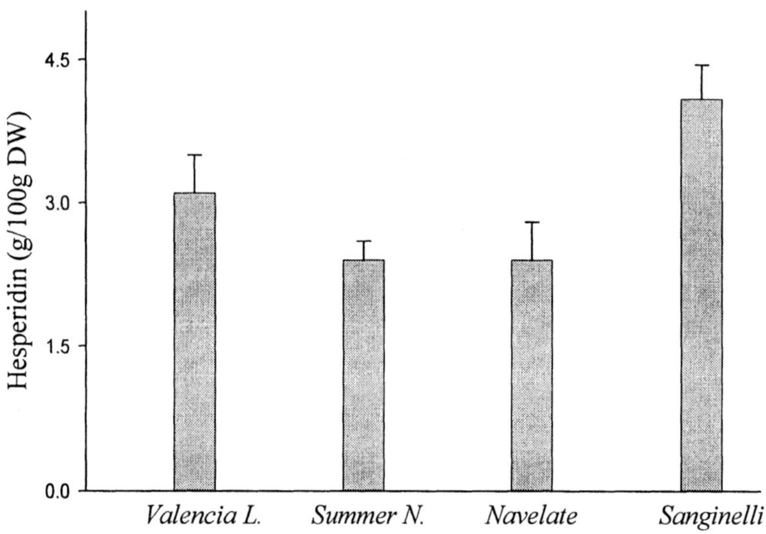

Figure 2. Levels of flavanone hesperidin in mature fruits of different varieties of Citrus sinensis. The data represent mean values ± SE (n =3) of this flavanone (g/100 g DW).

The highest concentrations of nobiletin and sinensetin were detected in *Citrus sinensis* cv. Valencia Late (11 and 6 mg/100 g DW, respectively).

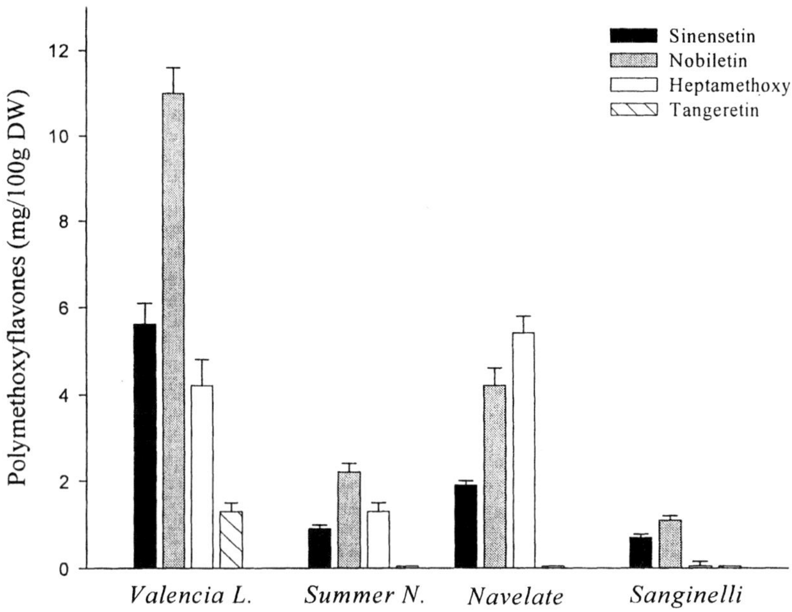

Figure 3. Levels of the polymethoxyflavones, sinensetin, nobiletin, heptamethoxyflavone and tangeretin (mg/100 g DW), in mature fruits of different varieties of Citrus sinensis. The data represent mean values ± SE (n=3).

Heptamethoxyflavone, on the other hand, was at its highest level in cv. Navelate (around 5 mg/100 g DW) (Figure 3).

Antifungal Properties of *Citrus* Flavonoids Against *Phytophthora* sp., *Penicillium* sp. and *Geotrichum* sp.

Several phenolic compounds have been described as taking part in the resistance mechanisms of genus *Citrus* to pathogens, among them coumarins, flavanones and flavones.

Coumarins are synthesized by the mechanically injured plant or in response to microbial infection, where they are thought to act as phytoalexins. Some species of *Citrus* when infected by phytopathogenic fungi have been shown to accumulate coumarins such as xanthyletin, seselin and scoparone, although the exact nature of the coumarins biosynthesized in this process varies within a species according to the pathogen in question (*8, 42-49*).

Less is known about the role which other constitutive phenolic compounds such as flavones and flavanones, play in the the defense mechanism of this genus. When the distribution of these compounds in *Citrus* fruits was studied, they were revealed to be mainly located in the peel: polymethoxyflavones in the flavedo and flavanones in the albedo (*40, 50-52*). For this reason, some authors consider that they may help protect the fruit from possible pathogenic attacks (*11, 53-56*).

Some of the polymethoxyflavones described above seem to be involved in the defense mechanism of *Citrus* sp. against *Phytophthora citrophthora*, *Penicillium digitatum* and *Geotrichum* sp. (*11*). Studies have shown that a non-terpene extract from the essential oil of sour orange inhibits *P. citrophthora* growth by 100%, while the same extract from clementine and sweet orange inhibits growth of the same fungus by 72 and 14%, respectively. *Penicillium digitatum* was totally inhibited (100%) by extracts from sweet *Citrus* species (clementine and sweet orange) and 77% inhibited by sour orange extract. *Geotrichum* sp. was more sensitive to a sour orange extract (57% inhibition) than to extracts from clementine and sweet orange (47 and 34% inhibition, respectively, compared with the control) (*11*).

The IC_{50} measured *in vitro* for the polymethoxyflavones isolated from tangelo Nova [(C*itrus reticulata* B) x tangelo Orlando (*Citrus reticulata* x *Citrus paradisi*)] or *Citrus sinensis* fruits against *Phytophthora citrophthora* revealed that nobiletin (IC_{50} = 0.59±0.07 mM) is more active than sinensetin, heptamethoxyflavone or tangeretin, which presented IC_{50} values of 0.91±0.05, 1.04±0.07 and 1.72±0.13 mM, respectively (*56*). A comparison of the IC_{50} value for tangeretin against *P. citrophthora* and that obtained against *Penicillium digitatum* (IC_{50} = 6.45±0.53 mM) (*55*) shows that this polymethoxyflavone is more effective against *Phytophthora.*

Changes in the levels of these same polymethoxyflavones are also observed *in vivo* when the fruits of *Citrus sinensis* (cv. Valencia late) are infected by *Phytophthora citrophthora,* which suggests that these secondary compounds participate in the defense mechanisms of citric species against pathogens. For example, when the level of infection in the fruit is very high, the concentrations of these polymethoxyflavones are higher than in uninfected fruit (increases of 48, 28, 26 and 24%, respectively for heptamethoxyflavone, nobiletin, sinensetin and tangeretin) (*12*). Their respective concentrations remain above control levels, though to a lesser extent, as the degree of infection by *P. citrophthora,* decreases (*12*). Contrary to that observed in the case of polymethoxyflavones during the infection processes of *Citrus sinensis* by *P. citrophthora*, the hesperidin and isonaringin contents fell by 13 and 67%, respectively, whereas the contents of their corresponding aglycons, hesperetin and naringenin, increased, suggesting the hydrolyzing effect of this fungus on the glycosylated flavanones. The *in vitro* study revealed that these compounds acted as antifungal agents, the most active being the aglycons (naringenin and hesperetin), followed by the polymethoxyflavones and flavanone glycosides (*12*).

The IC_{50} obtained for hesperidin isolated from tangelo Nova [(C*itrus reticulata* B) x tangelo Orlando (*Citrus reticulata* x *Citrus paradisi*)] or *Citrus sinensis* fuits against *Phytophthora citrophthora* was 19.6 ± 2.5 mM. This result suggests that, although they are more abundant in the fruit than polymethoxyflavones, flavanones are less active as fungistatic agents in the defense mechanism of *Citrus* species, as has also been observed in other plant materials (*55*).

All these flavonoids acted as fungistatic agents at the concentration assayed, causing a mycelial growth inhibition and marked abnormalities in hyphal size and morphology (collapse, irregular swelling and excessive branching) (Figure 4). The fact that higher concentration of these compounds are necessary to inhibit fungal growth when they are incorporated in the medium in *in vitro* assays, than *in vivo*, suggest that they have a synergistic effect when they act together, as has been suggested for other plant materials (*56*).

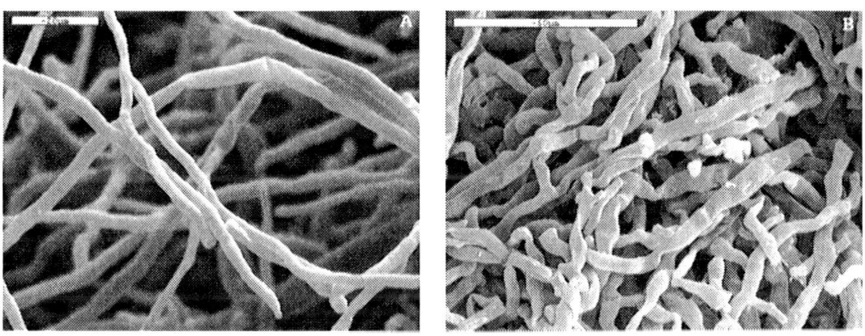

Figure 4.- SEM image of the changes in hyphal morphology and growth of P. citrophthora mycelium cultured in control PDA culture medium (A) x1200 and in the same PDA culture medium to which tangeretin (1.5 mM) (B) x1000 had been added.

Based on the results described above, we suggest that the constitutive secondary metabolites of *Citrus sinensis* studied (flavones and flavanones) may act as fungitoxins in the resistance mechanism against fungal attack, acting as the first and second lines of defense, respectively. However, this finding does not discount the fact that other secondary compounds induced after infection, such as coumarins, may also act in the defense mechanism of this plant material, as has been described in other *Citrus* species (*8*).

Increase Resistance Against Pathogens Fungi in *Citrus* by Modulation of Flavonoid Biosynthesis

The concentration of flavanones, polymethoxyflavones and scoparone in fruits of different *Citrus* sp. and *Citrus* hybrids can be increased by treatment with Brotomax, a supplemental nutritional product (Agrométodos, Spain) (*8, 57*). When recently set tangelo Nova fruit were treated with 0.3% Brotomax, there were no significant differences between the growth of treated and untreated fruit. However, hesperidin levels were 25% higher after 65 days in the treated fruit. Differences remained, though not so pronounced, after 96 and 120 days. The same treatment (0.3% Brotomax) also increased the biosynthesis and/or accumulation of polymethoxyflavones, and 96 days after treatment sinensetin and tangeretin levels were 33 and 22%, respectively, higher than control levels, while nobiletin and heptamethoxyflavone levels were 46% higher (*57*). Treatment with 0.5% Brotomax increased scoparone levels in the fruit of *Citrus paradisi*, *Citrus aurantium* and tangelo Nova compare with the levels observed in untreated fruit (*8*).

After confirming the modulating effect of Brotomax on the flavonoids levels of these *Citrus* fruits, a parallel study revealed that treated fruit offered a greater resistance to attack by *Phytophthora* sp. and *Penicillium* sp. (*8, 57*). On the other hand, it has been observed that the levels of flavanone, naringin, and the polymethoxyflavone, tangeretin, in *Citrus aurantium* fruits can be modulated by UV irradiation. The growth of *P. digitatum* on previously irradiated fruit was reduced by up to 45% with regard to non-irradiated fruit (*55*).

On the basis on these results, we suggest that Brotomax can be used in pre-harvest hormonal treatment and UV irradiation as a post-harvest treatment, as an alternative or in combination with the use of chemical fungicides, since such treatment induces resistance in *Citrus* sp. and *Citrus* hybrids by increasing the concentration of flavonoids.

These past and ongoing studies support the significant role of flavonoids in plant survival. The importance of these beneficial compounds in plant prosperity should not be over-shadowed by the growing interest in the impact of flavonoids and other phytochemicals on human health.

Acknowledgements

This work has was supported by Grant AGR/05, from the Consejería de Agricultura, Agua y Medio Ambiente from Murcia, Spain, and by Agrométodos S.A., from Madrid, Spain.

References

1. Horowitz, R.M.; Gentili, B. In *Citrus Science and Technology*; Nagy, S.; Shaw, P.E.; Velchuis, M.K. Eds.; AVI Publishing, Westport, CT, **1977**; Vol 1, pp 397-426.
2. Castillo, J.; Benavente-García, O.; Del Río, J.A. *Plant Physiology* **1992**, *99*, 67-73.
3. Castillo, J.; Benavente-García, O.; Del Río, J.A.. *J. Agric. Food Chem.* **1993**, *41*, 1920-1924.
4. Benavente-García, O.; Castillo, J.; Del Río, J.A. *J. Agric. Food Chem.* **1993**, *41*, 1916-1919.
5. Del Río, J.A.; Fuster, M.D.; Sabater, F.; Porras, I.; García-Lidón, A.; Ortuño, A. *J. Agric. Food Chem.* **1995**, *43*, 2030-2034.
6. Del Río, J.A.; Fuster, M.D.; Sabater, F.; Porras, I.; García-Lidón, A.; Ortuño, A. *Food Chem.* **1997**, *59*, 433-437.
7. Ortuño, A.; García-Puig, D.; Fuster, M.D.; Pérez, M.L.; Sabater, F.; Porras, I.; García-Lidón, A.; Del Río, J.A. *J. Agric. Food Chem.* **1995**, *43*, 1-5.
8. Ortuño, A.; Botía, J.M.; Fuster, M.D.; Porras, I.; García-Lidón, A.; Del Río, J.A. *J. Agric. Food Chem.* **1997**, *45*, 2740-2743.
9. Wollenweber, E.; Jay, M. In *The Flavonoids - Advances in Research since 1980*. Harborne, J. B. Ed.; Chapman and Hall, London, **1988**; pp 233 - 302.
10. Ooghe, W.C.; Ooghe, S.J.; Detavernier, C.M.; Huyghebaert, A. *J. Agric. Food Chem.* **1994**, *42*, 2191-2195.
11. Del Río, J.A.; Arcas, M.C.; Benavente-García, O.; Ortuño, A. *J. Agric. Food Chem.* **1998**, *46*, 4423-4428.
12. Del Río, J.A.; Gómez, P.; Báidez, G.A.; Arcas, M.C.; Botía, J.M.; Ortuño, A. *J. Agric. Food Chem.* **2004**, *52*, 1913-1917.
13. Chen, Y.T.; Zheng Jia, Z.J.; Ju, Y. *Free Radical Biol. Med.* **1990**, *9*, 19-21.
14. Salvayre, R.; Negre, A.; Affany, A.; Lenoble, M.; Douste-Blazy, L. *Prog. Clin. Biol. Res.* **1988**, *280*, 313-316.
15. Guengerich, F.P.; Kim, D.H. *Carcinogenesis* **1990**, *11*, 2275-2279.
16. Francis, A.R.; Shetty, T.K.; Bhattacharya, R.K. *Carcinogenesis* **1989**, *10*, 1953-1955.
17. Anon, *Food Dev.* **1982**, *16*, 29.
18. Gabor, M. In *Plant flavonoids in biology and medicine II: biochemical, cellular and medicinal properties*; Cody, V.; Middleton, E.; Harborne, J. B.; Beretz, A. Ed.; Alan R Liss, Inc., New York, **1988**; pp 1-15.
19. Emim, J.A.S.; Oliveira, A.B.; Lapa, A.J. *J. Pharmacol.* **1994**, *46*, 118-122.
20. Lonchampt, M.; Guardiola, B.; Sicot, N.; Bertrand, M.; Perdrix, L.; Duhault, J. *Arzneim. Forsch. Drug Res.* **1989**, *39*, 882-885.

21. Fujiki, H.; Horiuchi, T.; Yamashita, K.; Hakii, H.; Suganuma, M.; Nishino, H.; Iwashima, A.; Hirata, Y.; Sugimura, T. *Prog. Clin. Biol. Res.* **1986**, *213*, 429-440.
22. Berkarda, B.; Koyuncu, H.; Soybir, G.; Baykut, F. *Res. Exp. Med.* **1998**, *198*, 93-99.
23. Horowitz, R.M.; Gentili, B. U.S.A. Patent 3, 087, 821, **1963**.
24. Krbechek, L.; Inglett, G.; Holik, M.; Dowling, B.; Wagner, R.; Ritter, R. *J. Agric. Food Chem.* **1968**, *16*, 108-112.
25. Horowitz, R.M. In: *Plant flavonoids in biology and medicine: biochemical, pharmacological, and structure-activity relationships*; Cody, V.; Middleton, E.; Harborne, J.B. Ed.; Alan, R. Liss; New York, **1986**; pp 163-175.
26. Bär, A.; Borrego, F.; Benavente, O.; Castillo, J.; Del Río, J.A. *Food Sci. Technol.* **1990**, *23*, 371-376.
27. Berqvist, D.; Hallbrook, T.; Lindblad, B.; Lindhagen, A. *Vasa* **1981**, *10*, 253-260.
28. Benavente-García, O.; Castillo, J.; Sabater, F.; Del Río, J. A. *J. Agric. Food Chem.* **1997**, *45*, 4505-4515.
29. Robbins, R.C. In *Citrus Nutrition and Quality*; Nagy, S.; Attaway, J.A.; Ed.; American Chemical Society: Washington, Dc, **1980**, pp 43-59.
30. Middleton, E. Jr.; Kandaswami, C. *Biochem. Pharmacol.* **1992**, **43**, 1167-1179.
31. Chen, J.; Montanari, A.M.; Widmer, W.W. *J. Agric. Food Chem.* **1997**, *45*, 364-368.
32. Shimoi, K.; Masuda, S.; Furogori, M.; Esaki, S.; Kinae, N. *Carcinogenesis* **1994**, *15*, 2669-2672.
33. Kandaswami, C.; Perkins, E.; Soloniuk, D.S.; Drzewiecki, G.; Middleton, E. *Cancer Lett.* **1991**, *56*, 147-152.
34. Stapleton, A.E.; Walbot, V. *Plant Physiol.* **1994**, *105*, 881-889.
35. Bracke, M.E.; Bruyneel, E.A.; Vermeulen, S.J.; Vennekens, K.; Marck, V.V.; Mareel, M.M. *Food Technol.* **1994**, *48*, 121-124.
36. Midleton, E.; Drzewicki, G. *Biochem Pharmacol.* **1982**, *31*, 1449-1453.
37. Midleton, E. *Biochem. Pharmacol.* **1986**, *31*, 1449-1453.
38. Gabor, M. In: *Plant Flavonoids in Biology and Medicine: Biochemical, Pharmacological, and Structure-Activity relationships;* Cody, V.; Middleton, E.; Harborne, J.B.; Beretz, A. Ed.; Alan R. Liss Inc., New York, **1986**; Vol. 213, pp 471-480.
39. Kamiya, S.; Esaki, S.; Konishi, F. *Agric. Biol. Chem.* **1979**, *43*, 1529-1536.
40. Kanes, K.; Tisserat, B.; Berhow M.; Vandercook, C. *Phytochem.* **1992**, *32*, 967-974.
41. Jourdan, P.S.; McIntosh, C.A.; Mansell, R.L. *Plant Physiol.* **1985**, *77*, 903-908.
42. De Lange, J.H.; Vincent, A.P.; Du Plessis, L.M.; Van Wyk, P.J.; Ackerman, L.G.J. *Phytophylac.* **1976**, *8*, 83-84.

43. Baudoin, A.; Eckert, J.W. *Phytopathol.* **1985**, *75*, 174-179.
44. Khan, A.J.; Kunesch, G.; Chuilon, S.; Ravise, A. *Fruits* **1985**, *40*, 807-811.
45. Vernenghi, A. ; Ramiandrasoa, F. ; Chuilon, S. ; Ravise, A. *Fruits* **1987**, *42*, 103-111.
46. Afek, U.; Sztejnberg, A. *Phytopathol.* **1988**, *78*, 1678-1682.
47. Sulistyowati, L.; Keane, P.J.; Anderson, J.W. *Physiol. Mol. Plant Pathol.* **1990**, *37*, 451-461.
48. Kim, J.J.; Ben-Yehoshua, S.; Shapiro, B.; Henis, Y.; Carmeli, S. *Plant Physiology* **1991**, *97*, 880-885.
49. Stange, R.R. Jr.; Midland, S.L.; Eckert, J.W.; Sims, J.J. *J Nat. Prod.* **1993**, *56*, 1627-1629.
50. Machida, K.; Osawa, K. *Chem. Pharm. Bull.* **1989**, *37*, 1092-1094.
51. Mizuno, M.; Inhuma, M.; Ohara, M.; Tanaka, T.; Iwamasa, M. *Chem. Pharm. Bull.* **1991**, *39*, 945-949.
52. Ortuño, A., Arcas, M.C., Benavente-García, O., Del Río, J.A. *J. Agric. Food Chem.* **1999**, *66*, 217-220.
53. Ben-Aziz, A. *Science* **1967**, *155*, 1026-1027.
54. Huet, R. *Fruits* **1982**, *37*, 267-271.
55. Arcas, M.C.; Botía, J.M.; Ortuño, A.; Del Río, J.A. *Eu. J. Plant Pathol.* **2000**, *106*, 617-622.
56. Ortuño, A.; Arcas, M.C.; Botía, J.M.; Fuster, M.D.; Del Río, J.A. *J. Agric. Food Chem.* **2002**, 50, 2836-2839.
57. Del Río, J.A.; Arcas, M.C.; Botía, J.M.; Báidez, A.G.; Fuster, M.D.; Ortuño, A. In *Recent Res. Devel. Agric. Food Chem.*; Pandalai, S.G. Ed.; Research Signpost, India, **2000**; Vol. 4, pp 331-341.

Chapter 14

Modulation of Cholesterol and Triacylglycerol Biosynthesis by Citrus Polymethoxylated Flavones

Cholesterol-Lowering Properties of Citrus Flavonoids

John A. Manthey[1] and Elzbieta M. Kurowska[2]

[1]Citrus and Subtropical Products Laboratory, Agricultural Research Service, SAA, U.S. Department of Agriculture, Winter Haven, FL 33881
[2]KGK Synergize Inc., London, Ontario N6A 5R8 Canada

Citrus polymethoxylated flavones modulate the biosynthesis of cholesterol and triacylglycerols via multiple mechanisms. Tangeretin inhibits the activities of diacylglycerol acyltransferase and of microsomal triglyceride transfer protein, as well as activates the membrane peroxisome proliferator-activated receptor in human hepatoma *HepG2* cells. These modulatory effects subsequently inhibit the assembly and secretion of apolipoprotein B-containing lipoproteins, such as the very low-density lipoprotein (VLDL) and the low-density lipoprotein (LDL). Nobiletin, but not tangeretin, inhibited macrophage acetylated LDL metabolism linked to the action of the specific class A scavenger receptor. This inhibitory effect blocked the formation of macrophage foam-cells, which are essential to atherosclerotic plaque formation. In hamster feeding trials the polymethoxylated flavones dramatically lowered serum total cholesterol, LDL+VLDL cholesterol, as well as the levels of serum triacylglycerols. Total liver concentrations of tangeretin derivatives corresponded to hypolipidemic concentrations of intact tangeretin in earlier *in vitro* studies. If similar actions occur in humans, these compounds may be viable alternatives to the statin drugs to combat elevated cholesterol and triacylglycerols.

Citrus fruit are rich in polyphenols, particularly flavonoids and hydroxycinnamates, and in certain species, coumarins and psoralens (*1*). The flavonoids in citrus include several main classes of compounds including numerous flavanone glycosides, flavone glycosides and the highly methoxylated flavones, termed polymethoxylated flavones (PMFs) (Figure 1). These latter compounds lack glycosidation and contain few, if any, free phenolic hydroxyls. These chemical properties strongly influence the metabolism and oral bioavailability of the PMFs, as well as their interactions with other biological molecules. As lipophilic, planar molecules, PMFs are likely to exhibit significantly greater permeabilities across biological membranes than most glycosidated flavonoids and, as a consequence, are likely to exhibit a wide range of biological activities. Extensive biological testing of the PMFs in numerous enzyme inhibition assays, cell culture studies, and small animal trials has borne this out (*2*). However, with long-term dietary intake, many of the glycosidated flavonoids in citrus, *i.e.* hesperidin, naringin, diosmin, *etc.*, also show many similar biological actions, particularly pertaining to anticancer and anti-inflammation activities (*2*).

An important biological action for both the citrus flavanone glycosides, as well as for the PMFs, is the lowering of blood serum cholesterol (*3-11*). Hypolipidemic effects have also been observed for the nonglycosidated hesperetin and naringenin flavanone aglycones (*3*). These effects were first investigated in human hepatoma *HepG2* liver cells, using an assay measuring the production of atherogenic apolipoprotein B (apoB)-containing lipoproteins (apoB-Lp), such as the very low-density lipoprotein (VLDL) and the low-density lipoprotein (LDL). *HepG2* cells incubated with either hesperetin or naringenin exhibited lowered net secretion of LDL-associated apoB (*3*). The decreased apoB secretion occurred with a reduction in the levels of cellular cholesterol esters, whereas the cholesterol esterification decreased dose-dependently at flavonoid concentrations up to 200 μM (*3,4*). The IC_{50} values for the inhibition of apoB secretion were 43 μg/mL or 142.2 μM (hesperetin) and 48 μg/mL or 178.1 μM (naringenin) (*5*). Further studies also showed that naringenin and hesperetin inhibited the activities of the acyl CoA:cholesterol acyltransferases, ACAT1 and ACAT2, along with a selective inhibition of gene expression for ACAT2, and an inhibition of the microsomal triglyceride transfer protein (MTP) (*4*). Both hesperetin and naringenin increased the expression of the LDL receptor, an effect likely to increase cellular uptake and degradation of LDL (*4*). Naringenin was subsequently shown to inhibit the lipid assembly and subsequent secretion of apoB lipoproteins, primarily by decreasing triacylglycerol (TG) accumulation in the endoplasmic reticulum (*4*). The observed decreases in TG accumulation were linked to inhibition of the cellular MTP activity and gene expression (*6*).

Effects of the flavanone glycosides hesperidin and naringin on the levels of serum cholesterol and TGs have also been characterized in animal trials. Naringin fed to hypercholesterolemic rabbits did not significantly affect plasma cholesterol, but decreased the area of fatty streaks in thoracic aorta, and reduced

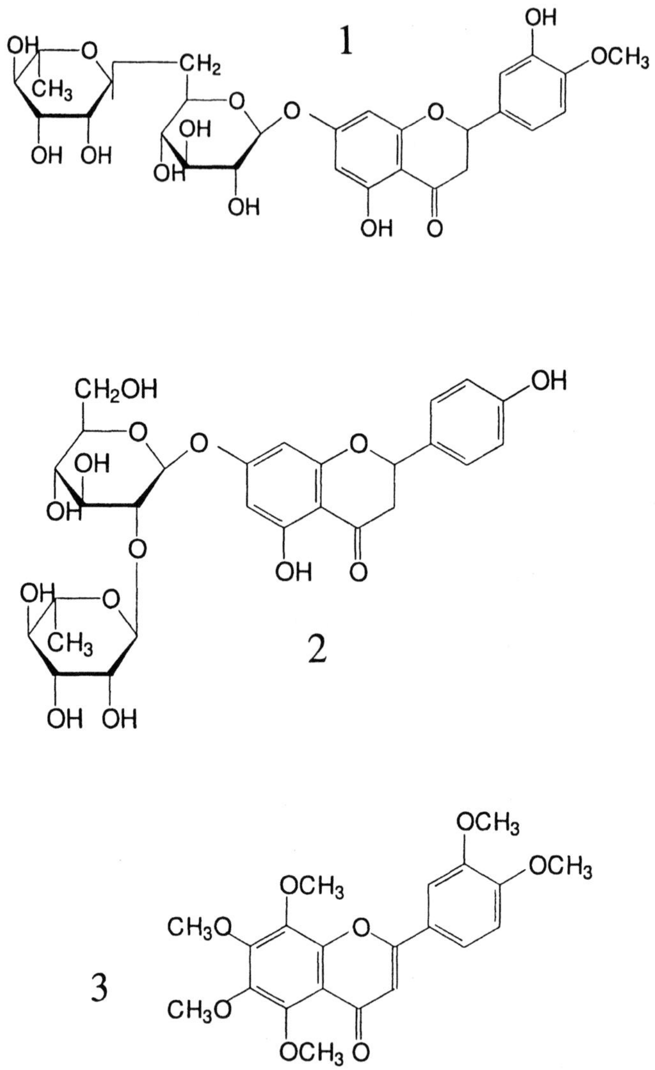

Figure 1. Structures of citrus PMFs and flavanone glycosides. 1, hesperidin;, 2, naringin; 3, nobiletin; 4, tangeretin; 5, heptamethoxyflavone; 6, sinensetin; 7, tetramethylscutellarein. *Continued on next page.*

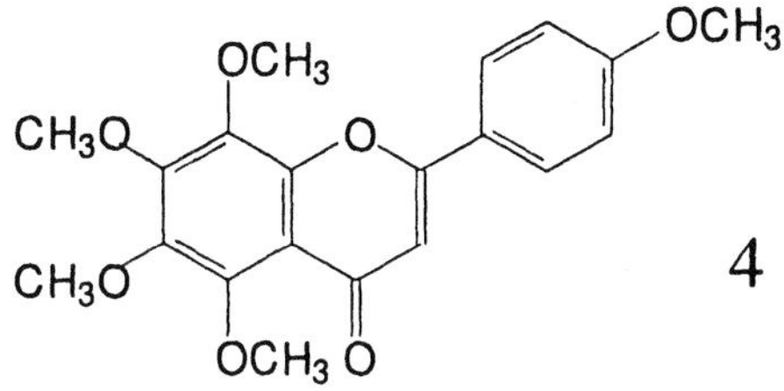

4

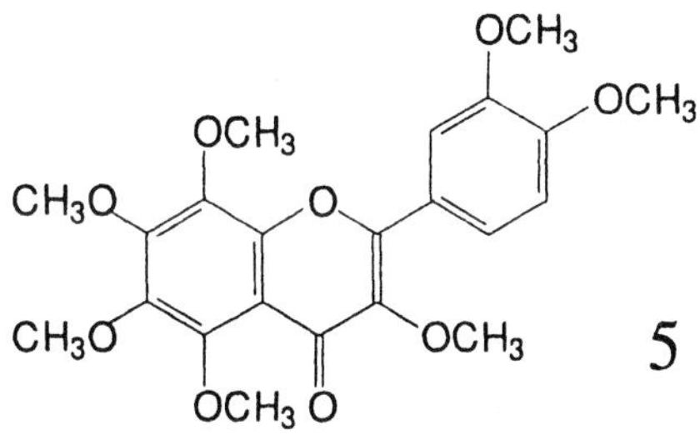

5

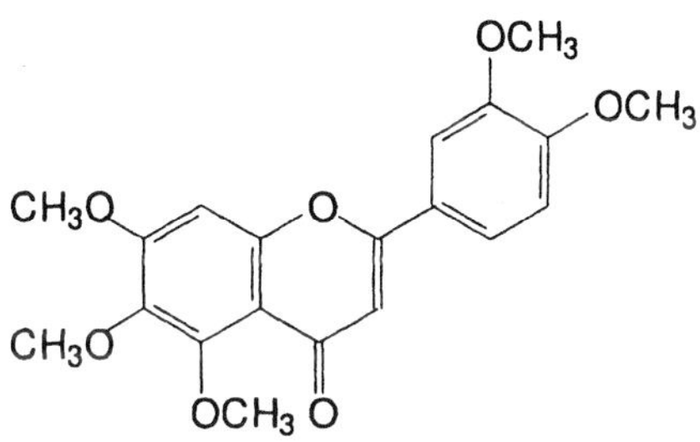

6

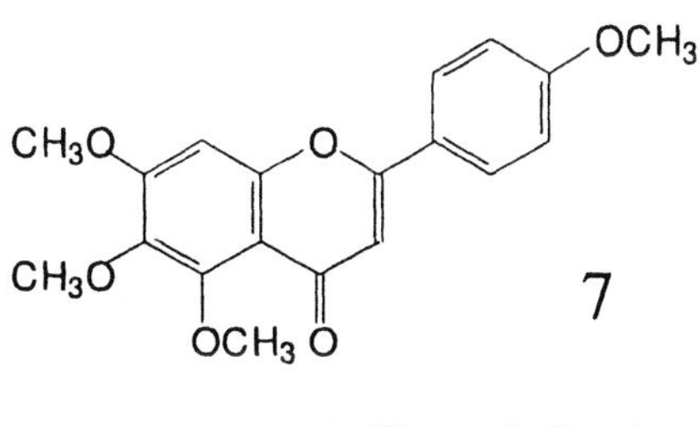

7

Figure 1. Continued.

subintimal foam cell infiltration on microscopic morphometry (7). Naringin inhibited the expression of the intercellular adhesion molecule -1 (ICAM-1) on endothelial cells of these treated animals. Attenuation of ICAM-1 similarly occurred in ischemic tissue treated with structurally related diosmin and hesperidin (*8*). In hypercholesterolemic rabbits, a diet containing 0.5% naringin produced dramatically lowered plasma total and LDL cholesterol and hepatic lipids. Male rabbits fed naringin exhibited lowered hepatic ACAT activities and exhibited sharply decreased levels of morphological damage in the vasculature induced by the high cholesterol diet (*9*). Similar decreases in hepatic ACAT activity and plasma cholesterol were detected in hesperidin- and naringin-fed rats maintained on a high cholesterol diet (*10,11*). An important distinction was observed between hesperidin and naringin in these animal studies. Significant decreases occurred in the levels of the plasma TGs in the naringin-fed rats, but not in the hesperidin-fed rats. Finally, male rats fed a high cholesterol diet along with 0.02% hesperetin, and alternatively a mixture of hesperetin metabolites (*m*-hydroxycinnamic acid, 3,4-dihydroxyphenylpropionic acid, and ferulic acid) had significantly reduced plasma TG and total cholesterol compared to the untreated controls (*12*). As part of a recent feeding trial, hypercholesterolemic hamsters were given a diet of a 3.0% hesperidin/naringin mixture. This diet produced a 28% decrease in serum total cholesterol, a 38% decrease in the serum VLDL and LDL cholesterol, an 18% decrease in the serum high density lipoprotein (HDL) cholesterol, and a 57% decrease in serum TGs (*13*). In contrast, this diet produced substantial increases in hepatic lipids, including, a 75% increase in total cholesterol, a 77% increase in free cholesterol, a 72% increase in cholesterol esters, but a 23% decrease in TGs. This latter effect on the TGs is in sharp contrast to the concurrent changes that occurred in the hepatic cholesterol and cholesterol conjugates.

In a recent human trial, a modified, water-soluble glucosyl hesperidin significantly lowered serum TGs in hypertriglyceridemic subjects, while no significant decreases occurred in total serum cholesterol (*14*). In contrast, administration of naringin to hypercholesterolemic humans produced only modest decreases in serum cholesterol and no decreases in plasma TGs (*15*). It would be interesting to determine what property of the soluble glucosyl hesperidin imparts the TG-lowering activity. Future trials with hesperidin would help determine if the activity of the modified glucosyl hesperidin is linked to the chemical constituents of the flavonoid aglycone, or to the increased solubility, and possibly to the increased bioavailability, of the modified, water-soluble glucosyl hesperidin.

In a similar manner, citrus PMFs exhibited lipid-lowering properties in cell culture studies as well as in small animal trials. Kurowska and Manthey (*5*) reported that PMFs isolated from orange oil inhibited apoB secretion by *HepG2* cells. IC_{50} values for these compounds were significantly lower than those of the flavanone aglycones, hesperetin (43 ppm) and naringenin (48 ppm). The three most active inhibitors were tangeretin (2.5 ppm), nobiletin (4.9 ppm), and 3,5,6,7,8,3',4'-heptamethoxyflavone (7.8 ppm).

Formulations containing PMFs were subsequently tested for lipid-lowering properties in hypercholesterolemic hamsters (*13*). Diets containing either 1.0% tangeretin or 1.0% of a 1/1 mixture of tangeretin and nobiletin had similar effects in lowering serum lipids. The 1.0% tangeretin diet produced a 25% decrease in serum total cholesterol, a 39% decrease in VLDL + LDL cholesterol, and a 48% decrease in serum TGs, while no change occurred in the high-density lipoprotein (HDL) cholesterol. In contrast, significant increases in liver lipids were observed, *i.e.* a 46% increase in total cholesterol, a 48% increase in free cholesterol, a 47% increase in cholesterol esters, but a 29% decrease in TG. A diet containing 0.25% of a 1/1 mixture of tangeretin and nobiletin showed the same trends, but produced smaller changes in the serum and liver lipids, with the important exception of serum TGs, which decreased by nearly the same levels associated with the higher percent PMF diets. A second hamster trial using a diet of a 1.0% PMF mixture produced similar changes in the serum lipids that occurred with the 1.0% tangeretin and 1.0% tangeretin/nobiletin diets.

A study was also conducted to identify and quantify tangeretin and nobiletin metabolites in blood serum, urine, and liver of hypercholesterolemic hamsters. HPLC-MS analyses of the metabolites in the blood serum showed the conversion of tangeretin into a series of dihydroxytrimethoxyflavone and monohydroxytetramethoxyflavone glucuronides. Only trace levels were detected of the aglycones and of unmodified tangeretin. The estimated total concentrations of all metabolites in the serum solids were 110 ppm, or an equivalent of 21 μM intact tangeretin. The occurrence of glucuronides in the liver and urine was similarly detected. Free aglycones ranged from 38 to 65% of the total metabolites in the liver, with the dihydroxytrimethoxyflavones constituting the major portions of these compounds. The total concentrations of all hepatic tangeretin metabolites were within the range of 25-106 ppm, an equivalent of 16-67 μM tangeretin in the fresh tissue. The total concentrations of PMF metabolites in the urine from hamsters fed 1.0% tangeretin, or 1.0 tangeretin/nobiletin diets were in the range from 11 to 21 mM. Nearly all of the metabolites in the urine were glucuronidated (*13*).

Ensuing biochemical studies of the lipid-lowering properties of the PMFs focused on the roles of tangeretin, for which the reduction of apoB secretion by *HepG2* cells was both rapid, and apoB specific (*16*). Figure 2 shows the inhibition time course resulting from exposure of the liver cells to 72 μM tangeretin for 0, 2, 4, and 8 hours. By 2 hours there was a nearly 50% reduction of apoB secretion, and no further medium accumulation of apoB occurred beyond 4 hours. The inhibition was not due to decreased viability of the tangeretin-treated cells, nor was it due to increased proteosomal degradation of extracellular apoB. *HepG2* cells incubated with 72 μM tangeretin for 24 h, then postincubated in tangeretin-free media, secreted apoB within 70 to 80% of the levels of the untreated cells, suggesting a partial reversibility of the apoB-lowering effect. Another important finding was that when the liver cells were incubated with ^{3}H-leucine, with and without tangeretin, there was no difference

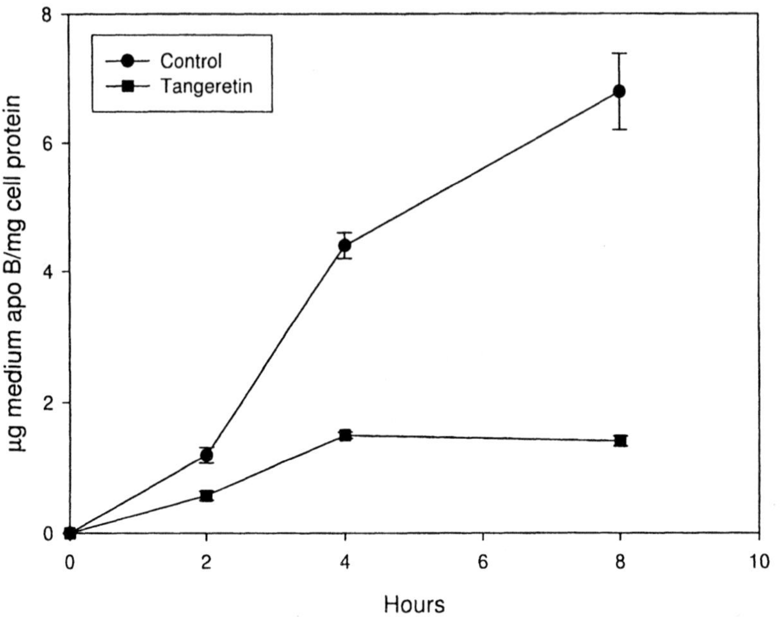

Figure 2. Inhibition time course resulting from exposure of HepG2 *liver cells to 72 µM tangeretin for 0, 2, 4, 8 hours. (Reproduced with permission from reference 16. Copyright 2004 AOCS.)*

in total trichloroacetic acid precipitable radioactivity, whereas, the sharp decrease that occurred for the apoB following this treatment indicated that the effects produced by tangeretin were specific for apoB.

One possible mechanism of blocking apoB-Lp secretion by liver cells is the inhibition of the synthesis of lipids necessary for its assembly and export. To test this mechanism, tangeretin was evaluated for its ability to inhibit lipid synthesis and accumulation in *HepG2* cells. This was done by measuring the effects of tangeretin on the cellular synthesis of cholesterol, cholesterol esters and TGs (*16*). Cells incubated with [1- ^{14}C]acetate or [1- ^{14}C]glycerol were treated for 24 h in the presence vs. absence of 72 □M tangeretin. Tangeretin reduced the rates of incorporation of radiolabeled precursors into cellular cholesterol, cholesterol esters and TGs by 45, 82, and 64%, respectively.

The inhibition of TG synthesis by naringenin, similar to that for tangeretin, was previously shown to strongly reduce the rate of early assembly and secretion of lipids into apoB-Lp (*3*,*4*). One of the critical control points in the assembly of lipids into apoB is the rate of TG synthesis, catalyzed by diacylglycerol acyltransferase (DGAT). By controlling the rate determining step between diacylglycerol and fatty acid CoA, DGAT controls the availability of TGs for lipid assembly into apoB and subsequent transport of lipoproteins out of the cell (*17*). To test whether tangeretin influences the activity of DGAT in liver cells, DGAT activity was measured after exposure of *HepG2* cells to tangeretin for 24 h (*16*). Tangeretin at 29 µM and 72 :M decreased the rates of incorporation of ^{14}C-palmitoyl-CoA into cellular TGs by DGAT by 35% and 39%, respectively. These results failed to show a strong dose dependency at these tangeretin concentrations, but did provide an indication that tangeretin is able to influence TG synthesis at this DGAT-catalyzed rate determining step.

A second important control point in the early assembly of lipids into lipoproteins involves the MTP, where the inhibition of this transfer protein has been shown to influence the secretion of apoB-Lp (*18*). Using the same basic protocol as before, tangeretin was tested for its effect on the MTP at 29 □M and 72 □M tangeretin. On incubation at these concentrations, the cellular MTP activity was inhibited by 22% and 35%, respectively (*16*).

A final mechanism investigated for tangeretin pertained to the activation of the peroxisome proliferator-activated receptor (PPAR), which in the liver, reduces the quantity of fatty acids available for the synthesis of TGs by enhancing beta-oxidation of fatty acids via the activation of acyl CoA oxidase and carnitine palmitoyl-CoA transferase (*19,20*). To evaluate this, liver cells were treated with tangeretin at 29 □M and 72 □M for 24 h and PPAR activity in homogenates of these treated cells was assessed by electophoretic mobility shift assays and autoradiography (*16*). The results showed that in the presence of tangeretin PPAR activation increased by 25% at 29 □M and by 36% at 72 □M. These results suggest that tangeretin-induced increases in PPAR activity might contribute to decreases in cellular accumulation of TGs *via* beta-oxidation, and represent a DGAT-independent mechanism of inhibiting TG synthesis. The mechanistic findings on the actions of tangeretin suggest that PMFs influence lipid synthesis, lipid assembly into apoB-Lp, and secretion of lipoproteins out of liver cells by multiple mechanisms. These mechanisms are summarized in Figure 3. The complex actions of PMFs are consistent with their effects on the plasma lipids observed in hypercholesterolemic hamsters (*13*). Clinical trials are in progress to determine if similar effects occur in humans following dietary intake of PMFs.

Other important cardioprotective actions of the citrus PMFs pertain to their effects on macrophages and vascular inflammation. Macrophages are intimately linked to many different chronic diseases including atherosclerotic plaque formation (*21*). In large part, the involvement of macrophages in atherosclerosis is their uptake of LDL and oxidized LDL, and their subsequent transformation into foam cells. Uptake of lipoproteins by macrophages is initiated by their binding to cell surface receptors followed by their internalization and catabolism (*22-24*). There are specificities in the receptors involved in the uptake of lipoprotein by macrophages, including the LDL receptor (*23*), and the class A scavenger receptors (SR-A), which selectively bind chemically modified LDL (*i.e.* oxidized LDL). Generation of oxidized LDL is largely driven by the action of lipoxygenases and the generation of superoxide anion (*25,26*). While the uptake of native, unmodified LDL by macrophage receptors is a highly

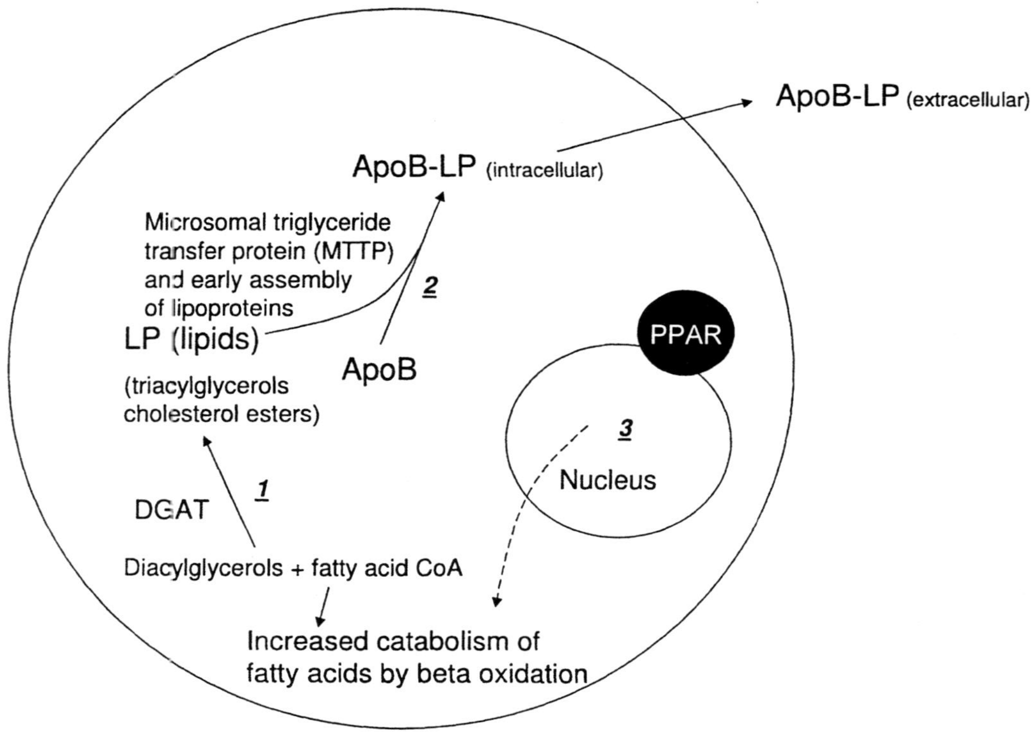

Figure 3. Summary of sites of activity of the PMFs in decreasing apoB secretion and TG synthesis. 1: Inhibition of diacylglycerol acyltransferase (DGAT). 2: Inhibition of MTP. 3: Activation of PPAR, and increased catabolism of fatty acids.

regulated event (*27*), the uptake of modified cholesterol of LDL by the SR-A receptors is unregulated, and is a primary event that drives atherosclerotic plaque formation (*28*).

The abilities of naringenin, hesperetin, tangeretin, and nobiletin, to mediate SR-A expression and metabolism were examined in cultured mouse J774A.1 macrophages (*29*). A known ligand of the SR-A receptor, acetylated LDL (acLDL), was used in these studies as a marker of the SR-A receptor activity (*30*). In macrophages, all four flavonoids inhibited cellular uptake of beta-VLDL by the LDL receptor, while only nobiletin inhibited macrophage-mediated metabolism of acLDL. This inhibition occurred without changes in the total levels of SR-A protein or in the expression of the receptor on the plasma membrane. Sites of action were speculated by Whitman *et al.* (*29*) to possibly include second-messenger signaling pathways involving phosphatidylinositol-3-OH kinase (*31*), the inhibitory/other subclass of guanine nucleotide binding proteins ($G_{i/o}$-proteins) (*32*), or similar pathways. Many flavonoids have a propensity to interact with nucleotide binding sites (discussed below), and a similar type of receptor/protein binding may be a mode of action of nobiletin in this particular receptor system. These results suggest, therefore, that nobiletin may prevent atherosclerosis *via* a number of mechanisms, the first by reducing plasma VLDL, LDL, and TGs, and by directly inhibiting macrophage-derived foam cell formation at the site of injury in vascular tissue.

Relevant to this discussion of the anti-atherosclerotic properties of PMFs are the findings that PMFs exhibit yet other biological actions that may prevent cardiovascular disease, particularly their inhibition of chronic inflammation. Again, many of these actions are attributable to the effects of PMFs on macrophages and on proinflammatory responses of activated monocytes. Manthey *et al.* (*33*) reported that PMFs suppress production of the tumor necrosis factor-α by lipopolysaccharide (LPS)-activated human monocytes. Also inhibited was the formation of the macrophage inflammatory protein-lα (MIP-lα) and interleukin-l0 (IL-10). IL-10 plays complex roles in lipid uptake by macrophage-derived foam cells and atherosclerotic plaque stabilization (*34*). The most active compound, 3,5,6,7,8,3',4'-heptamethoxyflavone (HMF), induced a substantial elevation of cAMP in activated monocytes. Similarities in the profiles of cytokine inhibition by PMFs to the profile of the known phosphodiesterase-4 inhibitor, 3-isobutyl-1-methylxanthine, suggest that PMFs inhibit cytokine production by suppression of phosphodiesterase-4. Further actions of PMFs on macrophages during inflammation were subsequently shown by nobiletin's inhibition of LPS-induced production of prostaglandin E2 in J774A.1 macrophages (*35*). Nobiletin inhibited gene expression of the pro-inflammatory IL-1α, IL-β, IL-6 and tumor necrosis factor-α in these LPS-activated macrophages. The inhibitory effects of nobiletin on the expression of the cycbooxygenase-2 and inducible NO synthase proteins, and of prostaglandin E2 release in mouse macrophage RAW 264.7 cells have also been reported (*35,36*). Inhibitory actions similar to these are likely to contribute to the anti inflammatory properties of PMFs, and possibly play roles in the prevention of cardiovascular disease.

While many of the biological activities of flavonoids, such as the PMFs, can be linked to their inhibition of enzymes involved in chronic diseases (*37*), the mechanisms of these inhibitions at the molecular level are unclear. Yet, the evidence of the binding of flavonoids suggests that these compounds, or their metabolites, attenuate cellular events *via* receptor binding, and thus influence cell activation processes. It would be logical to suggest that allosteric binding may contribute to the inhibition of a number of enzymes involved in inflammation and atherosclerotic plaque formation. Yet, specificity has been widely reported for the binding of many flavonoids to the ATP binding sites of a number of regulatory enzymes (kinases, ATPases, phosphodiesterases, etc.) (*37,38*). In the inhibition of phosphodiesterases, quantum chemical calculations have suggested that the competition between the pyrone ring of the flavonoids and the pyrimidine ring of cAMP occurs *via* $\pi \rightarrow \pi$ interactions between these molecules and the nucleotide binding sites (*38*). Similarities were also detected in the charge distributions of the pyrone rings of the flavonoids and the pyrimidine ring of cAMP, suggesting that similar interactions occur for the binding of flavonoids and cAMP with the nucleotide binding pocket.

Similar types of interactions between PMFs and nucleotide binding sites have been further indicated by the tight binding of these compounds to the several classes of human adenosine receptors. These receptors are involved in the immune, cardiovascular, and central nervous systems (*39,40*); thus, these systems are potential targets of action by agonists/antagonists of adenosine. The A_3 receptors have already been implicated in vascular effects, inflammation, and cancer (*41*), three areas where flavonoids show considerable activity (*2*). Structure/activity relationships for the binding of plant flavonoids to the three subtypes of adenosine receptors (A_1, A_{2A}, and A_3) have been extensively analyzed (*42*), where methylations of hydroxyl constituents typically increased binding to the three subclasses of receptors (*43*). These findings led to the study of the binding of citrus PMFs to the three subtypes of adenosine receptors. Most of the PMFs analyzed in this study exhibited affinities to the A_1 and A_{2a} receptors in the micromolar range, but showed little selectivity (*41*). Three of the PMFs, 3-hydroxy-5,7,3',4'-tetramethoxyflavone, sinensetin, and 5,7,3',4'-tetramethylquercetin exhibited binding constants, K_i, below 1 μM for their binding to the A_3 receptor.

The understanding of the biological actions of PMFs in the prevention of chronic diseases is still incomplete, but the wide range of actions detected for these compounds suggests that there are numerous sites of action with far ranging effects on cell activation and cell signaling processes. Thus far, data suggest that PMFs influence a variety of events relating to atherosclerosis and inflammation and their inhibition of these underlying disease states may prove useful for their eventual commercialization as either nutraceuticals or food ingredients with targeted pharmacological endpoints.

References

1. Berhow, M.; Tisserat, B.; Kanes, K.; Vandercook, C. Survey of Phenolic Compounds Produced in Citrus. Technical Bulletin 1856. U.S. Department of Agriculture, Agricultural Research Service, Peoria, IL 1998.
2. Manthey, J.A.; Guthrie, N.; Grohmann, K. *Curr. Med. Chem.* **2001**, *8*, 135-153.
3. Borradaile, N.M.; Carroll, K.K.; Kurowska, E.M. *Lipids* **1999**, *34*, 591-598.
4. Wilcox, L.J.; Borradaile, N.M.; De Dreu, L.E.; Huff, M.W. *J. Lipid Res.* **2001**, *42*, 725-734.
5. Kurowska, E.M.; Manthey, J.A. *Advances in Experimental Medicine and Biology* **2002**, *505* (Flavonoids in Cell Function), 173-179.
6. Borradaile, N.M.; De Dreu, L.E.; Barrett, P.; Hugh, R.; Murray, W. *J. Lipid Res.* **2002**, *43*, 1544-1554.
7. Choe, S.C.; Kim, H.S.; Jeong, T.S.; Bok, S.H.; Park, Y.B. .J. *Caradiovasc. Pharmacol.* **2001**, *38*, 947-955.
8. Korthuis, R.J.; Gute, D.C. *J. Vasc. Res.* **1999**, *36 (Suppl. 1)*, 15-23.
9. Jeon, S.-M.; Park, Y.B.; Choi, M.-S. *Clin. Nutr.* **2004**, *23*, 1025-1034.
10. Park, Y.-B.; Do, K.-M.; Bok, S.-H.; Lee, M.-K.; Jeong, T.-S.; Choi, M.-S. *Int. J. Vit. Nutr. Res.* **2001**, *71*, 36-44.
11. Choi, M.-S.; Do, K.-M.; Park, Y.-B.; Jeon, S.-M.; Jeong, T.-S.; Lee, Y.-K.; Bok, S.-H. *Annals of Nutrition and Metabolism* **2001**, *45*, 193-201.
12. Kim, H.-K.; Jeong, T.-S.; Lee, M.-K.; Park, Y.-B.; Choi, M.-S. *Clin. Chim. Acta* **2003**, *327*, 129-137.
13. Kurowska, E.M.; Manthey, J.A. *J. Agric. Food Chem.* **2004**, *52*, 2879-2886.
14. Miwa, Y.; Yamada, M.; Sunayama, T.; Mitsuzumi, H.; Tsuzake, Y.; Chaen, H.; Mishima, Y.; Kibata M.; *J. Nut. Sci. Vitamin.* **2004**, *50*, 211-218.
15. Jung, U.J.; Kim, H.J.; Lee, M.K.; Kim, H.O.; Park, E.J.; Kim, H.K.; Heong, T.S.; Choi, MS. *Clin. Nutrition.* **2003**, *22*, 561-568.
16. Kurowska, E.M.; Manthey, J.A.; Casachi, A.; Theriaubt, A.G. *Lipids*, **2004**, *39*, 143-151.
17. Farese, R.V., Jr.; Cases, S.; Smith, S.J. *Curr. Opin. Lipidol.* **2000**, *11*, 229-234.
18. Gordon, D.A.; Jamil, H. *Biochim. Biophys. Acta* **2000**, *1486*, 72-83.
19. Keller, J.M.; Collet, H.; Bianchi, A.; huin, C.; Bouillaud-Kremarik, P.; Becuwe, P.; Schohn, H.; Domenjoud, L.; Dauca, M. *Int. J. Dev. Biol.* **2000**, *44*, 429-442.
20. Rodríguez, J.C.; Gil-Gómez, G.; Hegardt, F.G.; Haro, D. *J. Biol. Chem.* **1994**, *269*, 18767-18772.
21. Castillo, A.; Tontonoz, P. *Ann. Rev. Cell Develop. Biol.* **2004**, *20*, 455-480.
22. Goldstein, J.L.; Anderson, R.G.; Brown, M.S. *Nature* **1979**, *279*, 679-685.
23. Goldstein, J.L.; Brown, M.S.; Anderson, R.G.; Russell, D.W.; Schneider, W.J. *Annu. Rev. Cell Biol.* **1985**, *1*, 1-39.

24. Brown, M.S.; Goldstein, J.L. *Proc. Natl. Acad. Sci. USA*, **1979**, *76*, 3330-3337.
25. Steinbrecher, U.P.; Parthasarathy, S.; Leake, D.S.; Witztum, J.L.; Steinberg, D. *Proc. Natl. Acad. Sci. USA* **1984**, *81*, 3883-3887.
26. Kuhn, H.; Belkner, J.; Zaiss, S.; Fahrenklemper, T.; Wohlfeil, S. *J. Exp. Med.* **1994**, *179*, 1903-1911.
27. Brown, M.S.; Goldstein, J.L. *Annu. Rev. Biochem.* **1983**, *52*, 223-261.
28. Steinberg, D.; Parthasarathy, S.; Carew, T.E.; Khoo, J.C.; Witztum, J.L. *N. Engl. J. Med.* **1989**, *320*, 915-924.
29. Whitman, S.C.; Kurowska, E.M.; Manthey, J.A.; Daugherty, A. *Atherosclerosis* **2005**, *178*, 25-32.
30. Cornicelli, J.A.; Butteiger, D.; Rateri, D.L.; Welch, K.; Daugherty, A. *J. Lipid Res.* **2000**, *41*, 376-383.
31. Whitman, S.C.; Daugherty, A.; Post, S.R. *J. Lipid Res.* **2000**, *41*, 807-813.
32. Sano, H.; Higashi, T.; Matsumoto, K. *J. Biol. Chem.* **1998**, *273*, 8630-8637.
33. Manthey, J.A.; Grohmann, K.; Montanari, A.; Ash, K.; Manthey, C.L. *J. Nat. Prod.* **1999**, *62*, 441-444.
34. Halvorsen, B.; Waehre, T.; Scholz, H.; Clausen, O.; Von der Thuesen, J.H.; Mueller, F.; Heimli, H.; Tonstad, S.; Hall, C.; Froland, S.; Biessen, E.A.; Damas, J.K.; Aukrust, P. *J. Lipid Res.* **2005**, *46*, 211-219.
35. Lin, N.; Sato, T.; Takayama, Y. *Biochem. Pharmacol.* **2003**, *65*, 2065,2071.
36. Murakami, A.; Nakamura, Y.; Torikai, K. *Cancer Res.* **2000**, *60*, 5059-5066.
37. Middleton, E., J.; Kandaswami, C. *Biochem. Pharmcol.* **1992**, *4*, 1167-1179.
38. Ferrell, J.E., Jr.; Chang Sing, P.D.G.; Loew, G.; King, R.; Mansour, J.M.; Mansour, T.E. *Molecular Pharmacol.* **1979**, *16*, 556-568.
39. Strickler, J.; Jacobson, K.A.; Liant, B.T. *J. Clin. Invest.* **1996**, *98*, 1773-1779.
40. Sajjadi, F.G.; Takabayashi, K.; Foster, A.C.; Domingo, R.C.; Firestein, G.S. *J. Immmunol.* **1996**, *156*, 3435-3442.
41. Jacobson, K.A.; Stefano, J.; Manthey, J.A.; West, P.L.; Ji, X.-D. *Advances in Experimental Medicine and Biology* **2002**, *505* (Flavonoids in Cell Function), 173-179.
42. Karton, Y.; Jiang, J.L.; Ji, X.-D.; Melman, N.; Olah, M.E.; Stiles, G.L.; Jacobson, K.A. *J. Med Chem.* **1996**, *39*, 2293-2301.
43. Hasrat, J.A.; De Bruyne, T.; DeBacker, J.P.; Vauquelin, G.; Vlietinck, A.J. *J. Pharm. Pharmacol.* **1997**, *49*, 1150-1156.

Chapter 15

The Health Benefits of Modified Citrus Pectin

Isaac Eliaz[1], John Guardino[1], and Kerry Hughes[2]

[1]Amitabha Medical Clinic and Healing Center, 7064 Corline Court, Suite A, Sebastopol, CA 95472
[2]EthnoPharm, P.O. Box 3222, Vallejo, CA 94590

Modified citrus pectin (MCP) is a dietary supplement derived from citrus pectin, which has been modified to produce a product of low molecular weight and low esterification. In contrast, extracted, unmodified citrus pectin contains molecules of many varying lengths and is highly esterified. Fragmented pectin of low molecular weight is more readily absorbed into the blood stream. Dietary supplement grade MCP is designed to provide these more absorbable pectins in order to deliver greater health benefits. Although clinical indications and effectiveness of MCP is still being studied, recent research suggests that MCP may have significant health benefits. In vitro, animal studies and human clinical trials have demonstrated applications in the prevention and treatment of cancer in reducing solid tumor growth, metastasis, and angiogenesis. Recent research also indicates that MCP may play an important therapeutic role as a chelator of heavy metals. The health benefits, including clinical indications, preclinical research, clinical data, dosage and safety of MCP are discussed in this review.

Historic Use Of Citrus Pectin

Although pectin has a long tradition for use in household cooking for gelling jams, it was not produced industrially until early in the 20th century. In the food and pharmaceutical technology industries, pectins are used as stabilizers and gelifiers (European identification code E440a [pectins] and E440b [amidated pectins]) (*1*). They are used for such diverse applications as yogurt, confectionery, and acid milk drinks. The natural image, functionality, and nutritional benefits of pectin have stimulated the development of new applications in the food, pharmaceutical and cosmetic industries. Much of the interest in the health benefits of citrus pectin was generated from the large body of research on fibers. After the initial wave of enthusiasm in dietary fiber diminished, citrus pectin as a dietary supplement or ingredient likewise became a less popular topic. Today, as functional foods are a fast growing segment of the food industry, new applications are being discovered for food ingredients. As a dietary aid, pectins have been proven to be efficacious in treating hyperlipidemia and in preventing cardiovascular disease (*1, 2, 8*).

Pectins have also been used in pharmaceutical because of their hydrophilicity. Upon absorption of water they become a thickening agent that can regularize the transit of gastric contents. In this way, they have been useful for the symptomatic treatment of vomiting in infants and for diarrhea (*1*). Specifically, citrus pectin has been shown to be able to improve small and large bowel mucosal structure, prolong intestinal transit and decrease diarrhea. It is also able to improve the colonic absorptive function when added in enteral liquid diet in preclinical studies (*23*).

History And Development Of Mcp

The history of the development of MCP begins with the research of Avraham Raz who was the first to discover and publish on the role of galectin-3 molecules in cancer. In one experiment, he and his colleagues found direct evidence of the role of galactoside-binding lectin in cancer. Recombinant galactoside-binding lectin was inserted into tumorigenic, weakly metastatic, fibrosarcoma cells, and this resulted in an increase in the incidence of lung metastasis in both syngeneic and nude mice. He concluded that these results demonstrated direct evidence for the relationship between galactoside-binding lectin, transformation and metastasis (*20, 21*).

Platt and Raz (*19*) were the first to test this theory, and designed a study to compare regular citrus pectin (CP) against MCP for its effect on lung tumors.

MCP injected into syngeneic mice resulted in a significant decrease in lung colonization while the injection of CP resulted in a significant increase. In a follow-up study, Inohara and Raz (*14*) investigated the effects of both CP and MCP on the cell-cell and cell-matrix interactions that are mediated by carbohydrate-recognition. They concluded that the carbohydrate recognition of galectin-3 may be the mechanism of cell-extracellular matrix interaction, and that this may be related to how the tumor cell grows, as well as the embolization of tumor cells.

Pienta and his collaborators then showed the efficacy of orally administered MCP on metastasis (*18*). Five years later, Strum et al. (*24*) performed the first pilot human clinical trial on MCP for its effect on prostate cancer (specifically the PSA doubling time). By this time, the chemistry and manufacturing of MCP had become more standardized, and elegant techniques had been developed to provide a more predictable, standardized MCP product. A second, phase II clinical trial investigating its effect on disease activity in prostate cancer patients with a significant response was completed (*11*).

Chemistry

Although pectin is found in the cell wall of all citrus fruits, the industrial product is extracted from citrus waste (with 30-35% pectins in the albedo, and a yield of about 10%) generated by fruit juice manufacturing. Chemically unaltered citrus pectin is a complex polysaccharide (long-chain carbohydrate) that has many branches and a high degree of methylation (Figure 1). Weakly methylated pectins have a degree of methylation up to 50 percent and those above 50% are considered highly methylated. The degree of methylation of unmodified citrus pectin is about 70-75 percent. Standard citrus pectin is industrially produced by inactivating enzymes with heat and dissolving dried citrus peels in a hot acidic aqueous solution. The extract is then centrifuged or filtered (and possibly digested with amylase to free it from starch) and precipitated by the addition of isopropanol. The precipitate is filtered, dried and ground (*1*).

There are generally two kinds of pectin polysaccharides, homogalacturonans and rhamnogalacturonans. Homogalacturonans are rare, as they are highly methoxylated and are mainly consisted of a chain of 1→4-linked α–D-galacturonic acid. Rhamnogalacturonans have a main chain with repeating α-L-rhamnose units. The configuration is as follows:

$$\rightarrow 4)\text{-}\alpha\text{-D-Gal}p\text{A-}(1\rightarrow 2)\text{-}\beta\text{-L-Rha}p\text{-}(1\rightarrow$$

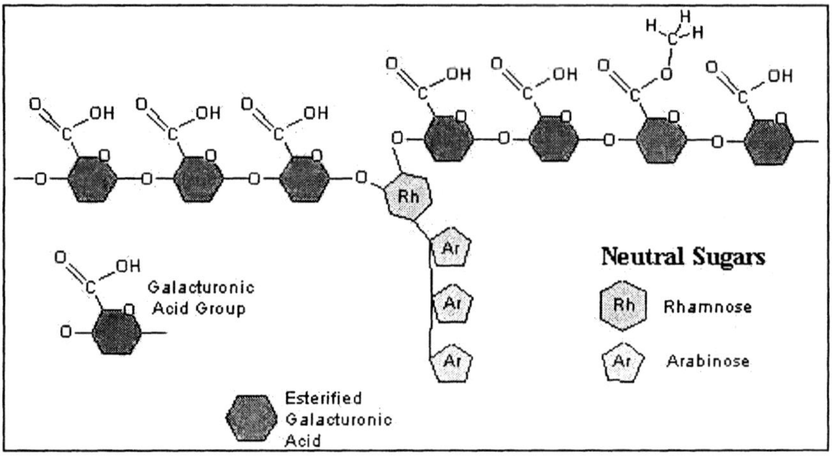

Figure 1. An illustration of unmodified citrus pectin

Some pectins may have polymers with almost purely galacturonic regions without the interruption of rhamnose units, and others that have a predictable repetition of rhamnose and galacturonic acid. Often, pectin polymers are macromolecules that have alternating non-substituted segments (smooth zones) and others that have segments with many substitutions (hairy zones) (*1*). Commercially available citrus pectin has extensive branching (hairy zones) and averages 10-100 kDa (*15*).

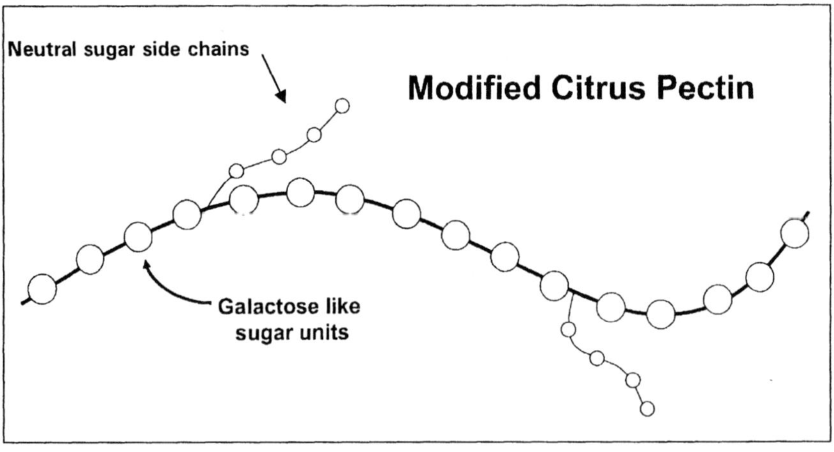

Figure 2. An illustration of a Modified Citrus Pectin chain with repeating galactose units.

There are many ways to alter citrus pectin in order to create different structural properties, which confer different functional properties. MCP was originally produced using a relatively crude technique of high-pH treatment of the main galacturonic chains followed by a low-pH treatment, resulting in an average molecular weight of approximately 10KDa. Since then, more sophisticated techniques have been developed using enzymatic degradation resulting in a more standardized product (*15*). MCP sold as a dietary supplement and researched clinically is generally manufactured using enzymatic degradation techniques. This results in an altered form of citrus pectin that is made up of lower molecular weight chain compounds with low methoxy content and increased water-solubility. Galactose is one of the polysaccharide components present in MCP, and it is this compound that is though to interact with galectin-3 (galactose-specific lectins) proteins on the cell wall surface of cancer cells.

Pharmacology

MCP has been found to have many of the same health benefits as regular citrus pectin, as it is of similar composition, but may be absorbed more readily into the blood stream. Some forms of MCP have been observed to lower cholesterol in clinical studies (*3, 16, 25*).

Two exciting areas of therapeutic research that are ongoing with MCP are its potential use for halting cancer metastasis and its use as a chelator of toxic metals. MCP's mechanism of action for the treatment of cancer involves its interference with both cell to cell and cell to cellular matrix interactions that are mediated by the carbohydrate binding galectin-3 molecules. The role of therapeutic agents that affect carbohydrate mediated recognition processes is an evolving field of cancer research. Many stages of cancer growth and progression have been found to involve these recognition processes. As metastasis is one of the key aspects in cancer that determines its survival, controlling cellular growth and progression before it reaches this point is an important treatment strategy. MCP's potential use as a therapeutic agent, for cancer is an important field of future study.

Galectins are present on a number of different types of cancer cells, including those of prostate, breast, colon, lymphoma, melanoma, glioblastoma and laryngeal epidermoid cancer. As cancer progresses in stages, galectin density has been observed to increase proportionally on the cell surface. When metastasis occurs, galectins are known to play a roll in cellular adhesion and the ability of the cancer cells to 'take root' in a new site in the body.

As it is rich in galactoside residues, MCP has a natural affinity for cancer cells with galectin-3 receptors. MCP molecules have the ability to bind to galectins (Figure 3) and inhibit the cancer from growing and developing to more advanced stages (*3, 22*). There is also evidence that MCP may also play a role in reducing solid tumor growth (*17*).

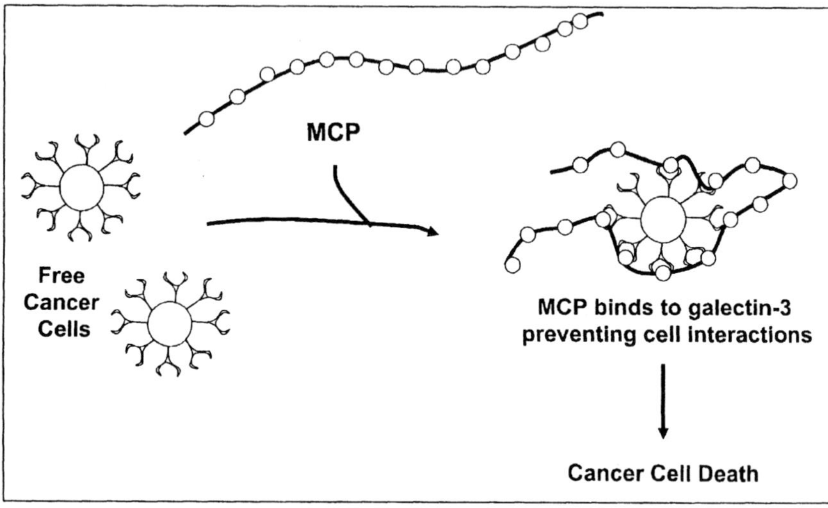

Figure 3. MCP binding to and blocking galectin receptors on a cancer cell, thereby preventing further cancer development.

Key Preclinical Studies

MCP has been found preclinically to mediate tumor growth, angiogenesis and metastasis presumably through the alteration in function of galectin-3. Preclinical work on MCP for its use in cancer has focused on melanomas, lung, breast and prostate cancer cell types. Specifically, the effect of MCP on in vivo tumor growth, angiogenesis, and metastasis was studied in athymic mice.

Breast Cancer and MCP in Mice and *in vitro:*

Nangia-Makker et al. (*17*) fed mice MCP in order to determine its effect on human breast cancer cells. Mice were given MCP orally and then injected orthotopically with human breast cancer cells (MDA-MB-435).

Tumor growth, angiogenesis, and spontaneous metastasis in vivo were significantly reduced with the administration of MCP.

Nangia-Makker et al. (*17*) tested MCP in vitro in experiments involving human umbilical vein endothelial cells (HUVEC) binding to galactin-3. When MCP was administered at a concentration of: 0.1%, it inhibited binding by 72.1%, and at a concentration of 0.25% inhibition was 95.8%. Chemotaxis of HUVEC towards galactin-3 was then measured, and it was found a 0.005% concentration was able to inhibit chemotaxis by 68%, and a 0.1% concentration was able to inhibit chemotaxis by 100%. Breast cancer cells expressing galactin-3 were inhibited in binding to HUVEC dose-dependently by MCP. These experiments found an inhibitory effect of MCP on suppressing tumor growth, angiogenesis and metastasis. The mechanism of action was presumed to be through the interference of galactin-3 function. However, quantitative absorption of MCP and into the bloodstream and corresponding dosage has not been established.

Colon cancer and MCP in mice:

MCP was tested for its effect on solid tumor growth in balb-c mice with colon-25 implanted tumors. MCP was administered in a low dose of 0.8 mg/ml or a high dose of 1.6 mg/ml in drinking water on a daily basis. When compared against control mice that were administered 1 ml distilled water, palpitation of the tumors showed a significant reduction in size in both treatment groups. The low dose treatment resulted in a 36% decrease in tumor size, while the high-dose treatment resulted in a 70% reduction in tumor size (*12*).

Prostate Cancer and MCP: *in vitro* and animal studies:

Hsieh and Wu (*13*) tested MCP for its effect on cell growth, cyclin/kinase, endogenous phosphoproteins and nm23 gene expression in human prostate cells. The effect of MCP on nm23 protein was investigated because of the reported inverse relationship between metastasis and nm23 gene expression in some cancer cells. MCP was added to the media of the cultured androgen-independent prostatic JCA-1 cells.

MCP was found to reduce cell growth, reduce [3H]thymidine incorporation into DNA, increase specific endogenous phosphoproteins (including cAMP-stimulated 52,000 protein), and suppress nm23 protein.

The reduced [3H]thymidine incorporation into DNA was correlated to the down-regulation of cyclin B and p34cdc2 expression.

Pienta et al. (*18*) studied the effect of MCP on the metastasis of prostate adenocarcinoma cells in rats. The rats were injected with one million MAT-LyLu cells on day 0, and then the mice were administered MCP in their drinking water from day 4 until day 30 at 0.0%, 0.01%, 0.1%, or 1.0% (wt/vol). Lung metastases were found in 15 out of 16 of the rats in the control group. In the treatment groups the numbers were reduced to 7 out of 14 rats in the 0.1% group, and 9 out of 16 of the rats in the 1.0% group. Primary tumors were not found to be reduced in any of the groups, therefore the authors concluded the MCP was inhibiting the spontaneous metastasis of prostate carcinomas in the Copenhagen rat.

Clinical Data

There has been limited clinical data for the therapeutic use of MCP, and those clinical studies that do exist have been mostly at a pilot level. However, one phase II clinical trial investigating the therapeutic effect in cancer was conducted (*10*). The indications for which MCP has been tested clinically have been for cancer and metastasis and for heavy metal chelation. The outcome measure used for determining MCP's effect in cancer has been measurements of the prostate specific antigen (PSA) doubling time in patients with recurrent prostate cancer after local ablation of the prostate with either surgery or radiation. Recent clinical studies demonstrated the use of MCP for the chelation of heavy metals from the body (*5, 7*).

Cancer Growth and Metastasis:

In a pilot clinical trial on the effect of MCP (Pecta-Sol®) on prostate cancer, Strum et al. (*24*) demonstrated beneficial effects on patient prostate specific antigen (PSA) doubling time. This pilot trial included subjects who had relapsed or failed prior cancer treatment. Subjects were given 15 grams daily of MCP (in three divided doses) and PSA doubling time was measured. A greater than 30% lengthening in the doubling time was found in 4 out of 7 of the patients. Patients who responded the most were those with a low starting PSA level. Three years after this study all participants were still alive for follow up.

In a phase II pilot clinical study in men with prostate cancer, MCP was again tested for its effect on PSA doubling time (PSADT).

This study recruited prostate cancer patients who had prostate-specific antigen velocity failure after localized treatment of radical prostatectomy, radiation or cryosurgery. The men were administered MCP (Pecta-Sol®), 15 g daily in divided doses for one year) and changes to their prostate-specific doubling time was recorded as primary outcome measures. Ten patients completed the study, and eight out of those ten patients responded to treatment. The PSA doubling time more than doubled in half of the patients in the experimental group, with increases ranging from 129-941% after 12 months of treatment. The authors concluded that MCP may lengthen the PSADT in men with recurrent prostate cancer (*11*).

Heavy Metal Detoxification:

MCP was given in a preliminary study to patients and found to increase urinary secretion of heavy metals, such as lead, mercury, cadmium and arsenic. The participants were given 15 grams daily of MCP for five days and then 20 grams on day six. Baseline readings of 24-hour urine samples were compared against 24-hour urine samples on day one and day six. The results of the study suggested that MCP encourages excretion of toxic metals with no apparent side effects (*7*). In an early study by Gralak et al. (*9*), the influence of MCP on Ca, Mg, Fe, Zn, Mn, and Cu absorption was studied in rats. When tested against other soluble and insoluble fiber sources, all but MCP increased fecal excretion and decreased the absorption of Ca, Mg, Fe, Mn, Zn and Cu. Therefore, MCP may be a chelator, capable of increasing the urinary excretion of heavy metals, but not reducing absorption of other essential minerals.

In another pilot human clinical trial, MCP was tested for its long-term effects on reducing total mercury body burden in five subjects. Baseline total body mercury body burden of the participants was estimated using a standard DMPS (2,3-Dimercapto-1-propanesulfonic acid) challenge technique of 250 mg *i.v.*, followed by 6 hours of urine collection. MCP (Pecta-Sol®) was then administered at a dosage of 15 grams daily. Total mercury body burden was then measured again after approximately 4 months and found to be significantly decreased in all subjects from a mean average of 52 mcg / g creatinine to 16 mcg / g creatinine after dietary intervention with MCP. A 69% drop for the population ($p=0.0313$), was found for the 5 participants of the study. Results appeared to improve over time. In light of the results from a prior study where MCP was able to chelate other toxic heavy metals, the authors concluded that it may also play a therapeutic role in the chelation of mercury. MCP was well tolerated and thought to act as a chelator, but controlled follow-up studies are needed to confirm this clinical use (*5*).

Dosage

In all the clinical trials to date, MCP has been used for both cancer and heavy metal detoxification studies at the level of 15 grams daily, taken in three divided doses. Manufacturers and dietary supplement distributors of MCP also recommend lower doses for cancer preventative purposes of 3-5 grams daily, in three divided doses, but there has been no clinical verification of this. For biopsy protection, 15 grams per day for one week before biopsy or surgery and 2-4 weeks after procedure has been recommended (*3, 5*).

Safety and Toxicology

MCP is a purified component of standard citrus pectin, which is officially recognized as GRAS (generally regarded as safe). MCP is also thought to have the same level of safety as unmodified pectin. Reported side effects have been rare but may include transient gastrointestinal discomfort or loose stool (*3, 5*).

Pregnancy and Lactation

Although no specific studies have been conducted on the safety of MCP for use in pregnant or lactating mothers, it is thought to have a similar tolerability and safety as citrus pectin that is used in foods. Food grade pectin is also thought to be safe for pregnant and lactating mothers. However, due to the lack of definitive safety data in pregnancy, MCP can't be safely recommended during pregnancy.

Clinical Indications

MCP has exhibited some activity for the following clinical indications. Additional research will be needed to optimize its therapeutic use in these areas:

For Cancer:

- To reduce the size or growth of primary tumors
- To prevent or slow metastasis
- To prevent or slow angiogenesis

Other Potential Health Benefits:

- For detoxification; to reduce heavy metal load
- For reducing cholesterol and possibly for arteriosclerosis
- For immunomodulation

Preliminary research suggests MCP has the potential to be useful at any stage of cancer, whether the goal is to reduce a primary tumor, and/or to prevent the progression and spread of disease. PSA doubling time has been used as a benchmark in clinical studies to determine the effectiveness of MCP in the treatment of cancer (*10, 11*).

As heavy metal load may also be a complicating concern in cancer patients, the use of MCP for the dual indications of halting cancer progression, as well as reducing heavy metal load, may be an interesting clinical application for future research (*5, 7*).

Conclusion

In conclusion, early research suggests that modified citrus pectin may be useful for treating a variety of ailments including cancer and chronic heavy metal toxicity. While the results of these studies have been very encouraging, further research will be necessary to confirm its health benefits, elucidate therapeutic mechanisms and determine optimum molecular weight and structure for specific treatments and preventative strategies.

References

1. Bruneton, J. *Pharmacognosy Phytochemistry Medicinal Plants.* Lavoisier Publishing: Paris, France, 1995.
2. Cerda JJ, Normann SJ, Sullivan MP, Burgin CW, Robbins FL, Vathada S, Leelachaikul P. *Circulation.* **1994**, *89*, 1247-53.
3. Eliaz, I. *Clin. Prac. Alt. Med.*, **2001**, *2*, 177-179.
4. Eliaz, I. Compositions and methods for treating mammals with modified alginates and modified pectins. US Patent 6,462,029, 2002.
5. Eliaz, I. Modified citrus pectin (MCP) in the treatment of cancer. Paper presented at: *The American Chemical Society Annual Meeting:* August 23, 2004; Philadelphia, PA. *unpublished.*
6. Eliaz, I., McCulloch, M. Methods for treating mammals with modified alginates and pectins. US Patent 6,274,566, 2001.

7. Eliaz, I. Rode, D. The effect of modified citrus pectin on the urinary excretion of toxic elements. *Fifth Annual Conference of Environmental Health Scientists: Nutritional Toxicology and Metabolomics*, Univeristy of California, Davis, 2003, *unpublished.*
8. Fernandez ML, Sun DM, Tosca MA, McNamara DJ. *Am. J. Clin. Nutr.* **1994**, *59*, 869-78.
9. Gralak, M. A.; Leontowicz, M.; Morawiec, M.; Bartnikowska, E.; Kulasek, G. W. *Arch. Animal Nut.* **1996**, *49*, 293-299.
10. Guess, B., R. Jennrich, et al. *Prostate.* **2003**, *54*, 88-94.
11. Guess BW, Scholz MC, Strum SB, Lam RY, Johnson HJ, and Jennrich RI. *Prostate Cancer Prostatic Dis.* **2003**, *6*, 301-4.
12. Hayashi, A.; Gillen, A.C.; Lott, J.R. *Altern. Med. Rev.* **2000**, *5*, 546-52.
13. Hsieh, T.C.; Wu, J.M. *Biochem. Mol. Biol. Int.* **1995**, *37*, 833-41.
14. Inohara, H.; Raz, A. *Glycoconj. J.* **1994**, *11*, 527-32.
15. Kidd, P. *Alternative Medicine Review.* **1996**, *1*, 4-10.
16. Lim BO, Lee SH, Park DK, and Choue RW. *Biosci Biotechnol Biochem.* **2003**, *67*, 1706-12.
17. Nangia-Makker P, Hogan V, Honjo Y, Baccarini S, Tait L, Bresalier R, and Raz A. *J Natl Cancer Inst.* **2002**, *94*, 1854-62.
18. Pienta, K.J.; Naik, H.; Akhtar, A.; Yamazaki, K.; Replogle, T.S.; Lehr, J.; Donat; T.L.; Tait, L.; Hogan, V.; Raz, A. *J. Natl. Cancer Inst.* **1995**, *87*, 348-53.
19. Platt D, and Raz A. *J Natl Cancer Inst.* **1992**, *84*, 438-42.
20. Raz A, Carmi P, Pazerini G. *Cancer Res.* **1988**, *48*, 645-9.
21. Raz A, Zhu DG, Hogan V, Shah N, Raz T, Karkash R, Pazerini G, Carmi P. *Int J Cancer.* **1990**, *46*, 871-7.
22. Raz, A, and Lotan, R. *Cancer Metastasis Rev.* **1987**, *6*, 433-452.
23. Roth JA, Frankel WL, Zhang W, Klurfeld DM, Rombeau JL. *J Surg Res.* **1995**, *58*, 240-6.
24. Strum S, Scholtz, M, McDermed J, et al. Modified citrus pectin slows PSA doubling time: a pilot clinical trial. Paper presented at: *The International Conference on Diet and Prevention of Cancer*; Finland 1999. *unpublished.*
25. Vargo D, Doyle R, Floch MH. *Am J Gastroenterol.* **1985**, *80*, 361-4.

Chapter 16

Obesity, Metabolic Syndrome, and the Benefits of Citrus

Ken Fujioka and Michael W. Lee

Nutrition and Metabolic Research Center, Scripps Clinic Division of Endocrinology, Diabetes, and Metabolism, 12395 El Camino Real, Suite 317, San Diego, CA 92130

Background on Obesity

The World Health Organization estimates that there are currently over 300 million obese adults worldwide.[1] In the United States, the prevalence of obesity among adults has doubled over the past twenty years, and is now at 31%.[2] Even more troubling is the tripling (to 16%) of obesity (commonly called pediatric overweight) among American children over the same twenty years.[3] Modernity has created the growing epidemic of obesity; left unchecked, this societal scourge of the 21st century threatens to undo and even reverse the gains made thus far in lifespan and health.[4]

Up to 365,000 adult deaths per year in the U.S. have been attributed to excess weight.[5] Obese individuals are more likely to develop a variety of medical conditions, such as coronary artery disease, stroke, sleep apnea, type II diabetes, osteoarthritis, and certain malignancies (e.g., breast and prostate cancer).[6] Total costs attributable to obesity in the United States amounted to nearly $100 billion in 1995.[7] Among adults, obesity is associated with a decline in health-related quality of life that is greater than the decline associated with 20 years of aging.[8]

Metabolic Syndrome

Concurrent with the increase in obesity is the rise in prevalence of a condition known as metabolic syndrome. As a multidimensional risk factor for both cardiovascular disease and type II diabetes, the diagnosis of metabolic syndrome is extremely useful in predicting which individuals will develop obesity-related medical conditions and complications. Nearly 1 in 4 adult

Americans has metabolic syndrome, and the prevalence is even higher in those over the age of 50 and in certain ethnic populations (e.g., Hispanic Americans).[9]

Metabolic syndrome is due in part to abdominal obesity and the concept of insulin resistance, which result in characteristic changes in waist circumference, blood pressure, glucose homeostasis, and cholesterol levels. In 2001, the third Adult Treatment Panel (ATP III) of the National Cholesterol Education Program (NCEP) stated that the diagnosis of metabolic syndrome is established when 3 or more of the following risk factors are present (Table 1):[10]

Table 1: ATP III Definition of Metabolic Syndrome[10] (Diagnosis is established when ≥3 risk factors are present)

RISK FACTOR	DEFINING LEVEL
Abdominal Obesity (Waist Circumference)	
Men	>40 inches (>102 cm)
Women	>35 inches (>88 cm)
Triglyceride Level	≥150 mg/dL
HDL (High Density Lipoprotein) Cholesterol	
Men	<40 mg/dL
Women	<50 mg/dL
Blood Pressure	≥130/≥85 mm Hg
Fasting Glucose	≥110 mg/dL (revised to ≥100 mg/dL in 2004)[11]

In 2005, the International Diabetes Federation published similar criteria for the diagnosis of metabolic syndrome, placing a more stringent emphasis on central/abdominal obesity.[12]

Treatment of Metabolic Syndrome

The principal therapy for metabolic syndrome is weight loss and increased physical activity.[11] Weight reduction and exercise improve every element of metabolic syndrome: they lower triglyceride levels, raise HDL cholesterol, and improve blood pressure and glucose. The landmark Diabetes Prevention Program study showed that 7% weight loss and regular physical activity reduced the risk of type II diabetes by 58% over a period of four years.[13]

Benefits of Citrus on Metabolic Syndrome Risk Factors

There is also evidence that specific dietary changes will improve the individual risk factors of metabolic syndrome. Both reduced sodium intake and the DASH (Dietary Approaches to Stop Hypertension) eating plan, which emphasizes fruits, vegetables, and lowfat dairy foods, have been shown to reduce blood pressure in clinical studies.[14] Incorporation of monounsaturated fats and moderation in alcohol consumption are recommended in order to decrease elevated triglyceride levels.[15]

Consumption of citrus foods has beneficial effects on metabolic syndrome risk factors as well; this chapter will now focus on the available evidence from human studies thus far.

Flavonoids and Citrus

Flavonoids are the products of plant metabolism and provide much of the color and flavor to fruits and vegetables. Due to their antioxidant properties, there is growing interest in the potential health benefits of flavonoids.[16] Several epidemiologic studies have shown a protective effect of flavonoid consumption in cardiovascular disease and cancer.[17,18] The six major classes of flavonoids are listed in Table 2. Citrus foods are a major source of flavanones, such as hesperetin (oranges) and naringenin (grapefruit).

Table 2: Major Classes of Flavonoids

FLAVONOID CLASS	EXAMPLES	FOOD SOURCES
Flavones	Apigenin Luteolin	Parsley, thyme, celery
Flavonols	Quercetin Myricetin	Onions, broccoli, apples Berries, tea
Flavanones	Naringenin Hesperetin	Citrus fruit
Catechins/Flavanols	Epicatechin Gallocatechin	Tea, apples, cocoa
Anthocyanidins	Cyanidin Pelargonidin	Cherries, grapes
Isoflavones	Genistein Daidzein	Soya beans

Orange Juice

In healthy subjects with hypercholesterolemia, consumption of 750 mL of orange juice was shown to increase HDL-cholesterol levels by 21% over a four-week period.[19] According to a pilot study at the Cleveland Clinic, intake of 16 ounces of orange juice daily for six weeks significantly reduced blood pressure.[20]

Grapefruit

Since being introduced in the 1930s as part of the "Hollywood Diet," grapefruit has developed a reputation in the general public as a weight loss food.[21] Due to its inhibition of the CYP3A family of P-450 enzymes in the liver and small intestine, grapefruit affects the metabolism of a variety of medications, including felodipine, cyclosporine, atorvastatin, and erythromycin.[22]

At the Scripps Clinic Nutrition and Metabolic Research Center, a three month study was conducted to investigate the effects of grapefruit on weight and metabolic factors.[23] Ninety-one subjects were randomized to the following groups:

- ½ of a fresh grapefruit three times a day
- 500 mg grapefruit capsules three times a day
- 8 ounces of grapefruit juice three times a day
- Placebo capsules three times a day

Thirty-one patients (34%) had metabolic syndrome according to ATP III criteria. Weight and blood pressure were measured at monthly intervals. Laboratory work included a 75-gram two-hour glucose tolerance test at the start and end of the study; elevated insulin and/or glucose levels during such testing signifies insulin resistance, which is a key feature of metabolic syndrome.

Results

Compared to the placebo group, subjects who consumed fresh grapefruit had a statistically significant 1.6 kilogram weight loss over three months (Figure 1). Of particular interest was the finding that subjects who had metabolic syndrome and received any form of grapefruit product (fresh fruit, capsules, or juice) also lost significantly more weight (0.9-2.5 kilograms) than subjects on placebo (Table 3). In addition, subjects with metabolic syndrome and intake of fresh grapefruit had a significant reduction in 2-hour insulin level compared to the placebo group, suggesting that insulin resistance was decreased by fresh grapefruit. Grapefruit juice also decreased 2-hour insulin levels, but this finding did not reach statistical significance relative to placebo. Interestingly, grapefruit capsules did not improve insulin resistance in this study (also Table 3).

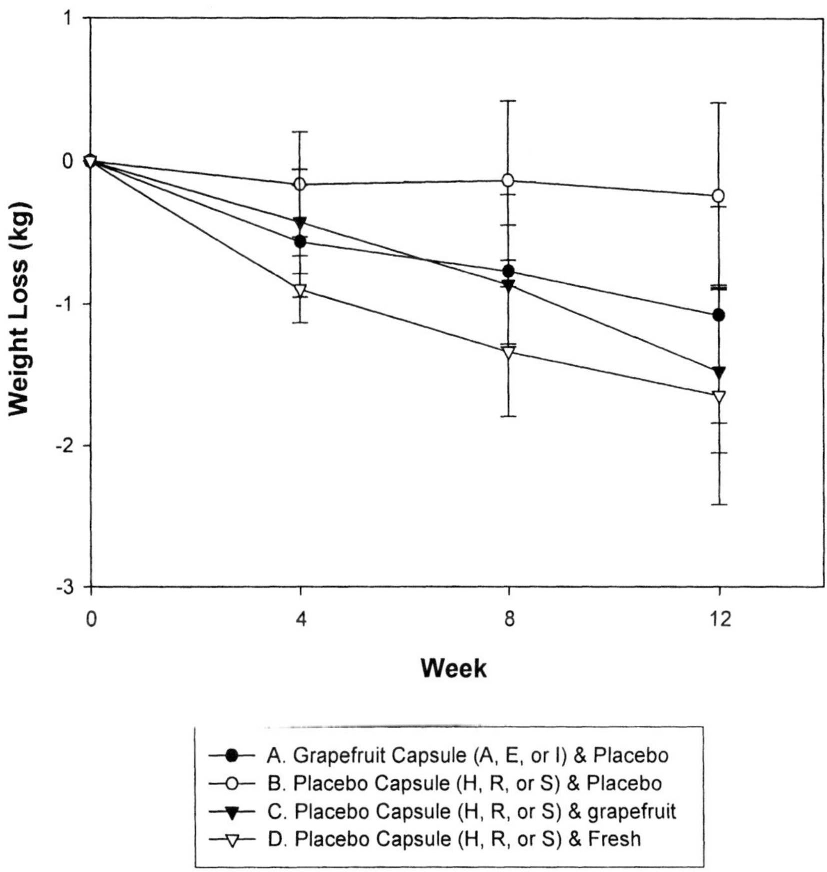

Figure 1: Weight Loss With Grapefruit Intake
(All Subjects, Regardless of Metabolic Syndrome Status)[23]
(Reproduced with permission from reference 23. Copyright 2005.)

Table 3: Weight and Insulin Changes in Subjects Over 12 Weeks of Treatment (Metabolic Syndrome Subgroup)[23]

Metabolic Syndrome Subgroup	A (Capsule)	B (Placebo)	C (Juice)	D (Fruit)
Weight (kg)	-1.9*	1.8	-2.5*	-0.9*
2-hour insulin (mcg/ml)	44	44	-59**	-76*

* Statistically significant relative to placebo ($p<0.04$)
**Statistically significant relative to a group other than the placebo group ($p<0.05$)
Source: Reproduced with permission from reference 23. Copyright 2005.

Conclusions

Based on the above studies, there is evidence that citrus foods may improve specific elements of metabolic syndrome. According to two small studies, orange juice increased HDL-cholesterol and reduced blood pressure. In our study, fresh grapefruit intake was shown to decrease weight and improve insulin resistance in obese and metabolic syndrome patients; consumption of fresh grapefruit and possibly grapefruit juice resulted in a reduction in 2-hour insulin levels. At this time, the mechanism by which fresh grapefruit improves insulin resistance is unknown. Further studies will be needed to determine how citrus exerts its beneficial effects. In this current climate of changing dietary guidelines, it would appear appropriate to recommend citrus as part of a healthy diet.

References

1. World Health Organization. Obesity and overweight: fact sheet. www.who.int/hpr/NPH/docs/gs_obesity.pdf
2. Flegal KM, Carroll MD, Ogden CL, Johnson CL. Prevalence and trends in obesity among US adults, 1999-2000. *JAMA* 2002;288:1723-1727.
3. Ogden CL, Flegal KM, Carroll MD, Johnson CL. Prevalence and trends in overweight among US children and adolescents, 1999-2000. *JAMA* 2002;288:1728-1732.
4. Olshansky SJ, Passaro DJ, Hershow RC, et al. A potential decline in life expectancy in the United States in the 21st century. *N Engl J Med* 2005;352:1138-1145.

5. Mokdad AH, Marks JS, Stroup DF, Gerberding JL. Actual causes of death in the United States, 2000. *JAMA* 2004;291:1238-1245.
6. Mun EC, Blackburn GL, Matthews JB. Current status of medical and surgical therapy for obesity. *Gastroenterology* 2001;120:669-681.
7. Wolf AM, Colditz GA. Current estimates of the economic cost of obesity in the United States. *Obes Res* 1998;6:97-106.
8. Sturm R. The effects of obesity, smoking, and drinking on medical problems and costs. Obesity outranks both smoking and drinking in its deleterious effects on health and health costs. *Health Aff (Millwood)* 2002;21:245-253.
9. Ford ES, Giles WH, Dietz WH. Prevalence of the metabolic syndrome among US adults: findings from the Third National Health and Nutrition Examination Survey. *JAMA* 2002;287:356-359.
10. NCEP Expert Panel on Detection, Evaluation and Treatment of High Blood Cholesterol in Adults: Executive Summary of the Third Report of the National Cholesterol Education Program (NCEP) Expert Panel on Detection, Evaluation and Treatment of High Blood Cholesterol in Adults (Adult Treatment Panel III). *JAMA* 2001;285:2486-2497.
11. Grundy SM, Brewer HB, Cleeman JI, Smith SC, Lenfant C, for the Conference Participants. Definition of metabolic syndrome: report of the National Heart, Lung, and Blood Institute/American Heart Association conference on scientific issues related to definition. *Circulation* 2004;109:433-438.
12. International Diabetes Federation. Press release, April 14 2005. www.idf.org/home.
13. Diabetes Prevention Program Research Group. Reduction in the incidence of type 2 diabetes with lifestyle intervention or metformin. *N Engl J Med* 2002;346:393-403.
14. Sacks FM, Svetkey LP, Vollmer WM, et al. Effects on blood pressure of reduced dietary sodium and the Dietary Approaches to Stop Hypertension (DASH) diet. *N Engl J Med* 2001;344:3-10.
15. American Diabetes Association: Dyslipidemia management in adults with diabetes (Position Statement). *Diabetes Care* 2004;27:S68-S71.
16. Ross JA, Kasum CM. Dietary flavonoids: bioavailability, metabolic effects, and safety. *Annu Rev Nutr* 2002;22:19-34.
17. Hertog MG, Feskens EJ, Hollman PC, et al. Dietary antioxidant flavonoids and risk of coronary heart disease: the Zutphen Elderly Study. *Lancet* 1993;342:1007-1011.
18. Knekt P, Kumpulainen J, Järvinen R, et al. Flavonoid intake and risk of chronic diseases. *Am J Clin Nutr* 2002;76:560–568.
19. Kurowska EM, Spence JD, Jordan J, et al. HDL-cholesterol-raising effect of orange juice in subjects with hypercholesterolemia. *Am J Clin Nutr* 2000;72:1095-1100.

20. Sprecher DL. JUICE (Juice Utilization Improves Cardiovascular Endpoints) study. Presented at the 51st Annual Scientific Session of the American College of Cardiology; Atlanta, GA; March 19, 2002.
21. Cunningham E, Marcason W. Is it possible to burn calories by eating grapefruit or vinegar? *J Am Diet Assoc* 2001;101:1198.
22. Wilkinson GR. Drug metabolism and variability among patients in drug response. *N Engl J Med* 2005;352:2211-2221.
23. Fujioka K, Greenway F, Sheard J, Ying Y. The effects of grapefruit on weight and insulin resistance: relationship to the metabolic syndrome. *J Med Food* 2005 (in press).

Chapter 17

Whither Grapefruit and Drug Interaction?

Basavaraj Girennavar[1], Shibu M. Poulose[1], Jennifer S. Brodbelt[3], Guddadarangavvanahally K. Jayaprakasha[1], Narayan G. Bhat[2], and Bhimanagouda S. Patil[1]

[1]Vegetable and Fruit Improvement Center, Department of Horticultural Sciences, Mail Stop 2119, Texas A&M University, College Station, TX 77843
[2]Department of Chemistry and Biochemistry, University of Texas at Austin, Austin, TX 78712
[3]Department of Chemistry, The University of Texas–Pan American, 1201 West University Drive, Edinburg, TX 78539

Co-consumption of grapefruit juice with common drugs such as calcium-channel blockers leads to increased bioavailability of drugs. Furocoumarins and flavonoids have been ascribed to be the primary components of grapefruit juice responsible for enhanced bioavailability of drugs by reversible and/or irreversible inhibition of CYP3A4 enzyme and P-glycoprotein. Grapefruit juice contains several furocoumarins such as bergamottin, dihydroxybergamottin, epoxy bergamottin, GF-I-1, GF-I-4 and GF-I-6. Levels of these compounds show a considerable variation among different grapefruit varieties. Elucidation of the levels of these compounds in different juice preparations will provide information for optimizing these compounds. Knowledge of furocoumarin levels in juice and the mechanisms of their interactions are expected to help in revising the dose of costly medications if co-administered with grapefruit juice or purified compounds.

Introduction

Grapefruit is considered a "store house" of health-promoting compounds, such as carotenoids, limonoids, flavonoids, pectin and vitamin C. Grapefruit juice carries the American Heart Association's "heart check" food mark (1). Based on current cell culture and animal studies, grapefruit has been shown to protect against a variety of chronic diseases and health conditions, such as atherosclerotic plaque formation (2), cancer (3-7), high blood cholesterol (8), and obesity (9). However, grapefruit juice consumption plummeted to decade low in 1999 (10) partially because of the reported interaction of grapefruit juice with commonly administered medications. While studying the effect of ethanol on felodipine absorption, Bailey and co-workers (11) demonstrated that a single glass of grapefruit juice used to mask the effect of ethanol also increased the bioavailability of felodipine significantly. After this first observation, the impact of grapefruit juice on drug bioavailability of several clinically important drugs has been evaluated by different groups around the world. The bioavailability of certain medications affected by the consumption of grapefruit juice is presented in Table 1. During the last decade, researchers have focused on the isolation of grapefruit juice components, elucidation of their mechanisms of interaction, and the determination of what type of drugs interact with the active compounds in grapefruit juice. The current status of research and clinical implications will be discussed in the chapter.

Bioavailability of drugs

Oral intake of drugs requires that the body must first absorb the active ingredient before it can act at the physiological site. The bioavailability of a drug depends on its solubility and membrane permeability (13) as well as the transport system of the organism and metabolism of the drug (14). A decisive criterion for the dosage of the drug depends upon its bioavailability. The extent of bioavailability is measured by the area under the blood concentration curve (15). Most drugs are recognized and processed by the body as xenobiotics. In many cases, the total drug available is limited by pre-systemic metabolism, either in the gut or in the liver which is also called "first pass metabolism". This greatly reduces the amount of drug that ends up in systemic circulation. Several factors influence the absorption of drug, such as both quantitative and qualitative components of food consumed along with drugs, as well as the time of food consumption relative to the intake of drugs. Intake of liquids and habitual consumption of coffee, tea, tobacco and alcohol also affect absorption.

Table 1. Potential interaction of known and anticipated medications with grapefruit juice (GFJ) bioactive components (12)*.

Drug Class	*Drug*	*Magnitude of Interaction*		
		Small/None	*Moderate*	*Large*
Statins (HMG-CoA Reductase inhibitors)	Fluvastatin	×		
	Provastatin	×		
	Cerivastatin		×	
	Atorvastatin		×	
	Simvastatin			×
	Lovastatin			×
Antibiotics	Clarithromycin	×		
Calcium-channel blockers	Diltiazem	×		
	Verapamil	×		
	Nifedipine			×
	Isradipine			×
HIV protease inhibitors	Indinavir	×		
	Sequinavir		×	
	Nelfinavir		×	
Immunosupressants	Cyclosporine		×	
	Tacrolimus		×	
Antihistamines	Fexofenadine	×		
	Cetirizine	×		
	Loratadine		×	
	Terfanadine			×
Antiarrhythmics	Quinidine	×		
	Amiodarone			×
Psychiatric medicines	Clozapine	×		
	Haloperidol	×		
	Warferin		×	
	Quetiapine		×	
Corticosteroids	Prednisone	×		
	Methiprednisolone		×	
Anxiolytics	Zolpidem	×		
	Temazepam	×		
	Triazolam		×	
	Buspirone			×

* Reproduced with permission of Lippincott Williams & Wilkins Publishers

Physical and mental stress, as well as chronological factors and pharmacokinetics, will affect the extent of drug absorbed. Climatic conditions, such as temperature, pressure and humidity, also affect the bioavailability. Dietary constituents such as grapefruit juice, NaCl and St. John's wort, significantly modify drug metabolism and transport, thus contributing to the variability in bioavailability (16).

Putative bioactive components of grapefruit juice

Grapefruit juice contains several bioactive compounds such as flavonoids, limonoids and coumarins. Some of the flavonoid aglycones such as naringenin, apigenin, hesperetin, quercetin and kaempferol are reported to inhibit microsomal CYP3A mediated oxidation of drugs in rat and human livers (17-18). Naringin is a major flavonoid and bitter principle of grapefruit juice (19), while it is scarcely detectable in orange juice (20). Early investigations considered naringin and its aglycone naringenin as possible compounds responsible for drug interactions (21). Nevertheless, when naringin was co-administered with felodipine *in vivo*, it did not show a clear influence on the pharmacokinetics of the drug (21). Therefore, the activity of flavonoids on CYP3A4 *in vivo* remains unclear.

Fukuda and coworkers reported the involvement of furocoumarins as the main component of grapefruit juice interacting with rat and human P450 CYP3A enzymes (22). Furocoumarins are compounds with a geranyl side chain(s). Grapefruit juice contains several furocoumarins and its derivatives which are considered as possible candidates for drug interactions (23). Until recently, six furocoumarins (Figure 1) have been reported from grapefruit juice (24) with differential inhibitory effect on CYP P450 enzymes. Bergamottin and 6',7' – dihydroxybergamottin are the major furocoumarins, whereas GF-I-1 and GF-I-4 are 100 times stronger inhibitors of microsomal CYP3A4 (24).

Effect of processing on juice furocoumarins content

In order to determine processing effects on furocoumarins, we compared the contents of three furocoumarins in commercially processed fresh grapefruit juice and hand-squeezed juice. The fruits were harvested from the Citrus Center, Texas A&M University Kingsville at Weslaco and grouped into two batches. One batch was hand-squeezed, and the other was processed at Texas Citrus Exchange (TCX) commercial juice plant under normal processing conditions.

Each batch contained 15 subsets, and each subgroup was repeatedly extracted three times with 100ml, 50ml and 50ml of ethyl acetate. The concentrated extract was reconstituted in methanol and analyzed by analytical HPLC with UV absorption detection at 240nm using aqueous methanol as the mobile phase. Results indicate that dihydroxybergamottin and bergamottin content were six and four times higher in hand squeezed juice than processed juice, respectively. There was no significant difference in the GF-I-1 content (Figure 2) (25).

Cytochrome P450 enzyme

Cytochrome P450 enzymes constitute a multigene family of principal detoxifying enzymes (26) that are involved in the oxidative metabolism of drugs and other xenobiotics (27). More than 60 key isoforms of cytochrome P450 are known, with hundreds of genetic variations, producing a wide variety of P450 enzymes. Several isoforms have been distinguished on the basis of their structure, substrate specificity or response to various types of inducers. Cytochrome P450 enzymes are located on the endoplasmic reticulum of cells throughout the body, but the highest concentration are found in the hepatocytes and small intestine (28). The cytochrome P450 enzyme system transforms lipophilic drugs to more polar compounds that can be excreted in urine (29). The metabolites are generally less active than the parent compound, but in some cases the metabolites can be toxic, carcinogenic or teratogenic (30). Among xenobiotic metabolizing cytochrome P450 enzymes, CYP1A2, CYP2C9, CYP2C19, CYP2D6 and CYP3A4 are the major drug metabolizing enzymes. Members of the CYP 3A subfamily are the most abundant cytochrome enzymes in humans, accounting for 30% of total cytochrome in liver and 70% of those in the gut (29). Induction and inhibition (30) are the most common causes of altered drug biotransformation during drug-drug and food-drug interaction. We used -*O*-dealkylation of ethoxyresorufin (EROD), benzyloxyresorufin (BROD) by CYP1B1 and hydroxylation of dibenzylfluorescein (DBF) by CYP3A4 as a measure of activity in purified human microsomal preparations. We found that highly purified furocoumarins from grapefruit juice such as GF-I-1, bergamottin and dihydroxybergamottin, strongly inhibited EROD and BROD activity of CYP1B1 at micromolar levels (Figure 3). Using a linear regression equation, the 50% inhibitory concentration (IC_{50}) values for individual compounds were calculated as previously described (31). In terms of the magnitudes of the IC_{50} values (Table 2), any value less than four micromoles was a strong indicator of the potential of the compounds to inhibit first pass metabolism (32).

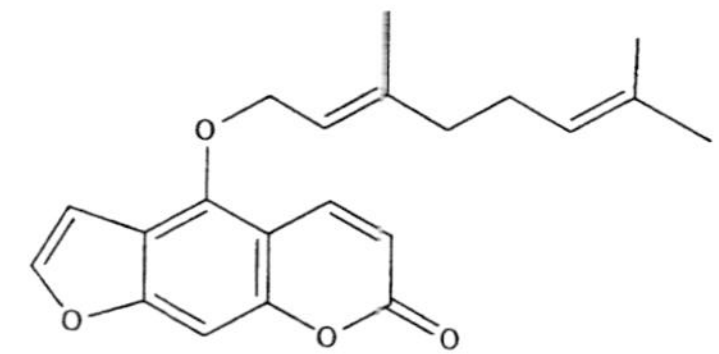

Bergamottin

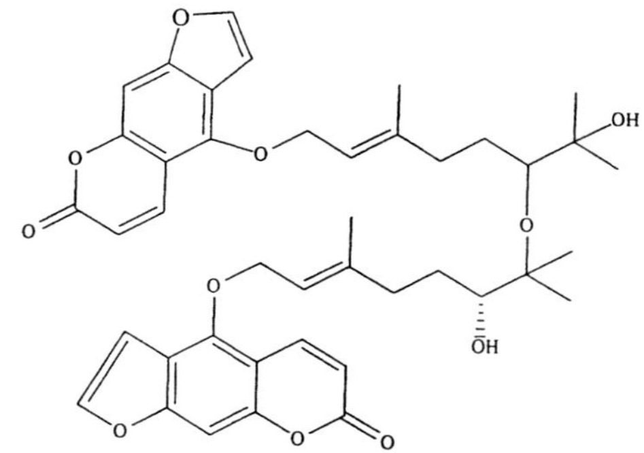

GF-I-1

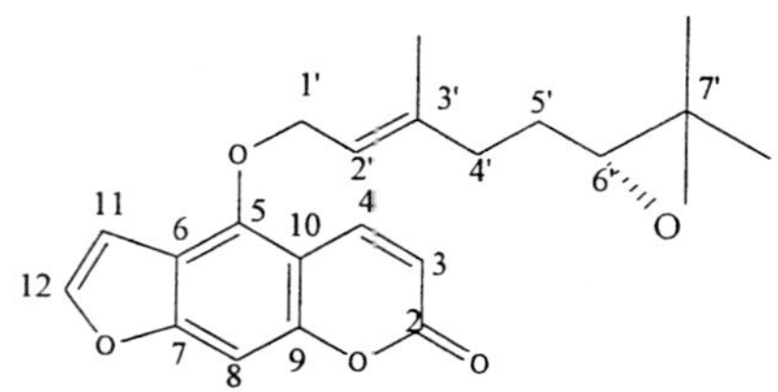

Bergamottin-6'-7'-epoxide
(GF-I-5)

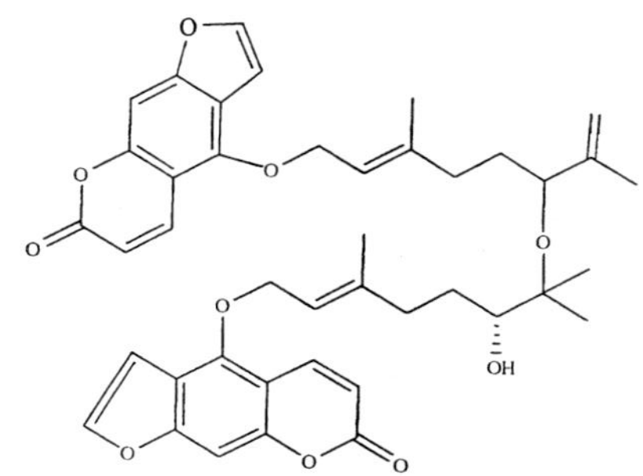

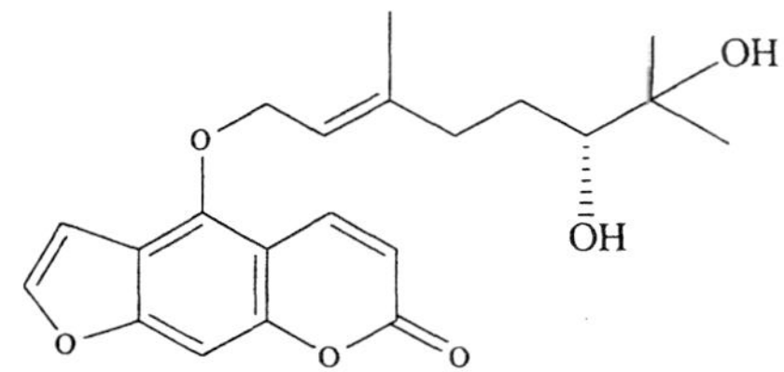

6'-7'-Dihydroxybergamottin

GF-I-4

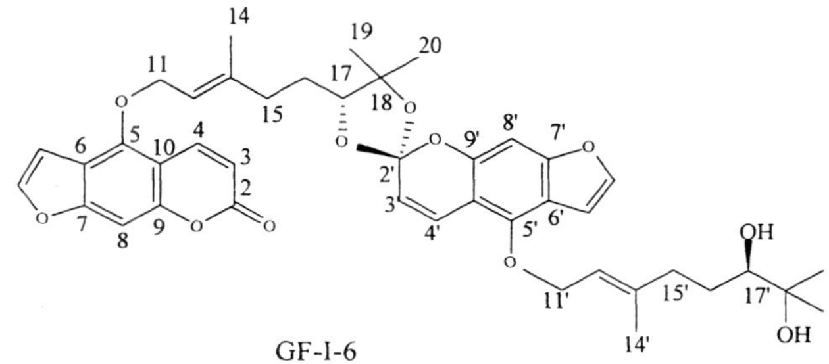

GF-I-6

Figure 1. Structure of furocoumarins found in grapefruit juice.

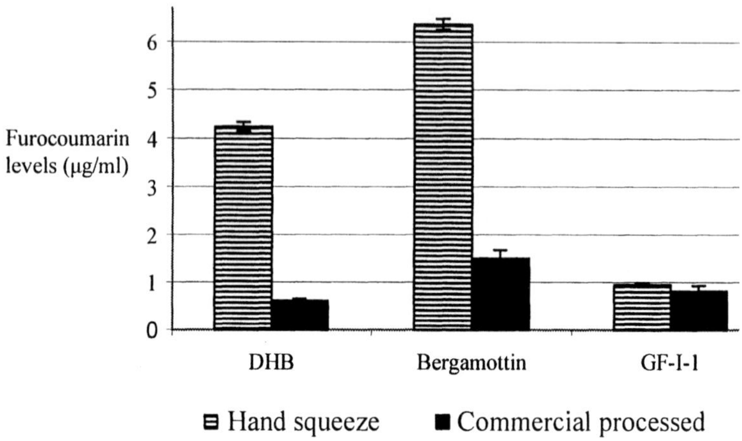

Figure 2. Processing effect on levels of furocoumarin in hand squeezed and commercial processed grapefruit juice. The results represent mean ± SD, n=15

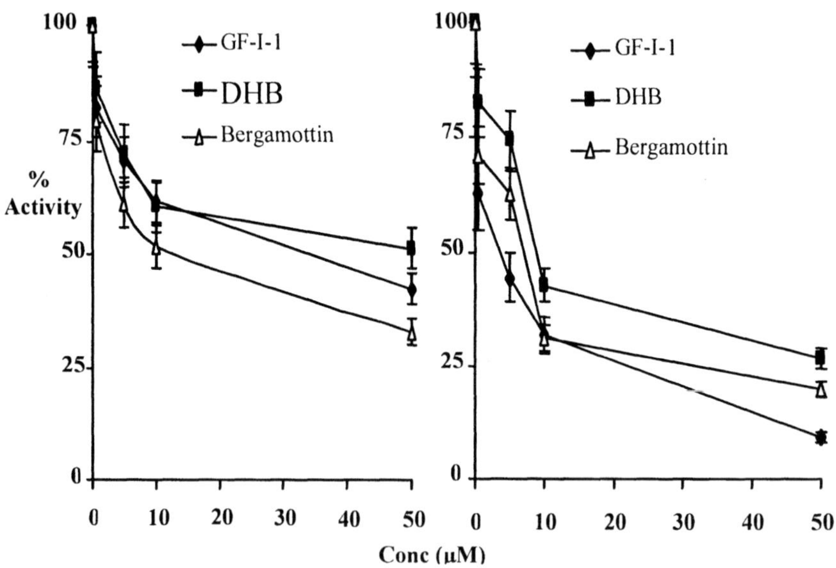

Figure 3. Percent –O-dealkylase activity of CYP1B1 with (a) ethoxy and (b) benzyloxy resorufin substrates. Expressed as percent mean ±SD, n=3. DHB = Dihydroxybergamottin.

Table 2. Effect of furocoumarins on CYP1B1 and CYP3A4 activity. The IC_{50} values are in micromoles (μM), expressed as mean ± SD, n=3.

	CYP1B1		CYP3A4
	ER	BR	DBF
Bergamottin	7.17±0.08	13.86±0.24	6.78 ± 0.091
DHB	8.89±0.07	56.37±0.69	3.26 ± 0.107
GF-I-1	3.56±0.12	33.56±0.72	1.21 ± 0.079

ER = Ethoxy resorufin BR =Benzyloxy resorufin DBF=Dibenzyl fluorescein
DHB =Dihydroxybergamottin

P-glycoprotein

P-glycoprotein is a membrane-localized efflux transporter that actively pumps out xenobiotics, including drugs from intercellular cytoplasm (33). This effect may result in limited bioavailability of drugs. P-glycoprotein appears to be part of a mechanism to protect the body from harmful substances. They are the part of first-pass metabolism, acting as "gate keepers" for absorption of drugs into the systemic circulation. It has been implicated as a primary cause of multi-drug resistance in tumors (34). An understanding of the physiological regulation of this and other transporters is key to designing strategies for therapeutic efficacy of drugs.

Mechanism of grapefruit juice drug interaction

Most lipophilic drugs are either metabolized by CYP3A or pumped back into gut lumen by the P-glycoprotein transporter (35). Thus, CYP3A and P-glycoprotein act in tandem as a barrier to the oral delivery of many drugs (36). Medications such as cyclosporine, ketoconazole (37) erythromycin, itraconozole (38) and diltizem (39) inhibit both intestinal and hepatic CYP3A4 reducing presystemic drug metabolism, resulting in an increase in the oral bioavailability of the absorbed drug. Many bioactive compounds from grapefruit juice such as furocoumarin (40) and flavonoids (19, 21, 23, 41, 42) interfere with CYP3A activity (Figure 4). Interestingly, grapefruit juice has no effect on the bioavailability of drugs when the drugs are administered intravenously (1), suggesting the involvement of intestinal CYP3A inhibition, not the hepatic CYP 3A inhibition as the major cause for increased oral bioavailability (43-46). Bergamottin, a major furocoumarin in grapefruit juice, reversibly inhibits the activities of CYP1A2, 2A6, 2C9, 2C19, 2D6, 2E1 and 3A4 in human liver microsomes (23). It also inactivates CYP3A4 after metabolic activation in a time- and concentration-dependent manner (23). Bergamottin-induced inactivation led to the loss of up to 50% of CYP 3A4 apoprotein, perhaps via apoprotein modification in the active site of the enzyme (23). Metabolites of bergamottin may undergo oxidation to form a reactive furanoepoxide that covalently binds to CYP 3A4 (28).

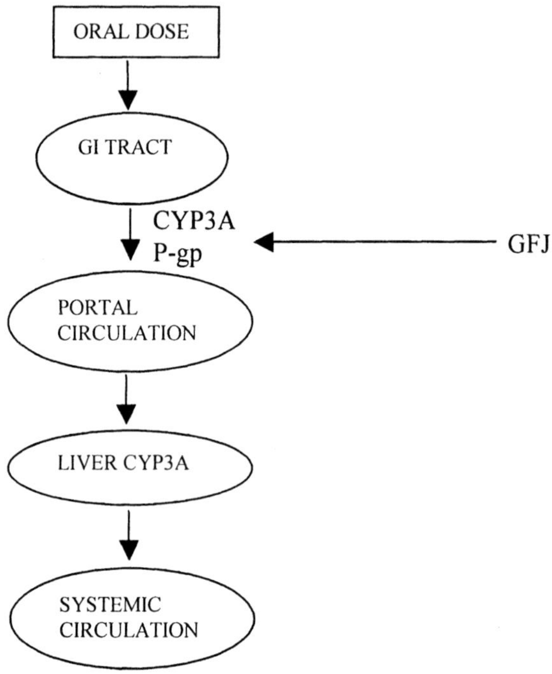

Figure 4. Sequence of events occurring during first-pass metabolism of orally administered drugs. Grapefruit Juice (GFJ) components may inhibit intestinal CYP3A, but have little or no effect on hepatic CYP3A (12) (Reproduced with permission of Lippincott Williams & Wilkins Publisher).

Grapefruit juice seems to interact with P-glycoprotein because P-glycoprotein and CYP3A have overlapping substrate specificities. Soldener and co-workers discovered that furocoumarins shown to activate P-glycoprotein in intestinal cell monolayer *in vitro* (47) resulting in an increased activity of P-glycoprotein. Thus, grapefruit juice might be expected to reduce the oral bioavailability of cyclosporine. Nevertheless, several clinical studies have shown an increase in oral bioavailability of cyclosporine, corroborating with the inhibition of P-glycoprotein (48-54). At surface the mechanism of interaction seems simple, but there is a need for thorough study on the mechanism of action.

Clinical implications

When grapefruit juice increases bioavailability of drugs by 3 to 15 fold (55), is it feasible to explore the possibilities of using grapefruit juice as a "super-pill" supplement ? It is a billion dollar question, especially in the context of costly and comprehensively used drugs, such as immunosuppressants (cyclosporine) and HIV protease inhibitors. Based on the extent of bioavailability obtained by single/double strength juice originating from white or red grapefruit variety, one can consider revising the dose of drugs. Considering the HIV epidemics and prices of anti-retroviral drugs, it is wise to explore the opportunities of grapefruit juice induced drug interaction. Alternatively, one can isolate or synthesize the furocoumarins and use them as a supplement to reduce the drug doses required for effectiveness.

Other food-drug and drug-drug interactions

The ability of dietary components to interact with drugs is not a new phenomenon. Interaction between vitamin K and leafy vegetables such as broccoli, brussel sproutes, cabbage and the blood thinning medication, warfarin, has been known for decades (56). St John's wort, one of the top selling dietary supplements often used for depression (57), reduces plasma levels of indinavir in healthy individuals when co-administered (58). Ruschitzka et al. reported an instance where co-administration of St. John's wort with cyclosporine resulted in rejection of a heart transplant because of insufficient levels of cyclosporine in plasma (59). Hyperforin, the main bioactive component of St John's wort, appears to have CYP3A enzyme induction (60) and selective serotonin reuptake inhibitor activity *in vitro*. Iron supplements are commonly consumed by elderly patients, and ferrous sulphate is often prescribed by physicians (61). Iron has been shown to decrease the bioavailability of tetracycline drugs (62) by binding to the functional groups of the drug. A partial list of food and drug interactions (63) is presented in Table 3.

Multiple drug use is common in the United States. More than 50% of individuals in a given week take at least one prescription drug, and more than 7% take at least five prescription drugs (64). Considering the serious adverse effects of drug-drug interactions, several approved drugs have been withdrawn from the market (65). Table 4 depicts some of the drugs withdrawn from the market during the last decade. Food-drug interactions are not limited to grapefruit juice. In the public interest, pharmaceutical companies should evaluate the compatibility of drugs with food before releasing. There are several drugs in the same category which are not affected by grapefruit juice (Table 1). There is need for educating/informing the pharmacist and physicians on the alternative medication instead of warning the public about the ill effects of grapefruit juice.

Table 3. Common food-drug interactions and their effects.

Foods	*Drugs*	*Effects*
Acidic food: pickles, vinegar, citrus fruits, cola drinks.	Erythromycin and penicillin	Ineffective dose
Potassium rich food: green leafy vegetables, bananas.	ACE inhibitors and diuretics	Irregular heat beat and palpitations
Vitamin K rich food: kale, spinach, cabbage, beef liver.	Anticoagulants	Counteracts drug effects
Caffeine	Histamine	Stomach irritation
Calcium rich food: almonds, pizza, ice cream, yogurt, milk.	Tetracycline	Effective dose of drug
Tyramine rich food: avocados, beer, raisins, soy sauce, sausage, chicken liver, mushrooms	Antihypertensives and MAO inhibitors	Nausea, headache, palpitations, elevated blood pressure.

Table 4. Examples of drugs withdrawn from U.S. Market as a result of drug-drug interaction.

Name of the drug	*Approved year*	*Withdrawn year*
Bromfenac	1997	1998
Mibefradil	1997	1998
Terfanidine	1985	1998
Cisapride	1993	2000
Cerivastatin	1997	2001

Conclusions

Grapefruit contains potential health promoting bioactive compounds beyond vitamin C; however, it is critical to understand the interaction of specific bioactive components with orally administered drugs. While studies on isolation and purification of specific furocoumarins are continued, animal and clinical trials need to be completed before any further recommendations can be made.

Abbreviations used

HPLC, High-performance liquid chromatography; CYP450, Cytochrome P450; GF-I-1, 4-[[6-hydroxy-7-[[1-[(1-hydroxy-1-methyl)ethyl]-4-methyl-6-(7-oxo-7*H*-furo[3,2-*g*][1]benzopyran-4-yl)-4-hexenyl]oxy-3,7-dimethyl-2-octenyl]-oxy]-7*H*-furo[3,2-*g*][1]benzopyran-7-one; GF-I-4, 4-[[6-hydroxy-7-[[4-methyl-1-(1-methylenyl)-6-(7-oxo-7H-furo[3,2-g][1]benzopyrran-7-one; GF-I-5, (R)-bergamottin-6',7'-epoxide; GF-I-6, 4-(6R,7-dihydroxy-3,7-dimethyl-5' 2E-octen-1-yloxy)-7H-furo[3,2g]chromene-spiro-7R, 2'- (4' ,4'-dimethyl-5' R-(3-methyl-5-(7-oxo-furo[3,2-g]chromen-4yloxy)-3E-penten-1-yl)-1' 3'-dioxolane). EROD, ethoxy reosrufin O-dealkylase; BROD, benzyloxy resorufin O dealkylase; DBF, dibenzyl fluorescein.

Acknowledgements

This work was supported by the USDA-IFAFS 2001-52102-11527, and Texas Producers Board Grant (2002-461555) and USDA-CSREES-Special grant # 2004-34402-14768.

References

1. Kane, C.G. *Mayo Clin Proc.* **2000,** *75*, 933-942.
2. Cirda, J. J.; Normann, S. J.; Sullivan, M. P.;Burgin, C.W.; Robbins, F. L.; Vathada, S. V.; Leelachaikul. *Circulation.* **1994,** *89*, 1247-1253.
3. So, F.V.; Githrie, N.; Chambers A.F.; Moussa M.; Carroll K.K. *Nutr Cancer.* **1996,** *26*, 167-181.
4. Poulose, S.M.; Harris, E.D.; Patil, B.S. *J. Nutrition* **2005,** *135*, 870-877.
5. Tian, Q.; Miller, E.D.; Ahmad, H.; Tang, L.; and Patil, B.S. *Nutrition and Cancer* **2001**. *40,* 180-184.
6. Liu, Y.; Ahmad, H.; Luo, Y.; Gardiner, D.T.; McKeehan, W.; Gunasekara, R.S.; Patil, B.S. **2002**. *J. Sci. Food and Agri., 82*, 469-477.

7. Liu, Y.; Ahmad, H.; Luo, Y.; Gardiner, D.T.; McKeehan, W.; Gunasekara, R.S.; Patil, B.S. *J. Agri. Food Chem.*, **2001**. *49*: 3051-3057.
8. Personal communication from Dr Pual Reddy.
9. Fujioka, K.; Greenway, F.; Sheard, J.; Ying, Y. *J Med Food* **2005.** (in press).
10. Fruit and Tree Nuts Outlook/FTS-314. *Economic Research Service USDA*. January 27, **2005.**
11. Bailey, D. G.; Spence, J. D.; Munoz, C.; Arnold, J. M. O. *Lancet.* **1991,** *337*, 268-269.
12. Greenblatt, D. J.; Patki, K. C.; Moltke, L. L. V.; Shader, R. I. *J Clin Psychopharmacol.* **2001,** *21*, 357-559.
13. Lipinski, C. A. *Journal of Pharmacology and Toxicological Methods.* **2000,** *44*, 235-249.
14. Waterbeemd, V. D.; Lennermas, H.; and Artursson, P. *Methods and Principles in Medicine Chemistry.* **2003,** Vol.18.
15. Ditter, L.; DiSanto, R. *The bioavailability of drug products.* **1978**, American Pharmaceutical Association, Washington DC pp.11-14.
16. Bhardwaj, R.K.; Glaeser, H.; Becquemont, L.; Klotz, U.; Gupta, S.K.;Fromm, M. F. *The Journal pharmacology and Experimental Therapeutics.* **2002,** *302*, 645-650.
17. Ha, H.R.; Chen, J.; Leuenburger, P.M.; Freiburghaus, A.U.; Follath, F. *Eur J Clin Pharmacol.* **1995,** *48*, 367-371.
18. Miniscalco, A.; Lundahl, J.; Regardh, C.G.; Edgar B.; Erikson U.G. *J. Pharmacol. Exp. Ther.* **1992,** *261*, 1195-1199.
19. Fuhr, U.; Klittich, K.; Staib, A. H. *Br J Clin Pharmacol.* **1993,** *35*, 431-436.
20. Ho, C.P.; Saville, D. J.; Coville F. P.; Wanwimolruk, S. *Pharmaceutica Acta Helvetiae.* **2000,** *74*, 379-385.
21. Bailey, D.G.; Arnold, J.M.; Munoz, C.; Spence, D.J. *Clin Pharmaco. Ther.* **1993,** *53*, 637-642.
22. Fukuda, K.; Ohta, T.; Yamazoe, Y. *Biol Pharm Bull.* **1997,** *20*, 560-564.
23. He, K.; Iyer K.R.; Hayes, R.N.; Sinz, M.W.; Woolf, T.F. and Hollenberg, P.F. *Chem Res Toxicol.* **1998,** *11*, 252-259.
24. Guo, L.Q.; Fukuda, K.; Ohta T.; Yamazoe Y. *Drug Metab dispos.* **2000**, *28*, 766-771.
25. Girennavar, B., Jayaprakasha, G. K., Pike, L. M., Patil, B. S. *J Agric and Food Chem* (communicated).
26. Nelson. D. R.; Koymas, L.; Kamataki, T.; Stegeman, J. J.; Feyereinsen, R.; Waxman, D. J.; Waterman. M. R.; Gotoh, O.; Coon, M. J.; Estabrook, R. W.; Gunsalus, I. C.; Nebert, D. W. *Pharmacogenetics.* **1996,** *6*, 1-42.
27. Degtyarenko, K. N. "Structural domains of P450-containing monooxygenase systems." *Protein Engineering,* **1995,** *8*, 737-747.
28. Zhang, Q. Y.; Dunbar, D.; Ostrowska, A.; Zeisloft, S.; Yang, JKaminsky, L. S. *Drug Metab Dispos.* **1999,** *46*, 49-53.
29. Meyer, J. M. and Rodvold, K. A. *Infect Med.***1996,** *13*, 463-464

30. Crespi, C. L.; Miller, V. P.; Penman, B. W. *Anal Biochem.* **1997,** *15*, 188-190.
31. Stahle, E. L.; Schloss, L.; Sundqvist V.A.; Brytting, M.; Hokeberg, I.; Cox, S.; Wahren B.,; Linde, A. *Antiviral Res.* **1998,** *40*, 105-112
32. Girennavar, B., Poulose, S. M., Jayaprakasha, G. K. Pikulski, M. Bhat, N. G. Brodbelt, J. S. and Patil, B. S. *J Bioorg and Med Chem* (communicated).
33. Thompson, S. J.; Koszdin, K.; Bernards, C. M. *Anesthesiology.* **2000,** *92*, 1392-1399.
34. Smith, C. D and Zilfou, J. T. *The J. Biol Chem.* **1995**, *270*, 28145-28152.
35. Patel, J.; Mitra, A. K. *Pharmacogenomics.* **2001**, *2*, 401-415.
36. Watkins, P. B. *Adv Drug Deliv Rev.* **1997,** *27*, 161-170.
37. Floren, L. C.; Bekersky, I.; Benet, L. Z. *Clin Pharmacol Ther.***1997,** *62*, 41-49.
38. Kivisto, K. T.; Lamberg, T. S.; Kantola, T.; Neuvonen, P. J *Clin Pharmacol Ther.* **1997**, *62*, 348-354.
39. Azie, N. E.;Brater, D. C.; Becker, P. A.; Jones, D. R.; Hall, S. D. *Clin Pharmacol Ther.* **1998,** *64*, 369-377.
40. Edwards, D. J.; Bellevue, F. H. III.; Woster, P. M. *Drug Metab Dispos.* **1996,** *24*, 1287-1290.
41. Bialey, D. G.; Kreeft, J. H.; Munoz, C.; Freeman, D. J.; Bend, J. R. *Clin Pharmacol Ther.* **1998,** *64*, 248-256.
42. Baily, D. G.; Dreeser, G. K.; Kreeft, J. H.; Munoz, C.; Freeman, J.; Bend, J. R. *Clin Pharmacol Ther.* **2000.** *68*, 468-477.
43. Ludhal, J.; Regardh, C. G.; Edgar, B.; Johnson, G. *Euro J Clin Pharmacol.* **1997,** *52*, 139-145.
44. Rashid, T. J.; Martin, U.; Clarke, H.; Waller, D. G.; Renwick, A. G.; Gerage, C. F. *Br J Clin Pharmacol.* **1995,** *40*, 51-58.
45. Kupferschmidt, H. H.; Fattinger, K. E.; Ha, H. R.; Follath, F.; Krahenbuhl, S. *Br J Clin Pharmacol.* **1998,** *45*, 355-359.
46. Kupferschmidt, H. H.; Ha, H. R.; Ziegler, W. H.; Mieir, P. J.; Krahenbuhl, S. *Clin Pharmacol Ther.* **1995,** *58*, 20-28.
47. Soldner, A.; Christians, U.; Susanto, M.; Wacher, V.J.; Silverman, J. A.; Benet, L. Z. *Pharmacology Research.* **1999,** *16*, 478-485.
48. Brunner, L. J.; Munar, M. Y; Vallian, J.; Wolfson, D. J.; Stennett, D. J.; Meyers, M. M.; Bennett, W. M. *Pharmacotherapy.* **1998,** *18*, 23-29.
49. Taniguchi, S.; Kobayashi H.; Ishii, M. *Arch Dermatol.* **1996,** *132*, 1249.
50. Yee, G. C.; Stanley, D. L.; Pessa, L. J.;Costa, T. D.; Beltz, S. E.; Ruiz, J.; Lowenthal, D. T. *Lancet.* **1995,** *345*, 955-956.
51. Emilia, G.; Long, G.; Bertesi, M.; Gandini, G.; Ferrara, L; Valenti, C. *Blood.* **1998,** *91*, 362-363.
52. Proppe, D. G.; Hoch, O. D.; McLean, A. J.; Visser, K. E. *Br J of Pharmacology.* **1995,** *39*, 337-338.
53. Johnston, A.; Holt, D. W. *Lancet.* 1995, *346*, 122-123.

54. Majeed, A.; Kareem, A. *Pediatr Nephrol.* 1996, *10*, 395-396.
55. Ameer, B.; Weintraub, R. A. *Clin Pharmacokinet.* **1997,** *33*, 103-121.
56. Greenblatt, D. J; Lisa, L.; Moltke, V. *J Clin Pharmacol.* **2005,** *45*, 127-132.
57. Teschi, B. J.; *Am J Obstet Gynecol.* **2003,** *188*, S44-S55.
58. Piscitelli, S. C.; Burstein, A. H.; Chaitt, D.; Alfaro, R. M.; Falloon, J. *Lancet.* **2000,** *355*, 547-548.
59. Ruschitzka, F.; Meier, P. J.; Turina, M.; Luscher, T. F.; Noll, G. *Lancet.* **2000,** *355*, 548-549.
60. Moore, L. B.; Goodwin, B.; Jones, S. A.Wisely. B.G.; Cosstte, J.; Singh, S.; Willson, T. M.; Collins, J. L.; Kliewer, S.A. *Proc Natl Acad Aci.* **2000,** *97*, 7500-7502.
61. Stewart, R. B.; Moore, M. T.; May, F. E. *J Clin Epidemiol.* **1991,** *44*, 1353-1359.
62. Campbell, N. R. C.; Hasinoff, B. B. *Br J Clin Pharmacol.* **1991,** *31*, 215-255.
63. Kim, G. John Hopkins Bayview Medical Center. **2001,** *15*.
64. Kaufman. D.; W.; Kelly. J. P.; Rosenberg. L.; Anderson. T. E.; Mitchell. A. A. *JAMA.* **2002,** *287*, 337-344.
65. Huang, S. M. *J Clin Pharmacol.* **2004,** *44*, 559-569.

Chapter 18

Grapefruit and Cancer: A Review

Kristine Cuthrell and Loïc Le Marchand

Cancer Research Center of Hawaii, University of Hawaii Epidemiology Program, 1236 Lauhala Street, Suite 407, Honolulu, HI 96813

Although a high citrus fruit intake has been associated with a decreased risk of certain cancers, especially aerodigestive cancers (1, 2), the effect of grapefruit (*citrus paridisi*) consumption on risk of cancer has rarely been examined separately in human studies. A number of *in vitro* and animal studies have been conducted with grapefruit juice, or its bioactive constituents, from which various mechanisms for an anticarcinogenic effect of grapefruit have been proposed. This review briefly summarizes the evidence from *in vitro*, animal and human studies focusing on grapefruit and/or grapefruit juice, and its unique bioactive compounds on thc dcvclopment of cancer. We also present preliminary findings from a controlled feeding study in which smokers consumed white grapefruit juice 3 times daily for a week and showed a decrease in the activity of a P450 liver enzyme (CYP1A2) that bioactivates carcinogens from cigarette smoke. This inhibiting effect on xenobiotic metabolizing enzymes may be one way through which grapefruit consumption may be protective against certain cancers (7).

Active Compounds in Grapefruit

A variety of biologically active compounds, including flavanones (naringin, hesperetin, eriodictyol) (4), furanocoumarins, such as bergamottin, and its metabolite, 6',7'-dihydroxybergamottin (6), terpenes (liminoids) (13), and polysaccharides in citrus pectin or modified citrus pectin (14), have been identified as potential contributors to the proposed anticarcinogenic effects of grapefruit. When researchers inadvertently discovered in 1989 that grapefruit juice significantly increased the oral bioavailability of felodipine, a calcium channel blocker drug (they were using grapefruit juice to mask the taste of ethanol, the intended test agent) (10), it created concern over potential clinical toxicity arising from this drug-food interaction. This observation also fostered a new interest in the mechanisms of action of the various bioactive compounds found in grapefruit (3). Further research identifed inhibition of the cytochrome P450 Phase I enzyme CYP3A4 by grapefruit juice as the mechanism for the increased bioavailability of a number of drugs that are also metabolized via this pathway (16); however, the specific compound(s) responsible for this effect, and the exact mode of action are still being investigated. Another Phase I enzyme, CYP1A2, has also been suggested to be inhibited by grapefruit juice *in vivo*, and by naringenin *in vitro* (9).

Both CYP3A4 and CYP1A2 are involved in the bioactivation of environmental procarcinogens, such as polycyclic aromatic hydrocarbons (PAHs), heterocyclic amines (HCAs), aflatoxin and nitrosamines (22). Further, metabolism of PAHs and HCAs by CYP3A4 have been shown to result in the formation of carcinogen-DNA adducts in human tissue (22, 23). This suggests a biological mechanism for the possible protective effect of grapefruit against certain cancers.

Naringin / Naringenin

Naringin is the most abundant flavonoid in grapefruit, constituting up to 10% of its dry weight with a concentration in juice of 450 μg/mL (3). It is the primary source of the bitter taste and unique aroma of grapefruit, and it is not found at any appreciable level in other citrus or fruit juices (3). Naringin is a glycoside which is hydrolyzed by the gut microflora to its corresponding aglycon, naringenin, when the sugar moiety is cleaved (5). Following the chance discovery that white grapefruit juice increased felodipine bioavailability, Bailey *et al.* (56) showed that grapefruit juice, but not orange juice, decreased by about 3-fold the plasma clearance of felodipine. This was followed by a number of studies (5, 18, 19, 21) focusing on naringin and naringenin, as the probable CYP3A4 inhibiting compounds in white grapefruit juice. Pink or red varieties of grapefruit contain less naringin and are, therefore, less bitter and, perhaps, less potent in anticarcinogenic effects (8).

Naringenin has been shown to have greater inhibitory effect on CYP3A4 activity than naringin in human microsomal liver cells (39% vs 6% inhibition) (55). However, even when naringenin was not present (it did not form at the pH used in the incubation procedure in this study), Edwards and Bailey (53) found that CYP3A4 concentrations in rat liver microsomes was reduced by 70% with grapefruit juice, and by a comparable amount with sour (Seville) orange juice (which contained 20% as much naringin). They concluded that some other compound(s) found in both grapefruit juice and sour orange was/were responsible for the effect. In addition to those *in vitro* studies in hepatic cells, a number of other studies, both *in vitro* (53, 55) and *in vivo* (15, 18, 21, 54), have now concluded that naringin and naringenin are not the main inhibitors of CYP3A4 in grapefruit juice (see below).

However, naringin may exert beneficial health effects through mechanisms other than the P450 enzyme pathway. It has recently been shown to protect against hydrogen peroxide-induced cytotoxicity and apoptosis in mouse leukemia P388 cells (59), as well as to protect against radiation-induced chromosome damage in mouse bone marrow by dose-dependent free radical scavenging of hydroxyl, superoxide and other radicals (60). Naringenin has been shown to exhibit cytotoxicity in a variety of human cancer cell lines (breast, stomach, liver, cervix, pancreas, colon and leukemia), as well as to inhibit tumor growth in Sarcoma S-180-implanted mice (63)

Clearly, the effects of naringin and naringenin in carcinogenesis are multifaceted and will require a substantial research effort to be fully elucidated.

Bergamottin and 6', 7'-dihydroxybergamottin

Bergamottin and its metabolite, 6', 7'-dihydroxybergamottin (DHB), are the furanocoumarins (also called psoralens) that are present at the highest concentration in fresh grapefruit (3). DHB was found by Schmiedlin-Ren *et al.* (20) to be at levels almost twice as high in reconstituted frozen concentrate grapefruit juice as in fresh squeezed juice, probably due to the addition of grapefruit oil during processing. These compounds were also found to vary significantly in concentration among different types and brands of grapefruit juice, but all were above the level required for 50% inhibition of CYP3A4 enzyme activity (IC_{50}). No reduction in CYP1A1 or CYP2D6 activity was noted, a finding previously observed *in vivo* (16). Because both bergamottin and DHB have been shown to be competitive inhibitors of CYP3A4 (6), it has been proposed that one or both might be responsible for the interaction between grapefruit and a number of medications that are also metabolized by CYP3A4.

While it appears that the major furanocoumarins in grapefruit peel oil and in grapefruit juice play a significant role in the inhibition of CYP3A4, *in vivo* experiments by Bailey *et al.* (21) and Goosen *et al.* (24) showed that grapefruit juice exhibits a greater effect than isolated bergamottin or DHB, suggesting that other compounds in grapefruit may act synergistically with these furanocoumarins to inhibit CYP3A4.

In a recent *in vitro* study (55) in human liver microsomes comparing the inhibitory effect of a number of flavonoids and furanocoumarins on CYP3A4 activity (measured by inhibition of quinine-3-hydroxylation), another furanocoumarin, bergapten, was found to be the most potent inhibitor (67%), followed by the flavonoid quercetin (55%) and naringenin (39%). Bergapten had an IC_{50} similar to that of bergamottin (25 μM and 22 μM, respectively), but was 10-fold less inhibitory than 6', 7'-dihydroxybergamottin (2 μM). It was also found to be 6-fold more potent than naringenin and 50-fold more potent than naringin. This finding lends support to the hypothesis that there are a number of compounds in grapefruit juice that appear to contribute to its P450 inhibitory effects.

Terpenes

Citrus fruits contain monoterpenes, such as *d*-limonene, and triterpenes, such as limonin and nomilin. While *d*-limonene is added to a number of food products as a flavoring agent, and to cleaning products because of its pleasant citrus fragrance (25), triterpenes have been identified as a contributing source of the bitter taste in citrus juices that adversely affect consumer acceptance (26).

Monoterpenes

Monoterpenes function physiologically as chemoattractants or chemorepellants, and are largely responsible for the distinctive fragrance of many plants (25). Limonene, the major monoterpene in citrus peel oils, has been shown to have chemopreventive activity against many cancer types in rodent models; specifically, *d*-limonene has been shown to inhibit chemically induced tumors of the breast (27-29), skin (30), liver (31), lung and forestomach (32,33), gastric mucosa (34) and colon (35). Limonene may have chemopreventive activity in both the initiation stage (by inducing Phase II enzyme glutathione-S-transferase) (36) and promotion stage (via cell remodeling/redifferentiation) (37) of carcinogenesis. It has also been shown to exhibit chemotherapeutic effects against established pancreatic and mammary tumors in rodents (38,39).

In an older, Southwestern U.S. population at elevated risk for squamous cell carcinoma (SCC) of the skin, citrus peel consumption - but not citrus fruit or juices - was associated with a decreased risk for this disease [odds ratio (OR) = 0.66, 95% CI = 0.45-0.95] (64). Citrus peel oil is > 90% *d*-limonene. Another study in the same population found an even greater reduced risk in subjects consuming both hot black tea, a source of polyphenols, and citrus peel (OR = 0.22, CI = 0.10-0.51, p for trend < 0.001) (65). The number of subjects consuming both hot tea and citrus peel was fairly small (cases = 23, controls = 38) in this study; however, the results were highly significant and were adjusted for age, gender and other factors affecting risk of skin SCC. The OR for those consuming iced black tea and citrus peel was 0.58 (CI = 0.30 –1.12, p = 0.04). Generally, iced tea is more dilute than hot tea, which may explain the weaker association.

Triterpenes

Limonoids are a group of structurally similar triterpene compounds found in citrus fruits. The limonoid aglycons, limonin and nomilin, have been shown to inhibit carcinogen-induction of tumors of the forestomach, lung, and skin in animal models (40-43). Chemically-induced colon carcinogenesis in rats has been shown to be significantly decreased (by 65%) by the citrus liminoids obacunone and limonin (49). Despite structural similarities among these compounds, nomilin has been shown by Lam *et al.* (43) to be more effective as an inhibitor during the initiation phase of skin carcinogenesis in the rodent model, whereas limonin was more active during the promotion phase (43), suggesting a different mode of action. Experiments on glutathione-S-transferase (GST) activity in mice found that while nomilin increased hepatic GST activity, limonin was ineffective (44). Miller *et al.* (26, 45, 46) using the hamster cheek pouch model for carcinogenesis, also observed different effects for these limonoids: Limonin was found to have significant activity in reducing tumor volume, whereas nomilin, classified as having partial activity, reduced tumor number.

Mixed limonoid glucosides, unlike the bitter aglycons, are tasteless and are found in high concentrations in commonly consumed citrus juices (320, 190, and 82 ppm average concentration in orange, grapefruit and lemon juice, respectively). Miller *et al.* noted that the more palatable glucosides of limonin and nomilin (limonin 17-δ-D-glucopyranoside and nomilin 17-δ-D-glucopyranoside) exhibited the same chemopreventive activity as their corresponding aglycons, indicating that perhaps a citrus juice containing more glucosides and less aglycons would taste sweeter and still retain antineoplastic activity (26, 45, 46). A recent report by Poulose *et al.* (48) found that citrus liminoid glucosides induced apoptosis in human neuroblastoma cells and exhibited free radical scavenging activity. Both Miller *et al.* and Poulose *et al.* found that changes to the A-ring of the liminoid nucleus resulted in a loss of anticancer activity, whereas changes to the D-ring appear to be tolerated without loss of effectiveness (26,48).

Modified citrus pectin

Modified citrus pectin (MCP) is a complex polysaccharide derived from the peel and pulp of citrus fruits. Citrus pectin is modified via alterations in pH and temperature into MCP, which has shorter, non-branched, galactose-rich, carbohydrates chains. These shorter polysaccharide units are able to bind to galactose-binding lectins (galectins) on the surface of some cancer cells, thereby blocking the cells from binding to each other. By inhibiting the adhesion of cancer cells, MCP appears to prevent the initial step leading to aggregation and metastasis (14). MCP has been shown to inhibit tumor growth, angiogenesis and metastasis of human breast and colon cancer cells injected into mice (11), and to significantly reduce prostate adenocarcinoma metastases, but not primary tumor growth, in Dunning rats (50). In a small clinical trial involving men with recurrent prostate cancer, prostate-specific antigen doubling time (PSADT) was increased by 30% in 7 out of 10 men taking 15 grams of MCP per day (12). Lengthening of PSADT corresponds to a slower tumor growth rate. Platt *et al.* (51) determined that MCP significantly decreased tumor metastases to the lung by greater than 90% in the highly metastatic B16-F1 mouse model. Given the generally poor prognosis for metastatic cancers, and the fact that MCP is a soluble fiber with no apparent adverse effects in humans, further research into the chemotherapeutic potential of MCP is of considerable interest.

Epidemiological Studies

Well over 100 epidemiological studies have examined the association of citrus fruit intake and cancer risk in the past 25 years; of 109 studies reviewed in a recent Australian report (52), 48 showed an inverse association, 57 no association and 4 a direct association for a variety of cancers. The majority of these studies were a case-control design; of the 11 cohort studies included, 8 found an inverse risk for cancer, 2 no association, and 1 a direct association. The most consistent protective effect from increased citrus consumption appears to be for cancers of the oropharynx, esophagus, lung and stomach, with reduced risk in the order of 40-50% (2, 52). We are aware of only one epidemiological study in the literature that specifically reported on the relationship between white grapefruit and risk of cancer in humans. Le Marchand *et al.* (8) found an OR for lung cancer of 0.5 (95% CI = 0.2-0.9, p for trend = 0.02) for the highest versus the lowest tertile of intake of white grapefruit in a population-based case-control study in Hawaii. The intertertial (33-67th percentile) intake range for white grapefruit was 0.0-9.0 grams/day. The OR's for the highest versus lowest tertile of intake of pink grapefruit (33-67th percentile: 0.0-9.0 g/d) and other citrus fruits (interquartile range 18.4-50.0 g/day) were also < 1.0, suggesting a possible protective effect, but these ORs were not statistically significant.

Feskanich *et al.* (66) reported a marginally significant decreased risk for lung cancer with increases of 1 serving/day of grapefruit [relative risk (RR) = 0.62, 95% CI = 0.37-1.04] or grapefruit juice (RR = 0.31, 95% CI = 0.31-1.01) in the Nurses Health Study cohort (females), but no significant association with lung cancer for any individual fruits, juices, or vegetables in the Health Professionals Follow-up Study (males). White and pink grapefruit were not evaluated separately in these two studies.

In a pooled analysis of prospective cohort studies looking at fruits, vegetables and lung cancer risk (71), statistically significant inverse associations were observed for 'oranges and tangerines' (RR = 0.74, 95% CI = 0.58-0.95, p for trend = 0.006) and for 'orange and grapefruit juice' (RR = 0.82, 95% CI = 0.71-0.94, p for trend = 0.01) comparing the lowest to the highest quartile of intake.

The release of an updated USDA carotenoid database in 1999 (15), followed by the first USDA flavonoid database (4) in 2003 has further emphasized the heterogeneity of the citrus fruit grouping (botanical classification: rutaceae) in terms of phytochemical composition. For example, pink grapefruit differs markedly in its composition from white grapefruit: Pink grapefruit is a moderately good source of the carotenoid lycopene which is not found in white grapefruit, but contains only trace amounts of the flavanone naringin, which is found abundantly only in white grapefruit. Moreover, pink grapefruit contains ~42 times more β-carotene than does white grapefruit (15). Several recent prospective cohort studies (67-69) have found a significant inverse association between β-cryptoxanthin intake and lung cancer. β-cryptoxanthin is found in moderately high amounts in frozen concentrated orange and tangerine juice, but only in trace amounts in grapefruit juice. Table I lists values for selected bioactive compounds found in citrus products.

If it is the case that the protective effect of these foods is due more to their non-nutritive bioactive compounds than to the more uniformly distributed vitamin C and folate, then, studies should evaluate associations for each citrus

Table I: Bioactive Constituents in Citrus Products*

Citrus Product:	*Vitamin C*[a]	*Folate*[b]	*Carotenoids*[c]	*Flavonoids*[d]	*Terpenes*	*Coumarins*
White Grapefruit:						
Raw, fresh	32 mg / 100 g	10 / 100 g	α-carotene: 80 mg / 100g β-carotene: 140 mg /100 g β-cryptoxanthin: n/a lutein & zeaxanthin: n/a	Hesperetin: 2 mg / 100g [e] Naringenin: 50 mg / 100g		Bergamottin: 0.4 mg / 100 g DHB: 0.4 mg / 100 g (20)
Juice, fresh	38 mg / 100 g	10 µg / 100 g		Eriodictyol: 1 mg/ 100 g Hesperetin: 3 mg/ 100 g Naringenin: 20 mg/ 100 g		DHB: commercial rep-29 µM hand-squeezed 23 µM (20)
Juice from conc.	134 mg / 100 g	15 µg / 100 g		Naringenin: 31 mg/100g [f]	Limonin: 1 mg / 100g Nomilin: 100 µg / 100 g (76) Liminoid glucoside: 19 mg / 100g (76)	Bergamottin: 0 mg / 100 g DHB: 0.8 mg /100 g 44.4 µM (20)
Pink/Red Grapefruit:						
Raw, fresh	31 mg / 100 g	13 µg / 100 g	α-carotene: 50 mg / 100 g β-carotene: 6030 mg / 100 g β-cryptoxanthin: 120 mg / 100 g lutein & zeaxanthin: 130 mg /100mg lycopene: 14620 mg / 100g	Naringenin: 11mg / 100 g Quercetin: 300 mg / 100 g		Bergapten: 1400 µg / 100 g (75)

Citrus Product:	*Vitamin C*[a]	*Folate*[b]	*Carotenoids*[c]	*Flavonoids*[d]	*Terpenes*	*Coumarins*
Juice, fresh	38 mg / 100 g	10 μg / 100 g		Eriodictyol: 0 mg / 100 g Hesperetin: 1 mg / 100 g Quercetin: 0 mg / 100 g	Limonin: 200μg / 100 g (76) Nomilin: 100 μg / 100 g (76)	DHB: Commercial prep- 13 μM hand-squeezed 16 μM (20)
Juice from conc.					Limonin: 2 ppm (76)	
Oranges:						
Raw, fresh	50 mg / 100 g	28 μg / 100 g	α-carotene: 160 mg/100 g β-carotene: 510 mg/100 g β-cryptoxanthin: 1220 μg / 100 g lutein & zeaxanthin: 1870 μg / 100 g	Hesperetin: 33 mg / 100g Naringenin: 11 mg / 100 g Quercetin: 1 mg / 100 g		
Sour orange juice				Quercetin: 0 mg / 100 g Eriodictyol: 15 mg / 100 g Hesperetin: 11 mg / 100 g Naringenin: 24 mg / 100 g Naringin: 1 mg/ 100 g (53)		
Juice, fresh	50 mg / 100 g	30 μg / 100 g	α-carotene: 20 mg / 100 g β-carotene: 40 mg / 100 g β-cryptoxanthin: 150 mg / 100 g lutein & zeaxanthin: 360 mg / 100 g	Eriodictyol: 0 mg / 100 g Hesperetin: 13 mg / 100 g Naringenin: 2 mg / 100 g	Limonin: 100 μg / 100 g Nomilin: 0 μg / 100 g (76)	

Continued on next page.

Table I: *Continued.*

Citrus Product:	*Vitamin C*[a]	*Folate*[b]	*Carotenoids*[c]	*Flavonoids*[d]	*Terpenes*	*Coumarins*
Juice, fresh (cont.)				Quercetin: 0 mg / 100 g Quercetin: 1 mg / 100 g Hesperidin: 73 mg / 100 g Naringin: 3 mg / 100 g (70)		
Juice, Fresh hybrid			α-carotene: 80 mg / 100 g β-carotene: 390 mg / 100 g β-cryptoxanthin: 3240 mg / 100 g lutein & zeaxanthin: 1050 mg / 100 g			
Juice from conc.	Frozen: 158 mg / 100 g Chilled: 33 mg / 100 g	Frozen: 147 μg / 100 g Chilled: 18 μg / 100 g	α-carotene: 20 mg / 100 g β-carotene: 240 mg / 100g β-cryptoxanthin: 990 mg / 100 g lutein & zeaxanthin: 1380 mg / 100 g	Frozen: Hesperetin: 26 mg / 100 g Naringenin: 3 mg / 100 g Chilled: Hesperetin: 4 mg / 100 g Naringenin: 1 mg / 100 g	Frozen: Liminoid glucosides: 32 mg / 100 g (26)	
Tangerines:						
Raw, Fresh	26 mg / 100 g	16 μg / 100 g	α-carotene: 140 mg / 100g β-carotene: 710 mg / 100 g β-cryptoxanthin: 4850 mg / 100 g lutein & zeaxanthin: 2430 mg / 100 g			

Citrus Product:	*Vitamin C*[a]	*Folate*[b]	*Carotenoids*[c]	*Flavonoids*[d]	*Terpenes*	*Coumarins*
Juice, fresh			α-carotene: 90 mg / 100 g β-carotene: 210 mg / 100 g β-cryptoxanthin: 1150 mg / 100 g lutein & zeaxanthin: 1660 mg / 100 g	Eriodictyol: 0 mg / 100 g Hesperetin: 10 mg / 100 g Naringenin: 1 mg / 100 g Quercetin: 0 mg / 100 g		
Juice, conc.			α-carotene: n/a β-carotene: 2270 mg/ 100 g β-cryptoxanthin: 27570 mg / 100 g lutein & zeaxanthin: n/a	Hesperetin: 22 mg / 100 g Naringenin: 4 mg / 100 g		
Citrus Peel:						
Orange				Hesperetin: 21 mg / 100 g Naringenin: 375 mg / 100 g (77)		

* Most values have been rounded to the nearest whole number; values other than uM have been converted to analyte per 100 grams.

[a] All vitamin C data were taken from the USDA National Nutrient Database for Standard Reference, Release 17, vitamin c (ascorbic acid)

[b] All folate data were taken from the USDA National Nutrient Database for Standard Reference, Release 17, Folate

[c] All carotenoid data were taken from the 1999 Updated USDA Carotenoid Database (15)

[d] All flavonoid data were taken from the 2003 USDA Flavonoid Database (4)

[e] The naringenin and hesperetin content in raw grapefruit is assumed to be from white grapefruit. The reference article did not specify white or pink grapefruit.

[f] The naringenin content in juice concentrate is assumed to be from white grapefruit juice. The reference article did not specify white or pink grapefruit.

fruit. Similarly, estimation of intake for the most promising and potent bioactive constituents would also be more informative than the current 'citrus fruits' or 'total fruits' groupings. Additionally, as genotyping has become less expensive and more widely used, investigations of how genetic polymorphisms modify the effects of these compounds may allow for a better biological understanding of the mechanisms involved.

Inhibition of CYP1A2 by White Grapefruit Juice: A Feeding Study

Because we found evidence for an inverse association between white grapefruit consumption and lung cancer in the case-control study described above (8), we explored the effect of this food on the activity of CYP1A2, an enzyme inducible by smoking that plays a major role in the bioactivation of PAHs and HCAs from tobacco smoke. We conducted a controlled-feeding study among 49 smokers in which subjects consumed 6 ounces (177 ml) of white grapefruit juice 3x a day for a week. During the week prior to consuming the grapefruit juice, subjects ate a non-inducing diet that excluded fruits, vegetables, caffeine, barbecued or grilled meat, spices and herbs, and alcohol. During the second week, participants consumed this non-inducing diet plus grapefruit juice. Subjects were regular smokers of $\geq$ 10 cigarettes a day. A single brand of juice (Safeway frozen concentrate) was purchased, from which 3 different case lots were mixed and reconstituted into one batch, then refrozen and thawed before serving. All meals were provided to the subjects who ate breakfast and lunch at an on-campus facility and were given a take-out dinner, as well as snacks and drinks. Subjects were asked to report any deviations from the diet protocol on a daily questionnaire. CYP1A2 activity was measured by caffeine phenotyping (72); caffeine dosing was given on day 7 of the non-inducing diet and on day 15, following 7 days of grapefruit consumption. Urine was collected during the fifth hour following caffeine dosage. We observed a mean 39% decrease ($p = 0.0004$) in CYP1A2 activity, as measured by the urinary metabolic ratio of (1,7-dimethyluric acid + 1,7-dimethylxanthine) : caffeine (17U + 17X/caf), following grapefruit juice consumption (see Figure 1). Results were adjusted for age, weight, sex and average number of cigarettes smoked per/day.

These results are consistent with the findings of Fuhr *et al.* (9) who reported a 23% decrease in the oral clearance of caffeine as measured by the saliva : plasma concentration ratio, and a 31% prolonged half-life in 12 subjects who consumed 300 ml of fresh grapefruit juice one-half hour prior to caffeine

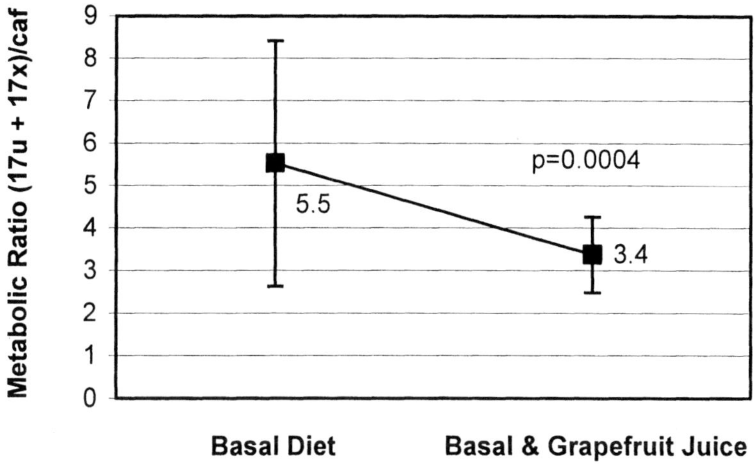

Figure 1. Mean CYP1A2 activity assessed among 49 smokers by caffeine metabolic ratio (1,7-dimethyluric acid + 1,7-dimethylxanthine) : caffeine = (17U + 17X/caf) after one week of non-inducing diet (basal) diet and after one week of the same diet plus 6 ounces of white grapefruit juice 3/x day. Error bars are standard error of the mean.

administration. Five of the ten subjects smoked 10 or more cigarettes per day. Smokers exhibited significantly higher oral caffeine clearance values (152 $\pm$ 49 s.d. ml min $^{-1}$) than nonsmokers (79 $\pm$ 28 s.d. ml min $^{-1}$) in periods without grapefruit juice administration, indicating higher baseline CYP1A2 activity. By s.d. ml min $^{-1}$) than nonsmokers (79 $\pm$ 28 s.d. ml min $^{-1}$) in periods without grapefruit juice administration, indicating higher baseline CYP1A2 activity. By contrast, in a sample of 10 nonsmoking subjects, Maish *et al.* (73) found no significant effect on caffeine metabolism overall, although they note that 4 subjects demonstrated a marked increase in the serum caffeine concentration-time curve with grapefruit juice administration.

CYP1A2 activity is known to vary widely between individuals and to be elevated in smokers (74). Since this enzyme plays an important role in the metabolic activation of a number of procarcinogens found in cigarette smoke, inhibiting this step through dietary modification might have beneficial implications for those who have as yet been unable or unwilling to quit smoking.

Conclusion

In summary, grapefruit and grapefruit juice have been the focus of a fairly intensive research effort following the discovery of a potentially harmful food-drug interaction in the late 1980s. It has been conclusively demonstrated in a number of *in vitro* and *in vivo* studies that grapefruit juice inhibits the activation of CYP3A4. We are aware of one other *in vivo* study (9) in addition to our own that demonstrated inhibition of CYP1A2 with grapefruit juice consumption. As these Phase I enzymes are responsible for the bioactivation of environmental procarcinogens, such as polycyclic aromatic hydrocarbons (PAHs), heterocyclic amines (HCAs), aflatoxin and nitrosamines, their inhibition could provide a mechanism for the possible protective effect of grapefruit against aerodigestive cancers.

Additionally, bioactive constituents, some of which are unique to grapefruit, such as naringin and its aglycon naringenin, as well as the terpenes and polysaccharides that are also found in other citrus fruits, have been found to have chemopreventative and/or chemotherapeutic activity. The observed effects include inhibition of the number and/or size of tumors, cytotoxicity for a variety of different cancer cell lines, and free-radical scavenging.

A number of epidemiological studies have found a reduced risk for cancers of the aerodigestive tract among individuals consuming high amounts of citrus fruit, usually with a greater protective effect than is found for total fruits (1). While the various citrus fruits are generally good sources of vitamin C and folate, they differ appreciably in their carotenoid and flavonoid content. Future research efforts in this area should focus on better quantifying non-nutritive bioactive compounds in the different varieties of citrus fruit, as well as assessing their mechanisms of action both *in vitro* and *in vivo*. It would also be of considerable interest for epidemiological studies to evaluate the association of specific citrus fruits and cancer risk, given their significantly different composition (e.g. white versus pink grapefruit).

Acknowledgements

The authors wish to thank Marie Kainoa Fialkowski for her invaluable assistance.

References

1. Vainio, H.; Bianchini, F., Eds.; *Fruits and Vegetables;* IARC Handbooks of Cancer Prevention; International Agency for Research on Cancer, World Health Organization, IARC Press, Lyon, France, **2003**; Vol. 8, 103-134.

2. World Cancer Research Fund, International Agency for Research on Cancer; *Food, Nutrition, and the Prevention of Cancer: a global perspective;* **1997**; 441-442.
3. Kane, G.C.; Lipsky, J.J.; *Mayo Clin. Proc.* **2000**, *75*, 933-942.
4. U.S. Department of Agriculture, Agricultural Research Service; *USDA Database for the Flavonoid Content of Selected Foods – 2003* URL http://www.nal.usda.gov/fnic/foodcomp.
5. Fuhr, U.; Kummert, A.L.; *Clin. Pharmacol. Ther.* **1995**, 58, 365-373.
6. Edwards, D.J.; Bellevue, F.H.; Woster, P.M. III; *Drug Metab. Dispos.* **1996,** 24, 1287-1290.
7. Rock, C.A.; Lampe, J.W.; Patterson, R.E.; *Annu. Rev. Pub. Health* **2000**, 21, 47-64.
8. Le Marchand, L.; Murphy, S.P.; Hankin, J.H.; Wilkens, L.R.; Kolonel, L.N.; *J Natl Cancer Inst.* **2000**, 92, 154-160.
9. Fuhr, U.; Klittich, K.; Staib, A.H.; *Br. J. Clin. Pharmacol.* **1993**, 35, 431-436.
10. Bailey, D.G.; Spence, J.D.; Edgar , B.; Bayliff, C.D.; Arnold, J.M.; *Clin. Invest. Med.* **1989,** 12, 357-362.
11. Nangia-Makker, P.; Hogan, V.; Honjo, Y.; Baccarini, S.; Tait, L.; Bresalier, R.; Raz, A..; *J. Natl. Cancer Inst.* **2002**, 94, 1854-1862.
12. Guess, B.W.; Scholz, M.C.; Strum, S.B.; Lam, R.Y.; Johnson, H.J.; Jennich, R.I.; *Prostate Cancer Prostatic Dis.* **2003**, 6, 301-304.
13. Lam, L.K.; Hasegawa, S.; *Nutr. Cancer* **1989**, 12, 43-47.
14. Alternative Medicine Review; *Monograph: Modified Citrus Pectin* Thorne Research, Inc., **2000**, 5, 573-575, www.thorne.com.
15. Holden, J.M.; Eldridge, A.L.; Beecher, I.; Buzzard, M.; Bhagwat, S.; Davis, C.S.; Douglass, L.W.; Gebhardt, S.; Haytowitz, D.; Schakel, S.; *J. Food Comp. and Analysis* **1999**, 12, 169-196.
16. Lown, K.S.; Bailey, D.G.; Fontana, R.J.; Janardan, S.K.; Adair, C.H.; Fortlage, L.A.; Brown, M.B.; Guo, W.; Watkins, P.B.; *J. Clin. Invest.* **1997**, 99, 2545-2553.
17. Ubeaud, G.; Hagenbach, J.; Vandenshrieck S.; Jung, L.; Koffel, J.C.; *Life Sci.* **1999**, 65, 1403-1412.
18. Bailey, D.G.; Arnold, J.M.; Munoz, C.; Spence, J.D.; *Clin. Pharmacol. Ther.* **1993**, 53; 637-642.
19. Bailey, D.G.; Arnold, J.M.; Strong. H.A.; Munoz, C.; Spence, J.D.; *Clin. Pharmacol. Ther.* **1993**, 54, 589-594.
20. Schmiedlin-Ren, P.; Edwards, D.J.; Fitzsimmons, M.E.; He, K., Lown, K.S., Woster, P.M., Rahman, A..; Thummel, K.E., Fisher, J.E.; Hollenberg, P.F.; Watkins, P.B.; *Drug Metab. Dispos.* **1997**, 25, 1228-1233.
21. Bailey, D.G.; Kreeft, J.H; Munoz, C.; Freeman, D.J.; Bend, J.R; *Clin. Pharmocol. Ther.* **1998**, 64, 248-256.

22. Keshava, C.; McCanlies, E.C.; Weston, A.; *Am. J. Epidemiol.* **2004**, 160, 825-841.
23. Lightfoot, T.J.; Coxhead, J.M.; Cupid, B.C.; *Mutat. Res.* **2000**, 472, 119-127.
24. Goosen, T.C.; Cillié, D; Bailey, D.G.; Yu, C.: He, K.; Hollenberg, P.F.; Woster, P.M.; Cohen, L.; Williams, J.A..; Rheeders, M.; Dikstra, P.; *Clin. Pharmacol. Ther.* **2004,** 76, 607-617.
25. Crowell, P.L.; *J. Nutr.* **1999**, 129, 775S-778S.
26. Miller, E.G.; Porter, J.L.; Binnie, W.B.; Guo, I.Y.; Hasegawa, S.; *J. Agric. Food Chem.* **2004**, 52, 4908-4912.
27. Elson, C.E.; Maltzman, T.H.; Boston, J.L.; Tanner, M.A., Gould, M.N.; *Carcinogenesis* **1988**, 9, 331-332.
28. Maltzman, T.H.; Hurt, L.M.; Elson, C.E.; Tanner, M.A.; Gould, M. N.; *Carcinogenesis* **1989**, 10, 781-783.
29. Elegbede, J.A.; Elson, C.E.; Qureshi, A.; Tanner, M.A.; Gould, M.N.; *Carcinogenesis* **1984,** 5, 661-664.
30. Elegbede, J.A.; Maltzman, T.H., Verma, A.K.; Tanner, M.A.; Gould, M.N.; *Carcinogenesis* **1986**, 7, 2047-2049.
31. Giri, R.K.; Parija, T.; Das, B.R.; *Oncol. Rep.* **1999**, 5, 1123-1127.
32. Wattenberg, L.W.; Coccia, J.B.; *Carcinogenesis* **1991**, 12, 115-117.
33. Wattenberg, L.W.; Sparnins, V.L.; Barany, G.; *Cancer Res.* **1989**, 49, 2689-2692.
34. Yano, H.; Tatsuta, M.; Iishi, H.; Baba, M.; Sakai, N.; Uedo, N.; *Int. J. Cancer* **1999**, 82, 665-668.
35. Kawamori, T.; Tanaka, T.; Hirose, M.; Ohnishi, M.; Mori, H.; *Carcinogenesis*, **1996**, 17, 369-372.
36. Elegbede, J.A.; Maltzman, T.H.; Elson, C.E.; Gould, M.N.; *Carcinogenesis*, **1993**, 14, 1221-1225.
37. Jirtle, R.L.; Haag, J.D.; Ariazi, E.; Gould, M.N.; *Cancer Res.* **1993**, 53, 2849-3853.
38. Haag, J.D.; Lindstrom, M.J.; Gould, M.N.; *Cancer Res.* **1992**, 52, 4021-4026.
39. Stark, M.J.; Burke, Y.D.; McKinzie, J.H.; Ayoubi, A.S.; Crowell, P.L.; *Cancer Lett.* **1995,** 96, 15-21.
40. Lam, L.K.T.; Hasegawa, S.; *Nutr. Cancer* **1989**, 12, 43-47.
41. Lam, L.K.T.; Zhang, J.; Hasegawa, S. *Food Technol.* **1994,** 48, 104-108.
42. Lam, L.K.T.; Zhang, J.; Hasegawa S.; Schut, H.A.J.; In *Food Phytochemicals for Cancer Prevention I. Fruits and vegetables*; Huang, M.-T., Osawa, T., Ho, C.-T., Rosen, R.T., Eds.; American Chemical Society: Washington, DC, 1994, pp 209-219.
43. Lam, L.K.T.; Hasegawa, S.; Bergstrom, C.; Lam, S.H.; Kenney, P. In *Citrus Limonoids Functional Chemicals in Agriculture and Foods*; Berhow, M., Hasegawa, S., Manners, Gl, Eds.; American Chemical Society: Washington, DC, 2000; pp 185-200.

44. Lam, L.K.T.; Li, Y.; Hasegawa, S.; *J. Agric. Food Chem.* **1989**, 37, 878-880.
45. Miller, E.G.; Fanous, R.; Rivera-Hidalgo, F.; Binnie, W.H.; Hasegawa, S.; Lam, L.K.T.; *Carcinogenesis* **1989**, 10, 1535-1537.
46. Miller, E.G.; Gonzales-Sanders, A.P; Couvillon, A.M.; Wright, J.M.; Hasegawa, S.; Lam, L.K.T.; *Nutr.Cancer* **1992**, 17, 1-7.
47. Miller, E.G.; Gonzales-Sanders, A.P.; Couvillon, A.M.; Binnie, W.H.; Hasegawa, S.; Lam, L.K.T.; *Food Technol.* **1994**, 17, 110-114.
48. Poulose, S.M.; Harris, E.D.; Patil, B.S.; *J. Nutr.* **2005**, 135, 870-877.
49. Tanaka, T.; Kohno, H.; Tsukio, Y.; Honjo, S.; Tanino, M.; Miyake, M.; Wada, K.; *BioFactors* **2000**, 13, 213-218.
50. Pienta, K.J.; Naik, H.; Akhtah, A.; Yamazaki, K.; Replogle, T.S.; Lehr, J.; *J. Natl .Cancer Inst.* **1995**, 87, 348-353.
51. Platt, D.; Raz, A.; *J. Natl. Cancer Inst.* **1992,** 18, 438-442.
52. Baghurst, K.; *The Health Benefits of Citrus*; Horticultural Australia, Ltd.: Sydney, AU, 2003; pp 13-14, www.auscitrus.org.au .
53. Edwards, D.J.; Bernier, S.M.; *Life Sci.* **1996**, 59, 1025-1030.
54. Bailey, D.G.; Dresser, G.K.; Kreeft, J.H.; Munoz, C.; Freeman, D.J.; Bend, J.R.; *Clin. Phamacol. Ther.* **2000**, 64, 468-477.
55. Ho, P-C; Saville, D.J.; *J. Pharm. Pharmaceut. Sci.* **2001,** 4, 217-227.
56. Bailey, D.G.; Spence, J.D.; Munoz, C.; Arnold, J.M.O.; *Lancet* **1991,** 337, 268-269.
57. Ueng, Y-F; Chang, Y-L, Oda, Y.; Park, S.S.; Liao, J-F; Lin, M-F; Chen, C-F; *Life Sci.* **1999**, 65, 2591-2602.
58. Fuhr, U.; Maier A.; Keller, A.; Steinijans, V.W.; Sauter, R.; Staib, A.H.; *Int. J. Clin. Pharmacol. Ther.* **1995,** 33, 311-314.
59. Kanno, S.; Shouji, A.; Asou, K.; Ishikawa, M.; *J. Phamacol. Sci.* **2003**, 92, 166-170.
60. Jagetia, G.C.; Venkatesha, V.A.; Reddy, T.K.; *Mutagenesis* **2003**, 18, 337-342.
61. Choi, Y.J.; Kang, J.S.; Park, J.H.; Lee, Y.J.; Choi, J.S.; Kang, Y.H.; *J. Nutr.* **2003**, 133, 985-991.
62. Schwarz, D.; Kisselev, P.; Roots, I.; *Eur J Cancer* **2005**, 41, 151-158.
63. Kanno, S.; Tomizawa, A.; Hiura, T.; Osanai, Y.; Shouji, A.; Ujibe, M.; Ohtake, T.; Kimura, K.; Ishikawa, M.; *Biol. Pharm. Bull.* **2005,** 28, 527-530.
64. Hakim, I.A.; Harris, R.B.; Ritenbaugh, C.; *Nutr. Cancer* **2000**, 37, 161-168.
65. Hakim, I.A.; Harris, R.B.; *BMC Dermatology* **2001**, 1,3. www.biomedcentral.com/1471-5945/1/3.
66. Feskanich, D.; Ziegler, R.G.; Michaud, D.S.; Giovannucci, E.L.; Speizer, F.E.; Willett, W.C.; Colditz, G.A.; *J. Natl. Cancer Inst.* **2000**, 92, 1812-1823.
67. Männistö, S.; Smith-Warner, S.A.; Spiegelman, D.; Albanes, D.; Anderson, K.; van den Brandt, P.A.; Cerhan, J.R.; Colditz, G.; Feskamich, D.;

Freudenheim, J.L.; Giovannucci, E.; Goldbohm, R.A.; Graham, S.; Miller, A.B.; Rohan, T.E.; Virtamo, J.; Willett, W.C.; Hunter, D.J.; *Cancer Epidemiol. Biomark. Prev.* **2004**, 13, 40-48.

68. Yuan, J-M; Stram, D.O.; Arakawa, K.; Lee, H-P; Yu, M.C.; *Cancer Epidemiol. Biomark. Prev.* **2003**, 12, 890-898.
69. Voorrips, L.E.; Goldbohm, A.; Brants, H.A.M.; van Poppel, G. A. F. C.; Sturmans, F.; Hermus R.J.J.; van den Brandt, P.A.; *Cancer Epidemiol. Biomark. Prev.* **2000**, 9, 357-365.
70. Careri, M.; Elviri, L.; Mangia, A.; *Rapid Commun. Mass Spectrom.* **1999**, 13, 2399-2405.
71. Smith-Warner, S.A.; Spiegelman, D.; Yaun, S-S; Albanes, D.; Beeson, L.; van den Brandt. P.A.; Feshanich, D.; Folsom, A.R.; Fraser, G.E.; Freudenheim. J.L.; Giovannucci, E; Goldbohm, R.A.; Graham, S.; Kushi, L.H.; Miller, A.B.; Pietnen, P.; Rohan, T.E.; Speizer, F.E.; Willett, W.C.; Hunter, D.J.; *Int. J Cancer* **2003**, 107, 1001-1011.
72. Butler, M.A.; Lang, N.P.; Young, J.F.; Capraso, N.E.; Vineis, P.; Hayes, R.B.; Teitel, C.H.; Massengill, J.P.; Lawsen, M.F.; Kadlubar, F.F.; *Pharmacogenetics* **1992**, 2, 116-127.
73. Maish, W.A.; Hampton, E.M.; Whitsett, T.L.; Shepard, J.D.; Lovallo, W.R.; *Pharmacotherapy* **1996**, 16, 1046-1052.
74. Chung, W-G; Kang, J-H; Park, C-S; Cho, M-H; Cha, Y-N; *Clin. Pharmacol. Ther.* **2000**, 67, 258-266.
75. Ho, P.C.; Saville, D.J.; Coville,, P.F.; Wanwimolruk, S.; *Pharm. Acta. Helv.* **2000**, 74, 379-385.
76. Manners, G.D.; Breksa, A.P.; Schoch, T.K.; Hidalgo, M.B.; *J Agric. Food Chem.* **2003**, 51, 3709-3714.
77. Justesen, U.; Knuthsen, P.; Leth, T.; *J. Chromatog. A.* **1998**, 799, 101-110.

Consumer Trends

Chapter 19

Trends in Consumer Attitudes toward Food and Health: From Food Biotechnology to Personalized Nutrition

David B. Schmidt

Executive Vice President, International Food Information Council, 1100 Connecticut Avenue, NW, Suite 430, Washington, DC 20036

Scientific knowledge of the health benefits of citrus and other food components is developing rapidly. For example, consumers cite oranges and orange juice more than any other food as the ones that come to mind in promoting health. Consumers obtain nutrition information from a variety of resources, including the media, food labels, and health professionals, which can contribute to confusion and frustration. In addition, information from the human genome is providing us with tremendous potential to improve the quality of human nutrition in the future. The term "nutrigenomics" has now been coined to describe a new concept in "personalized nutrition" where an individual's DNA profile will be used to better determine which foods or nutrients they should consume more or less of due to their increased risk for a particular disease or health condition. Using International Food Information Council's six years of consumer attitudinal research on functional foods and "personalized nutrition," as well as 2004 data updating consumer attitudes toward food biotechnology, this paper will provide readers the tools to effectively address the challenges and opportunities in communicating the health benefits of citrus and other food components to consumers.

More than 2000 years ago, Hippocrates said, "Let food be thy medicine." This concept underlies the definition of "functional foods" used by the International Food Information Council (IFIC): any food or food component that may provide a health benefit beyond basic nutrition. Citrus products are already at the center of a number of consumer trends indicating increased interest in beneficial food components for health promotion.

While citrus products have not been developed using biotechnology to date, consumer awareness and acceptance of foods produced through biotechnology remain stable despite major publicity on various unrelated animal diseases and food safety issues, according to a survey conducted in 2004 by Cogent Research (*1*) and commissioned by the International Food Information Council (IFIC).

A majority of consumers would be likely to purchase foods modified through biotechnology to be protected from insect damage and require fewer pesticide applications (66%), or to have improved taste or freshness (54%). Additionally, consumers who have heard or read about biotechnology are significantly more likely to purchase biotech food products for these benefits.

Full survey results and consumer information can be found on the IFIC Web site (http://ific.org). The survey was conducted January 2-11, 2004 by Cogent Research, Cambridge, MA, and consisted of approximately 1,000 telephone interviews among a nationally representative sample of adults 18 and older in the continental United States.

IFIC is also keeping a finger on the pulse of consumer attitudes toward functional foods, such as citrus products, with its most recent quantitative survey, conducted in March 2002. Cogent Research of Cambridge, Massachusetts, conducted telephone surveys with 1,004 randomly selected U.S. adults. Those surveys provided data that build on the quantitative data collected in 1998 and 2000.

Consumers find health professionals (47%) such as physicians and dietitians the most believable sources for food and nutrition information with the media at 23%. Family/friends/self were listed as most believable by 10%, the government at 9%, and only 1% listed food labels as the most believable source in an open-ended format. Past consumer research (*2*) has confirmed that consumers rely on a wide variety of information sources on food such as citrus and health and look for confirmation from each source before changing purchase behavior.

In an analysis of news media coverage of food safety and nutrition known as *Food for Thought V*, commissioned by the IFIC Foundation May through July 2003, functional foods represented the leading source of benefits mentioned in print and broadcast reports.

Continuing the trend since 1998, almost all consumers (94 percent) agree that certain foods have health benefits that go beyond basic nutrition and may reduce the risk of disease or other health concerns. Consumers express little familiarity with terms commonly used to describe this concept, including "functional foods" (62 percent like it, whereas 27 percent dislike it). Even less well liked is "nutraceuticals" (only 34 percent like it; 49 percent dislike it). Still, 85 percent of Americans are either "very interested" or "somewhat interested" in learning more about functional foods. (*3*) This level of interest has been consistently strong since 1998.

As in 1998 and 2000, a majority of consumers believe they have a "great amount" of control over their own health (68 percent). They overwhelmingly believe that food and nutrition play "a great role" in maintaining or improving overall health (71 percent), and the proportion is even greater than the proportion of individuals who believe that exercise (63 percent) or family health history (41 percent) is a key determinant of health. Although more than half (54 percent) of the respondents are reducing the amounts of certain foods or food components in their diets, 35 percent (compared to 36 percent in 2000 and 28 percent in 1998) (*3*) are adding foods or beverages for their health benefits, particularly vegetables, fruits including citrus, and water.

Citrus is at the top of the top 10 foods that consumers identify as having a health benefit beyond basic nutrition. [oranges or orange juice (9 percent), broccoli (9 percent), fish or fish oil (9 percent), green leafy vegetables (9 percent), carrots (8 percent), garlic (7 percent), fiber (6 percent), milk (6 percent), oats/oat bran/oatmeal (6 percent), and tomatoes (6 percent)] The foods in the top five have remained constant since 1998 and are consistently associated with America's top health concerns: cardiovascular disease and its factors, including heart disease/heart attack, high blood pressure, stroke, and high cholesterol, which remain the top collective concern of Americans (41 percent). Cancer continues to concern almost a third (30 percent) of consumers. Other health concerns that consumers mention include weight (17 percent), diabetes (17 percent), and nutrition/diet (12 percent). Overall, 44 percent of consumers associate foods or food components with a reduced risk of cancer, often naming fruits and vegetables. A slightly larger number of consumers (53 percent) associate foods with heart health, including fish or fish oil, garlic, and fiber.]

Almost two-thirds (63 percent) of Americans say they are eating at least one food to receive a functional health benefit. Although these results are not significantly different from those from the survey conducted in 2000 (59 percent), they do represent a significant increase from the results obtained in the survey (*3*) conducted in 1998 (53 percent).

When asked about specific associations between food and health, awareness of the connection between calcium and osteoporosis remains high, as was the case in 2000 (79 percent). The increasing popularity of orange juice fortified with calcium may contribute to this high awareness. Fewer Americans are aware of the association between antioxidants and cancer (54 percent), and fewer still know about the heart health benefits of soy protein (35 percent). Those who had heard of these associations were asked how much they had heard: 64 percent had heard "a lot" about the calcium-osteoporosis relationship, whereas only 34 percent had heard "a lot" about antioxidants cancer relationship and 23 percent had heard "a lot" about soy protein-heart disease relationship. Therefore, in addition to fewer consumers actually hearing about the last two relationships, those consumers are also hearing only "a little" about them.

The relatively recent determinations of relationships between soy protein and heart disease and between antioxidants and cancer may help to explain why belief in the efficacies of these relationships is lower than that for the efficacy of the calcium-osteoporosis relationship. Compared to the results for 2000, fewer consumers (59 percent) believe in the efficacy of the soy protein/heart disease relationship. Slightly more believe in the efficacy of the antioxidant-cancer relationship (66 percent).

It's a different story for calcium-osteoporosis relationship, with 91 percent of consumers believing in the efficacy of the relationship. The differences in the levels of belief in the effectiveness of these relationships lie first in the length of exposure to the information—the health benefits of calcium have been discussed in detail for many years, and calcium-fortified orange juice is now widely available. Also, a wide range of communicators from health professionals to journalists to government officials have extolled the health benefits of calcium against osteoporosis. In addition, Americans are less familiar with food sources of soy protein and antioxidants, and some consumers who did not like the taste of early soy products are unaware of new ones. Additionally, lower levels of belief in the efficacy of an association may be related to hearing relatively less about the association.

For functional foods to deliver their potential public health benefits, consumers need a clear understanding of and a strong level of confidence in the scientific criteria that are used to document health effects and claims. When communicating about functional foods, it is important to translate quality science into understandable and usable messages that meet consumer needs. The following are specific communication strategies: (1) Cite the need for credible, scientific criteria as the basis for messages about functional foods and the development of new food products. (2) Accentuate the "good news" about food. (3) Place new research findings into context with the overall body of scientific evidence. (4) Discuss the benefits of particular components within the context of familiar foods and overall eating patterns. (5) Do not overstate potential benefits, and ensure that any claims made on- or off-label are based on reasonable and responsible information.

A paradigm shift has occurred over time where the old model of research focusing on disease being treated by physicians has been updated and sometimes replaced by a focus on wellness where the media and other health professionals become additional sources for consumers who often make their own health decisions. It is no surprise then that consumers are very receptive to the idea of personalized nutrition or "nutrigenomics."

Cogent Research conducted in December 2002 (*2*) a total of six focus groups with consumers in three markets, including Los Angeles, CA, Dallas, TX and Washington D.C. All participants were required to meet specific screening criteria developed by Cogent Research and IFIC. These criteria provided us with a mix of general consumers who agree that foods can provide health benefits that go beyond general nutrition. They clearly see the benefits to their overall health, specifically, being able to potentially avoid the diseases and other health problems to which they are genetically predisposed.

Participants liked being able to have some control over their destiny. One woman felt that people would "make more wise choices about your life if you know these things in advance." Another woman stated that she "could avoid certain foods that could be triggers."

Although participants see the benefits of such an advance in the arena of food and health, they had a few concerns:

Privacy: Many participants were concerned with the confidentiality of the results of the DNA profile. They were afraid that insurance companies would look at the results and refuse to cover them if the results show they were likely to have a health problem that is expensive to treat. One group also discussed the possibility of discrimination, in general, based on one's genetics.

Expense: The cost of such DNA profiling was a concern for many participants. They would like the cost of the test and subsequent recommendations to be covered by insurance and/or available to everyone regardless of economic status.

Depression: Some participants expressed that the knowledge of what diseases or other health problems they are likely to get later in life would be depressing. Many stated that they would like to know, but not until they are older because they feel the knowledge "could hinder your life."

Unnecessary worry: A few participants mentioned that the results could be wrong and you could spend your life worrying unnecessarily and trying to avoid a certain disease or health problem that you are not actually predisposed to.

Limitations: A few participants mentioned that focusing on modifying one's diet ignores the other factors that influence one's health such as lifestyle and environment.

The terms "Personalized Nutrition" and "Individualized Nutrition" were both rated extremely positively by participants. While 22 of the 48 participants preferred Personalized Nutrition, 18 of the 48 preferred Individualized Nutrition. However, many participants found it difficult to choose one over the other. Those who had a strong preference for one over the other had the same rationale regardless of which one they liked best – (personalized/individualized) speaks to them more as an individual or as a person. In the end, it comes down to word preference.

"Nutrigenomics" and "Nutritional Genomics" received generally negative ratings. Participants mentioned both terms were difficult to understand. Nutrigenomics, in addition, was "scary" to some participants. They also mentioned the term sounds "mathematical and "like a disease." Each term was chosen as "best" by only one participant.

When asked if they see a connection between functional foods and personalized nutrition, participants were hesitant to respond. In most groups, one consumer would note that a personalized nutrition plan might include eating functional foods. However, it did not appear as if the connection was immediately evident to most.

The best advice for helping consumers to reap the health benefits of foods is to eat moderate portions of foods from the various groups in the Food Guide Pyramid, as well as increase the variety of foods consumed from each of these groups. Citrus products are uniquely positioned to benefit from increasing focus on food and health, as they are both an important natural source of functional components as well as convenient and popular vehicles for additional fortified components. After all, "variety is the spice of life!"

These consumer insights provide an opportunity for increasing awareness and education on the potential health benefits of citrus. It is important to understand that consumers don't rely on just one source of information on food and health, so an effort that targets multiple sources of information that complement each other would be most effective.

References

1. *Support for Food Biotechnology Stable Despite News on Unrelated Food Safety Issues*, URL http://www.ific.org/research/biotechres03.cfm; Cogent Research and commissioned by the International Food Information Council (IFIC) January 2-11 2004
2. *Functional Foods: Attitudinal Research (2002),* URL http://www.ific.org/research/funcfoodsres02.cfm; Cogent Research and commissioned by the International Food Information Council (IFIC) March 2002
3. *Functional Foods. Attitudinal Research (2000)*,URL http://www.ific.org/research/funcfoodsres00.cfm; Cogent Research and commissioned by the International Food Information Council (IFIC) May/June 2000

Indexes

Author Index

Ahmad, Hassan, 130
Andrade, Juan E., 161
Báidez, Ana, 175
Bertram, Heinz-Jürgen, 70
Bhat, Narayan G., 34, 219
Breksa, Andrew P., III, 95
Brennecke, Stefan, 70
Brodbelt, Jennifer S., 1, 34, 52, 219
Bulku, Ellida, 144
Burgess, John R., 161
Chapkin, Robert S., 121
Cuthrell, Kristine, 235
Dandekar, Deepak V., 18
Davis, Barry D., 52
Del Río, José A., 175
Eliaz, Isaac, 199
Frías, Víctor, 175
Fujioka, Ken, 211
Gibbins, Reed P., 82
Girennavar, Basavaraj, 52, 219
Gómez, Pedro, 175
Guardino, John, 199
Hasegawa, Shin, 95
Hughes, Kerry, 199
Jacob, Robert A., 95
Jayaprakasha, Guddadarangavvanahally K., 34, 52, 219
Kindel, Günter, 70
Kohno, Hiroyuki, 104
Krammer, Gerhard E., 70
Kurowska, Elzbieta M., 186
Le Marchand, Loïc, 235
Lee, Michael W., 211
Leonardi, Tety, 121
Li, Jiaxing, 130
Liu, Yingxue C., 121
Lupton, Joanne R., 121
Mackie, Kimberly, 130
Manners, Gary D., 95
Manthey, John A., 186
McIntosh, Jame E., 82
Miller, Edward G., 1, 82
Murakami, Akira, 104
Murphy, Mary E., 121
Ohigashi, Hajime, 104
Ortuño, Ana, 175
Patil, Bhimanagouda S., 1, 18, 34, 52, 82, 121, 130, 144, 219
Pike, Leonard M., 18, 121
Pikulski, Michael, 52
Polson, Maria, 130
Poulose, Shibu M., 219
Quiroga, Walter, 130
Ray, Sidhartha D., 144
Schmidt, Claus O., 70
Schmidt, David B., 254
Singh, Rakesh K., 18
Stöckigt, Detlef, 70
Sugie, Shigeyuki, 104
Suzuki, Rikako, 104
Tanaka, Takuji, 104
Taylor, Samuel E., 82
Toledo, Romeo T., 18
Turner, Nancy D., 1, 121

Vanamala, Jairam, 121
Wang, Naisyin, 121
Weber, Berthold, 70
Yano, Masamichi, 104
Yu, Jun, 18
Zhang, Junmei, 52
Zinkovsky, Daniel, 144

Subject Index

A

Acetaminophen
  potential to generate hydroxyl radical, 157
  proanthocyanidins counteracting hepatotoxic properties, 156
  toxicity to liver, 144, 145–146
  See also Drug-induced cell death
Aglycones
  structures of limonoid, from citrus, 36*f*
  See also Limonoids
Analytical methods
  bioactive compounds in citrus and human tissues, 10–11
  identification and analysis of limonoids, 45–46
Anthocyanins, bioavailability, 97–98
Antiarrhythmics, potential interaction with grapefruit juice components, 221*t*
Antibiotics, potential interaction with grapefruit juice components, 221*t*
Anticancer activity
  limonoids, 83–84
  See also Cancer
Antifungal properties, *Citrus* flavonoids against *Phytophthora* sp., *Penicillium* sp., and *Geotrichum* sp., 179–181
Antihistamines, potential interaction with grapefruit juice components, 221*t*
Antioxidant defense system
  dietary deficiency of vitamin E and selenium in rats as model, 162, 164, 166
  effects of naringenin consumption and oxidative stress on total weight, weight gain, parametrial fat mass and food intake at week 6, 167*t*
  effects of naringenin consumption on oxidative stress in rats, 166, 168*f*, 169
  flavonoids structural requirements for antioxidant activity, 164, 165*f*
  formation of reactive oxygen species (ROS), 162
  grapefruit juice consumption in humans, 169–172
  multifaceted endogenous, 162, 163*f*
  naringenin consumption and lipid oxidation in rats, 169
  oxidative stress by urinary 8-epi-protaglandin $F_{2\alpha}$, 172, 173*f*
  potential health benefits of non–nutrient substances, 164
  proposed mechanisms for flavonoids, 164
  ruby red grapefruit juice (RRGJ) and consumption effects, 171*t*
  total peroxyl radical antioxidant potential (TRAP) determination of dietary flavonoids and t–BHQ, 165*t*
  vitamin C concentrations and grapefruit consumption in humans, 172
Anxiolytics, potential interaction with grapefruit juice components, 221*t*
Apigenin
  physiological responses to dietary treatment, 125, 126*t*
  proliferation and apoptosis effects, 127
Azoxymethane-induced rat colon tumorigenesis

absorption and biotransformation of nobiletin, 115
animals, chemicals, and diets, 106
cyclooxygenase (COX) enzymes, 115
dietary feeding of nobiletin, 114
experimental procedure, 106, 107*f*
general observation, 109
incidence and multiplicity of intestinal neoplasms, 109, 110*f*, 111*f*
induction of apoptosis, 114–115
long-term experiment of effect of nobiletin, 105–106
materials and methods, 106, 108
measurement of proliferating cell nuclear antigen (PCNA) and apoptotic indices in colonic neoplasms, 108
measurement of prostaglandin E_2 (PGE_2) level, 108
PCNA and apoptotic indices in colonic neoplasms, 114, 116*f*, 117*f*
PGE_2 production, 115
polyamine content and PGE_2 level in colonic mucosa, 109, 112*f*, 113*f*
polyamine level, 108
potential mechanisms, 115, 118
statistical evaluation, 108
suppression effect on cell proliferation activity, 114

B

Bergamottin and 6',7'-dihydroxybergamottin
grapefruit, 237–238
structures, 224*f*, 225*f*
Bioactive compounds
analytical challenges and opportunities, 10–11
grapefruit, 2, 220
hydrolysis and metabolism/conjugation, 127–128
optimization through pre- and post-harvest factors, 9–10
plant-derived, from citrus, 2
See also Supercritical carbon dioxide (SC-CO_2) extraction
Bioavailability
anthocyanins, 97–98
drugs, 220, 222
limonoids, 97–98
Biological activity
flavonoids, 105
limonoids, 19, 96–97
Biological reactive intermediates (BRIs), formation, 145
Biosynthesis
flavanones and polymethoxyflavones, 175, 176*f*
flavonoids in *Citrus* species, 177–179
limonoids, 83
modulation of flavonoid, and resistance against pathogens fungi, 182
Biotechnology, food, 255
Biotransformation, flavonoids, 53
Bitterness, limonoids, 83
Blood chemistries
assays, 89*t*
screening limonoids in rats, 88–90
Box–Behnken design, supercritical fluid extraction, 25
Breast cancer
citrus limonoids, 85
modified citrus pectin (MCP), 204–205
4-Bromoflavone
effect on glutathione S-transferase (GST) activity, 135, 136*f*
effect on quinone reductase (QR) activity, 135, 137–138
See also Flavonoids

Brotomax treatment, flavonoid levels in *Citrus* sp., 182

C

Calcium, osteoporosis, 256, 257
Calcium-channel blockers, potential interaction with grapefruit juice components, 221*t*
Cancer
  chemopreventative activity of citrus limonoids, 3–4, 83–84
  citrus flavonoids, 5–7
  consumer awareness of food and health, 256
  discovery of galectin-3 in, 200
  epidemiological studies for grapefruit, 240–241, 246
  grapefruit consumption, 236, 240–241, 246
  growth and metathesis with MCP, 206–207
  modified citrus pectin (MCP), 240
  National Cancer Institute, 2
  pharmacology of MCP, 203–204
  See also Azoxymethane-induced rat colon tumorigenesis; Colon cancer; Grapefruit and colon cancer; Modified citrus pectin (MCP)
Carbon dioxide
  ideal supercritical fluid solvent, 22–23
  See also Supercritical carbon dioxide (SC-CO_2) extraction
Cardiovascular disease. polymethoxylated flavones (PMF), 195–196
Carotenoids
  bioavailability, 97–98
  citrus products, 242*t*, 243*t*, 244*t*, 245*t*
  plant-derived bioactive molecules, 2
Caspase-activated DNA-fragmentation
  agarose gel-electrophoresis, 148
  inhibition by citrus flavonoids, 153–154, 155*f*
Cell death. *See* Drug-induced cell death
Cell proliferation
  carcinogenesis, 114
  grapefruit and colon cancer, 124, 126–127
  index proliferating cell nuclear antigen (PCNA), 105, 108
  PCNA and apoptotic indices in colonic neoplasms, 114, 116*f*, 117*f*
  See also Azoxymethane-induced rat colon tumorigenesis
Cholesterol levels
  citrus limonoids, 84–85, 90
  effect of grapefruit juice consumption, 171*t*
Chronic disease, flavonoids inhibiting enzymes, 196
Citrus
  benefits for metabolic syndrome risk factors, 213
  bioactive compounds in, and human tissues, 10–11
  bioactive compound source, 35
  bioactive molecules, 2
  consumers identifying benefits, 256
  crop on global level, 2
  drug interactions, 7–8
  flavonoids, 213*t*
  health-promoting properties, 35
  isolation of limonoid aglycones and glucosides, 42*t*, 43*t*
  oils of fruits, 71
  structures of limonoid aglycones from, 36*f*
  See also Metabolic syndrome; Polymethoxyflavones
Citrus pectin
  fibroblast growth factor (FGF), 8
  historic use of, 200

illustration of unmodified, 202*f*
See also Modified citrus pectin (MCP)

Citrus species as flavonoid source
antifungal properties of *Citrus* flavonoids against *Phytophthora* sp., *Penicillium* sp. and *Geotrichum* sp., 179–181
biosynthesis of flavonoids in *Citrus*, 177–179
biosynthetic pathways to flavonoids, 175
changes of polymethoxyflavone levels for infected *Citrus*, 180–181
chemical structures of flavanones and polymethoxyflavones, 176*f*
flavanone glycosides, 175
flavones, 176
flavonoids in, 175
levels of hesperidin in mature fruits of *C. sinensis* varieties, 178*f*
levels of sinensetin, nobiletin, heptamethoxyflavone and tangeretin in *C. sinensis* varieties, 179*f*
modulating flavonoid biosynthesis for increased resistance, 182
scanning electron microscopy (SEM) of hyphal morphology changes and growth of *P. citrophthora mycelium*, 181*f*

Classes, flavonoids, 213*t*

Clinical data
cancer growth and metathesis with modified citrus pectin (MCP), 206–207
heavy metal detoxification, 207–208

Clinical indications, modified citrus pectin (MCP), 208–209

Cogent Research, participants controlling health destiny, 257–258

Collisional activated dissociation (CAD), flavonoids, 54–55

Colon cancer
bioactive compounds protecting against promotion stage, 122
diet and lifestyle, 122
modified citrus pectin (MCP), 205
mortality rates in Japan, 105
See also Azoxymethane-induced rat colon tumorigenesis; Grapefruit and colon cancer

Colorado potato beetle, limonoids for management, 3

Commercial interest, limonoids, 85–86

Consumer interest
citrus, 256
concerns about food and health, 258–259
confidence in scientific criteria, 257
food and health awareness, 256
functional foods, 255–256

Corticosteroids, potential interaction with grapefruit juice components, 221*t*

Coumarins
citrus products, 242*t*, 243*t*, 244*t*, 245*t*
phytochemicals in citrus, 53

Critical point, temperature and pressure, 20

Cytochrome P450 enzymes
drug-drug and food-drug interactions, 223, 226*f*
inhibition of CYP1A2 by white grapefruit juice, 246–247
inhibition of CYP3A4 by grapefruit juice, 236

D

Deoxyribonucleic acid (DNA)
agarose gel-electrophoresis probing caspase-activated DNA fragmentation, 148

citrus flavonoids preventing genomic destruction in liver and kidneys, 153–154, 155*f*
fragmentation assay, 147
fragmentation or laddering, 157–158
hesperidin and rutin preventing DNA fragmentation, 152, 154*f*
See also Drug-induced cell death
Depression, food and health concern, 258
Design of experiment (DOE), supercritical fluid extraction, 25–27
Detoxification enzymes
involvement of hesperidin and rutin, 158
See also Phase II detoxification enzymes
Diacylglycerol acyltransferase, polymethoxylated flavones inhibiting, 192–193, 194*f*
Diclofenac
potential to generate hydroxyl radical, 157
toxic effects, 156–157
toxicity to kidneys, 144, 145–146
See also Drug-induced cell death
Diet, National Cancer Institute, 2
Dosage, modified citrus pectin (MCP), 208
Drug-induced cell death
acetaminophen (APAP) and liver toxicity, 144, 145–146
agarose gel-electrophoresis probing caspase-activated deoxyribonucleic acid (DNA) fragmentation, 148
animals, chemicals, and diets, 146
APAP-induced oxidative stress in liver, 150, 152*f*
citrus flavonoids and acute liver and kidney injuries, 145–146
citrus flavonoids and APAP-induced genomic DNA fragmentation in liver, 152, 154*f*
citrus flavonoids and diclofenac (DCLF)-induced genomic DNA fragmentation in kidney, 152, 154*f*
DCLF and kidney toxicity, 144, 145–146
DCLF-induced oxidative stress in kidney, 150, 153*f*
determination of hepatotoxicity and nephrotoxicity, 147
DNA fragmentation or DNA-laddering, 157–158
estimation of lipid peroxidation, 147
experimental procedure, 146
flavonoids counteracting cytotoxic properties of xenobiotics, 156
glutathione scavenging free radicals and peroxides, 158
hesperidin and rutin preventing DNA fragmentation, 152, 154*f*
hesperidin and rutin preventing genomic destruction in liver and kidney, 153–154, 155*f*
inhibition of caspase-activated-DNAse activity, 153–154, 155*f*
materials and methods, 146–148
mechanisms of actions of flavonoids, 155–156
prevention of APAP-induced liver injury by hesperidin and rutin, 148, 149*f*
prevention of APAP-induced oxidative stress in liver by hesperidin and rutin, 149, 151*f*
prevention of DCLF-induced kidney injury by hesperidin and rutin, 148, 150*f*
prevention of DCLF-induced oxidative stress in kidney by hesperidin and rutin, 149, 151*f*
quantitative apoptotic DNA fragmentation assay, 147
reactive oxygen species (ROS) generation, 145, 157

reversal of APAP and DCLF-induced depletion of total glutathione levels in liver and kidney by hesperidin and rutin, 150, 152*f*, 153*f*
toxicity of DCLF (Voltaren), 156–157

Drug interactions
bioavailability of drugs, 220, 222
citrus and, 7–8
clinical implications, 229
cytochrome P450 enzyme and drug metabolism, 223, 226*f*
food-drug interactions, 229, 230*t*, 231
mechanism of, with grapefruit juice, 227–229
P-glycoprotein protecting body, 227
potential, with grapefruit juice (GFJ) bioactive compounds, 221*t*
sequence of events during first-pass metabolism of oral drugs, 228*f*
withdrawn drugs from U.S. market for drug-drug interactions, 230*t*
See also Grapefruit

E

Electrospray ionization mass spectrometry (ESI–MS)
flavonoids, 54, 55, 57
limonoids, 46
rutin, 56*f*

Epidemiological studies, grapefruit, 240–241, 246, 248

Expense, food and health concern, 258

Experimental design
screening limonoid toxicity, 86–87
supercritical fluid extraction, 25–27

Extraction
limonoid aglycones, 37–39
limonoid glucosides, 39, 41, 44
See also Limonoids; Supercritical carbon dioxide (SC-CO_2) extraction

F

Fibroblast growth factor , citrus pectin, 8

Flash chromatography
process, 46–47
purification of limonoids by, 47–48
separation apparatus, 47*f*

Flavanones, chemical structure, 176*f*

Flavone glycosides
chemical structures, 188*f*, 189*f*
lowering blood serum cholesterol, 187
See also Polymethoxylated flavones (PMFs)

Flavones
Citrus, 176
polymethoxyflavone structure, 74*t*
See also Polymethoxylated flavones (PMFs)

Flavonoids
absorption and metabolism, 164
analysis of, biotransformation products, 66
beneficial roles, 5–7
bioavailability, 97–98
biological activities, 105
biosynthesis in *Citrus*, 177–179
biotransformation, 53
Brotomax treatment of *Citrus* sp., 182
CAD (collisional activated dissociation), 54–55
CAD mass spectra for deprotonated rhoifolin and isorhoifolin, 58*f*
CAD mass spectra of isomeric diglycosyl flavonoids, 60*f*
challenges in supercritical carbon dioxide extraction, 27

citrus products, 242*t*, 243*t*, 244*t*, 245*t*
Citrus species as source, 175–177
counteracting cytotoxic properties of xenobiotics, 156
determination of glycosylation site, 59
dissociation patterns of complexes containing cobalt and rhoifolin, 62, 63*f*
dissociation routes for complexes, 61
effect of, on glutathione S-transferase (GST) activity, 135, 136*f*
effect of, on NAD(P)H:quinone reductase (QR) activity, 135, 137–138
electrospray ionization (ESI), 54
electrospray ionization–mass spectrometry (ESI–MS) of, 55, 57
ESI–MS of rutin, 56*f*
fragmentation patterns of complexes of rhoifolin, 60, 62*f*
high performance liquid chromatography–tandem mass spectroscopy (HPLC–MS/MS) applications, 64–65
interest in human health benefits, 19
major classes, 213*t*
mechanisms of actions in cellular processes, 155–156
metal complexation, 58–60
methods for low level detection, 53–54
phytochemicals in citrus, 53
plant-derived bioactive molecules, 2
proposed antioxidant mechanisms, 164
protecting against promotion stage of colon cancer, 122
specificity in binding to ATP binding sites, 196
structures of isomeric, 53*f*
structures of rhoifolin and isorhoifolin, 58*f*
tandem mass spectrometry (MS/MS), 54–55
tandem mass spectrometry of, 57–64
tuning fragmentation patterns, 62, 64
See also Antioxidant defense system; *Citrus* species as flavonoid source; Hesperidin; Nobiletin; Rutin; Supercritical carbon dioxide (SC-CO_2) extraction
Food and health, concerns, 258–259
Food biotechnology, consumer interest, 255
Food-drug interactions
common, 229, 230*t*, 231
See also Drug interactions
Food guide pyramid, health benefits of food, 259
Food sources, flavonoids, 213*t*
Free radicals, formation examples, 145
Functional foods
consumer interest, 255–256
definition, 255
Furanocoumarins, grapefruit, 237–238
Furocoumarins
effect of processing on juice content, 222–223
effect on cytochrome P450 enzymes activity, 227*t*
grapefruit juice, 222
levels in hand squeezed and commercial grapefruit juice, 226*f*
structures, 224*f*, 225*f*

G

Galectins, cancer cells, 203–204
Geotrichum sp., antifungal properties of *Citrus* flavonoids against, 179–181
Gibberellic acid, limonin and naringin, 9
Glutathione
  possible involvement of hesperidin and rutin, 158
  scavenging free radicals and peroxides, 158
  See also Drug-induced cell death
Glutathione S-transferase (GST)
  effect of flavonoids on GST activity, 135, 136*f*
  enhanced detoxification of carcinogens, 131–132
  sample preparation and enzyme activity, 134–135
Grapefruit
  antioxidant effects of juice consumption in humans, 169–172
  bergamottin and 6',7'-dihydroxybergamottin, 237–238
  bioactive compounds, 2, 220, 236–240
  bioactive constituents in pink/red grapefruit, 242*t*, 243*t*
  bioactive constituents in white grapefruit, 242*t*
  drug interactions, 7–8
  effect of processing on juice furocoumarins content, 222–223
  epidemiological studies, 240–241, 246, 248
  experimental for extraction from seeds, 23–24
  flavonoids, 213
  flavonoids in, and juice, 6
  furanocoumarins, 237–238
  Hollywood Diet, 214
  inhibition of enzyme CYP1A2 by white grapefruit juice, 246–247
  juice change during storage, 9–10
  liquid chromatography–tandem mass spectrometry analysis, 64, 65*f*
  mechanism of juice-drug interaction, 227–229
  modified citrus pectin (MCP), 240
  monoterpenes, 238–239
  naringin/naringenin, 236–237
  putative bioactive components of juice, 222
  structure of furocoumarins in, juice, 224*f*, 225*f*
  supercritical fluid extraction from, seeds, 25–26
  terpenes, 238–240
  triterpenes, 239–240
  weight loss, 8, 214, 215*f*
  See also Colon cancer; Drug interactions; Grapefruit and colon cancer
Grapefruit and colon cancer
  aberrant crypt foci, proliferation and apoptosis, 124
  apigenin, 127
  comparing responses of experiments, 127
  experimental timelines and carcinogen treatment, 124
  experiment II results, 125, 126*t*
  experiment I results, 124–125
  experiments I and II, 122–123
  hesperidin, 127
  irradiated grapefruit pulp, 127
  isolated bioactive compounds vs. untreated grapefruit, 127–128
  isolated naringin, 126–127
  materials and methods, 122–124
  naringenin, 127
  physiological responses to dietary treatments, 125*t*, 126*t*
  potential contribution of limonin, 126

statistics, 124
untreated grapefruit pulp vs. isolated limonin, 126
See also Colon cancer

H

Hamster cheek pouch model, naringin, 7
Harvest factors, optimization of bioactive compounds through pre- and post-, 9–10
Heavy metal detoxification, modified citrus pectin (MCP), 207–208
Hepatic dysfunctions, phytochemicals inhibiting, 145–146
Heptamethoxyflavone
Brotomax treatment and level of, 182
cardiovascular disease, 195
chemical structure, 176*f*, 189*f*
levels in mature fruits of *Citrus sinesis* varieties, 179*f*
Hesperetin
cholesterol- and triacylglycerol-lowering, 6
health-promoting activity, 6
inhibition of apolipoprotein B (apoB) secretion, 187
Hesperidin
bioavailability, 97
biosynthetic pathway, 175
Brotomax treatment of *Citrus* sp., 182
chemical structure, 176*f*, 188*f*
effect on glutathione S-transferase activity, 135, 136*f*
effect on quinone reductase (QR) activity, 135, 137–138
levels in mature fruits of *Citrus sinesis* varieties, 178*f*
physiological responses to dietary treatment, 125, 126*t*
possible involvement with detoxification enzymes, 158
prevention of acetaminophen-induced oxidative stress in liver, 149, 151*f*
prevention of diclofenac-induced oxidative stress in kidney, 149, 151*f*
proliferation and apoptosis effects, 127
protection of acetaminophen-induced liver injury, 148, 149*f*
protection of diclofenac-induced kidney injury, 148, 150*f*
protection of genomic DNA integrity, 152, 154*f*
reversal of acetaminophen- and diclofenac-induced depletion of glutathione levels, 150, 152*f*, 153*f*
serum cholesterol and triacylglycerol (TG), 187, 190
serum TGs in human trial, 190
structure, 53*f*
studying influence on liver and kidney injuries, 145–146
See also Drug-induced cell death; Flavonoids
High performance liquid chromatography (HPLC)
flavonoids by HPLC–tandem mass spectrometry, 64–65
identification and analysis of limonoids, 45–46
See also Polymethoxyflavones
HIV protease inhibitors, potential interaction with grapefruit juice components, 221*t*
Hollywood Diet, grapefruit, 214
Homogalacturonans, pectin polysaccharide, 201, 202*f*
Human consumption
antioxidant effects of grapefruit juice, 169–172
limonoids, 85–86

Human tissues, bioactive compounds in citrus and, 10–11

I

Immunosuppressants, potential interaction with grapefruit juice components, 221*t*
Individualized nutrition, term, 258
Insect control, citrus limonoids, 3
Insulin, grapefruit consumption, 214, 216*t*
Interactions. *See* Drug interactions
International Food Information Council (IFIC)
  consumer attitudes, 255
  functional food definition, 255
  screening criteria by Cogent Research and, 257–258
Irradiated grapefruit pulp, colon cancer development, 127
Isorhoifolin
  collisional activated dissociation (CAD) spectrum, 58*f*
  structure, 58*f*
  See also Flavonoids

J

Juice. *See* Grapefruit

K

Kidney. *See* Drug-induced cell death

L

Lactation, modified citrus pectin (MCP), 208
Lemon, non-volatiles of peel oils, 71
Limitations, food and health concern, 258
Limonene, monoterpene in citrus peel oils, 238–239
Limonin
  bitterness, 83
  conditions for supercritical fluid extraction, 25–26
  early colon cancer protection with isolated, 126, 127
  effect of feeding mode on extraction, 28*t*
  effect on glutathione S-transferase (GST) activity, 138, 139*f*
  experimental diet composition, 123*t*
  physiological responses to dietary treatment, 125*t*
  response surface analysis, 29*f*
  structure, 26*f*, 36*f*
  See also Supercritical carbon dioxide (SC-CO_2) extraction
Limonin glucoside (LG)
  conditions for supercritical fluid extraction, 25–26
  effect of feeding mode on extraction, 28*t*
  response surface analysis, 30*f*
  structure, 26*f*, 40*f*
  yield from citrus varieties, 45*t*
  See also Supercritical carbon dioxide (SC-CO_2) extraction
Limonoate A-ring lactone
  citrus tissues, 95–96
  structure, 96*f*
Limonoid glucosides
  citrus juices, 239–240
  extraction and purification, 39, 41, 44
  isolation and purification from citrus seeds, 44
  structures, 40*f*
  yield, 45*t*

Limonoids
- aglycones and glucosides from citrus varieties, 42*t*, 43*t*
- anticancer activity, 83–84
- anticarcinogenic activity, 132
- basic research, 83
- beneficial roles of citrus, 2–5
- bioactive compounds in citrus, 2, 53, 95–96
- bioavailability, 97–99
- biological activity, 19, 96–97
- biosynthesis pathways, 83
- bitterness, 83
- cancer treatment, 4
- challenges in supercritical carbon dioxide extraction, 27
- commercial interest, 85–86
- effect of, on glutathione S-transferase (GST) activity, 138, 139*f*
- extraction and purification of limonoid aglycones, 37–39
- extraction and purification of limonoid glucosides, 39, 41, 44
- flash chromatography, 46–48
- future work, 99
- general structure, 132, 133*f*
- identification and analysis, 45–46
- inhibiting HIV-1 replication, 5
- isolation and purification of limonoid glucosides from citrus seeds, 44
- limonin-like unknown, 98–99
- management of Colorado potato beetle, 3
- potential health benefits, 84–85
- protecting against promotion stage of colon cancer, 122
- structure-function relationship, 35, 37
- structures, 96*f*
- structures of limonoid aglycones from citrus, 36*f*
- structures of limonoid glucosides, 40*f*
- triterpenes in citrus fruits, 239
- yield of limonoid glucosides, 45*t*
- *See also* Supercritical carbon dioxide (SC-CO_2) extraction; Toxicity screening study

Lipid oxidation, effect of naringenin consumption in rats, 169

Lipids, blood, effect of grapefruit juice consumption, 171*t*

Lipoproteins, microsomal triglyceride transfer protein (MTP), 187, 193, 194*f*

Liquid chromatography/electrospray ionization mass spectrometry (LC/ESI–MS), limonoids, 46

Liquid chromatography/mass spectroscopy (LC/MS). *See* Polymethoxyflavones

Liquid chromatography/nuclear magnetic resonance (LC/NMR). *See* Polymethoxyflavones

Litters, screening limonoids in rats, 90, 91*t*

Liver. *See* Drug-induced cell death

Lycopene, storage of grapefruit juice, 9

M

Macrophages, actions of polymethoxylated flavones (PMF), 193, 195

Mass spectrometry
- bioactive compounds, 11
- identification and analysis of limonoids, 46

Media coverage, food safety and nutrition, 255

Metabolic syndrome
- benefits of citrus on risk factors for, 213
- definition, 212*t*
- diagnosis, 211–212
- flavonoids and citrus, 213

grapefruit, 214
orange juice, 214
risk factors, 212*t*
treatment, 212
weight and insulin changes, 216*t*
weight loss with grapefruit intake, 214, 215*f*

Metal complexation
CAD (collisional activated dissociation) for rhoifolin complex, 62*f*, 63*f*, 64*f*
collisional activated dissociation (CAD), 60, 61
determination of glycosylation site, 59
dissociation routes, 61
flavanoid ions, 58–60
rutin, 56*f*, 57
silver complexation, 59
tunable fragmentation patterns, 60, 62
See also Flavonoids

Mice. *See* Drug-induced cell death

Modified citrus pectin (MCP)
binding to and blocking galectin receptors, 203–204
breast cancer and MCP in mice, 204–205
cancer growth and metathesis, 206–207
cancer metathesis, 203
chelator of toxic metals, 203
chemistry, 201–203
clinical data, 206–208
clinical indications, 208–209
colon cancer and MCP in mice, 205
dosage, 208
heavy metal detoxification, 207–208
history and development, 200–201
illustration of MCP chain with repeating galactose units, 202*f*
inhibiting adhesion of cancer cells, 240
pharmacology, 203–204
preclinical studies, 204–206
pregnancy and lactation, 208
prostate cancer and MCP, 205–206
safety and toxicology, 208
solid tumors, 8

N

Naringenin
cancer chemopreventive potential, 6–7
decreasing triacylglycerol (TG) accumulation, 187
effect of consumption on lipid oxidation in rats, 169
effect on total weight, weight gain, parametrial fat mass and food intake, 167*t*
effects of consumption on oxidative stress in rats, 166, 168*f*, 169
grapefruit, 236–237
grapefruit flavonoid, 6
inhibition of apolipoprotein B (apoB) secretion, 187
inhibition of diacylglycerol acyltransferase (DGAT), 192–193, 194*f*
inhibition of TG synthesis, 192–193
physiological responses to dietary treatment, 125, 126*t*
See also Antioxidant defense system

Naringin
biosynthetic pathway, 175
cancer chemopreventive potential, 6–7
chemical structure, 26*f*, 176*f*, 188*f*
cholesterol- and triacylglycerol (TG)-lowering, 6
conditions for supercritical fluid extraction, 25–26
early colon cancer protection with isolated, 126–127

effect on glutathione S-transferase activity, 135, 136*f*
effect on quinone reductase (QR) activity, 135, 137–138
experimental diet composition, 123*t*
grapefruit, 236–237
grapefruit flavonoid, 6
hamster cheek pouch model, 7
physiological responses to dietary treatment, 125*t*
serum cholesterol and TG, 187, 190
See also Supercritical carbon dioxide (SC-CO_2) extraction
Narirutin, bioavailability, 97
National Cancer Institute (NCI), program on diet and cancer, 2
Neohesperidin
biosynthetic pathway, 175
chemical structure, 53*f*, 176*f*
health-promoting activity, 6
See also Flavonoids
Nephrotic dysfunctions, phytochemicals inhibiting, 145–146
News media, food safety and nutrition, 255
Nobiletin
absorption and biotransformation, 115
azoxymethane (AOM)-induced lesions, 105
Brotomax treatment and level of, 182
cardiovascular disease, 195
chemical structure, 74*t*, 107*f*, 176*f*, 188*f*
^{1}H nuclear magnetic resonance (NMR) spectrum, 77*f*
identification by LC/NMR, 76
inhibiting cancer cell proliferation, 5
levels in mature fruits of *Citrus sinesis* varieties, 179*f*
metabolites in hamster blood serum, urine and liver, 191
physiological responses to dietary treatment, 125, 126*t*
study of effect on AOM-induced rat colon carcinogenesis, 105–106
suppressing production of prostaglandin (PG) E_2, 105, 115
See also Azoxymethane-induced rat colon tumorigenesis; Flavonoids
Nomilin
bitterness, 83
effect on glutathione S-transferase (GST) activity, 138, 139*f*
Nucleotide binding sites, interactions of polymethoxylated flavones with, 196
Nutrigenomics, term, 258
Nutrition, functional foods, 255–256
Nutritional genomics, term, 258

O

Obesity
background, 211
See also Metabolic syndrome
Oral carcinogenesis, citrus limonoids, 84
Oranges
bioactive compounds, 2
bioactive constituents in, 243*t*, 244*t*
bioactive constituents in peel, 245*t*
flavonoids, 213
See also Citrus
Osteoporosis, calcium, 256, 257
Oxidative stress, imbalance of pro-oxidants, 145

P

Pathogens, modulating flavonoid biosynthesis for resistance against, 182
Pectin
  chemistry, 201–203
  See also Modified citrus pectin (MCP)
Penicillium sp., antifungal properties of *Citrus* flavonoids against, 179–181
Personalized nutrition
  connection between functional foods and, 258–259
  term, 258
P-glycoprotein
  protecting body, 227
  See also Drug interactions
Pharmacology, modified citrus pectin (MCP), 203–204
Phase II detoxification enzymes
  effect of flavonoids on GST activity, 135, 136*f*
  effect of flavonoids on QR activity, 135, 137–138
  effect of limonoids on GST activity, 138, 139*f*
  glutathione S-transferase (GST) and NAD(P)H:quinone reductase (QR), 131–132
  materials and methods, 134–135
  sample preparation and enzyme activity, 134–135
  treatment of animals, 134
Phytochemicals, inhibiting hepatic and nephrotic dysfunctions, 145–146
Phytophthora sp.
  antifungal properties of *Citrus* flavonoids against, 179–181
  scanning electron microscopy (SEM) of hyphal morphology and growth of *P. citrophthora mycelium*, 181*f*
Polyamine content
  cell proliferation activity, 114
  colonic mucosa, 109, 112*f*, 113*f*
  method, 108
  See also Azoxymethane-induced rat colon tumorigenesis
Polymethoxylated flavones (PMFs)
  accumulation of triacylglycerol (TG), 187
  anti-atherosclerotic properties, 195–196
  apolipoprotein B (apoB)-containing lipoproteins, 187
  biochemical studies of lipid-lowering properties, 191–192
  chemical structures, 74*t*, 176*f*, 188*f*, 189*f*
  chromatogram and total ion content (TIC) from LC/MS experiment, 72*f*, 73*f*
  citrus peel oils, 71
  class A scavenger receptors (SR-A), 193, 195
  defense mechanism of *Citrus* sp. against pathogens, 180–181
  effects on macrophages and vascular inflammation, 193, 195
  experimental, 76, 78
  HPLC/MS analyses, 78
  HPLC/NMR analyses, 78
  interactions with nucleotide binding sites, 196
  LC/NMR spectrum of nobiletin, 76, 77*f*
  lipid-lowering properties in hypercholesterolemic hamsters, 191
  lipid-lowering proteins in cell culture studies, 190
  lowering blood serum cholesterol, 187
  mechanisms of inhibition, 196
  mediating SR-A expression and metabolism, 195
  nobiletin, 74*t*, 176*f*, 188*f*
  plant material, 76

prevention of chronic diseases, 196
sinensetin, 74*t*, 176*f*, 189*f*
sites of activity in decreasing apoB secretion and TG synthesis, 194*f*
tangeretin, 74*t*, 176*f*, 189*f*
tetramethylscutellarein, 74*t*
two-dimensional plot from LC/NMR experiment, 71, 75*f*
Preclinical studies
breast cancer and modified citrus pectin (MCP) in mice, 204–205
colon cancer and MCP in mice, 205
prostate cancer and MCP, 205–206
Pregnancy, modified citrus pectin (MCP), 208
Preharvest and postharvest factors, optimization of bioactive compounds, 9–10
Pressure, critical point, 20
Pressure-temperature diagram, pure compound, 20*f*
Privacy, food and health concern, 258
Process flow diagram, supercritical fluid extraction, 26*f*
Prostaglandin E_2 (PGE_2)
colon carcinogenesis and, production, 105, 115
See also Azoxymethane-induced rat colon tumorigenesis
Prostate cancer
clinical trial, 206–207
modified citrus pectin (MCP), 205–206
Psoralens, grapefruit, 237–238
Psychiatric medicines, potential interaction with grapefruit juice components, 221*t*
Purification
limonoid aglycones, 37–39
limonoid glucosides, 39, 41, 44
limonoids by flash chromatography, 47–48
See also Limonoids

Q

Quercetogetin, chemical structure, 176*f*
Quinone reductase (QR)
effect of flavonoids on QR activity, 135, 137–138
protection from carcinogens, 132

R

Rats. *See* Antioxidant defense system; Azoxymethane-induced rat colon tumorigenesis; Grapefruit and colon cancer; Toxicity screening study
Reactive nitrogen species (RNS), formation, 145
Reactive oxygen species (ROS)
antioxidant defense system, 162, 163*f*
formation, 145
Response surface analysis
limonin, 29*f*
limonin glucoside (LG), 30*f*
supercritical fluid extractions, 28–30
Rhamnogalacturonans, pectin polysaccharide, 201, 202*f*
Rhoifolin
collisional activated dissociation (CAD) spectrum, 58*f*
structure, 58*f*
See also Flavonoids
Rutin
electrospray ionization mass spectra, 56*f*, 57
possible involvement with detoxification enzymes, 158
prevention of acetaminophen-induced oxidative stress in liver, 149, 151*f*

prevention of diclofenac-induced oxidative stress in kidney, 149, 151*f*
protection of acetaminophen-induced liver injury, 148, 149*f*
protection of diclofenac-induced kidney injury, 148, 150*f*
protection of genomic DNA integrity, 152, 154*f*
reversal of acetaminophen- and diclofenac-induced depletion of glutathione levels, 150, 152*f*, 153*f*
structure, 53*f*
studying influence on liver and kidney injuries, 145–146
See also Drug-induced cell death; Flavonoids

S

Safety, modified citrus pectin (MCP), 208
Scavenger receptors class A (SR-A), actions of polymethoxylated flavones (PMF), 193, 195
Screening study. *See* Toxicity screening study
Selectivity, definition, 21
Silver complexation
flavonoids, 59
See also Metal complexation
Sinensetin
Brotomax treatment and level of, 182
chemical structure, 74*t*, 176*f*, 189*f*
levels in mature fruits of *Citrus sinesis* varieties, 179*f*
Solid tumors, citrus pectin, 8
Solubility isotherm
extraction at high pressure, 22
typical, 21*f*
Solvent, carbon dioxide as ideal supercritical fluid, 22–23
Statins, potential interaction with grapefruit juice components, 221*t*
Storage, grapefruit juice, 9–10
Structure-function relationship, limonoids, 35, 37
Supercritical carbon dioxide (SC-CO_2) extraction
Box–Behnken design, 25*f*
carbon dioxide as ideal solvent, 22–23
challenges in, of limonoids and flavonoids process, 27
comparing upward and downward flows, 28
critical point for compound, 20
design of experiment (DOE), 25–27
effect of feeding mode on extraction, 28*t*
experimental, 23–24
limonin, limonin glucoside (LG), and naringin structures, 26*f*
natural products, 19–22
pressure-temperature diagram for pure compound, 20*f*
process flow diagram, 26*f*
response surface analysis, 28–30
schematic diagram, 24*f*
selectivity manipulations, 21
typical solubility isotherm, 21*f*
Supercritical fluids
natural product extraction, 19–22
See also Supercritical carbon dioxide (SC-CO_2) extraction

T

Tamoxifen, citrus flavonoid and therapeutic effect of, 5
Tandem mass spectrometry
collisional activated dissociation (CAD), 57, 58*f*
dissociation routes, 61

flavanoid biotransformation products, 66
flavonoids, 54–55
fragmentation patterns, 57
high performance liquid chromatography–MS/MS flavonoid applications, 64–65
identification and analysis of limonoids, 46
metal complexation of flavonoid ions, 58–60
rhoifolin and isorhoifolin, 57, 58*f*
silver complexation, 59
tunable fragmentation patterns, 60, 62
See also Flavonoids
Tangeretin
activation of peroxisome proliferators-activated receptor (PPAR), 193, 194*f*
biochemical studies of lipid-lowering properties, 191–192
Brotomax treatment and level of, 182
chemical structure, 74*t*, 176*f*, 189*f*
inhibiting cancer cell proliferation, 5
inhibiting lipid synthesis and accumulation in liver cells, 192
inhibition of diacylglycerol acyltransferase (DGAT), 192–193, 194*f*
levels in mature fruits of *Citrus sinesis* varieties, 179*f*
metabolites in hamster blood serum, urine and liver, 191
See also Citrus flavonoids
Tangerines, bioactive constituents in, 244*t*, 245*t*
Temperature
critical point, 20
solubility isotherm at constant, 21*f*
Terminology, food and health, 258–259
Terpenes
citrus fruits, 238–240
citrus products, 242*t*, 243*t*, 244*t*, 245*t*
limonoid glucosides, 239–240
limonoids, 239
monoterpenes, 238–239
triterpenes, 239–240
Tetramethylscutellarein
chemical structure, 189*f*
polymethoxyflavone structure, 74*t*
Thin layer chromatography (TLC), identification and analysis of limonoids, 45, 46
Toxicity, modified citrus pectin (MCP), 208
Toxicity screening study
blood assays, 89*t*
blood chemistries, 88–90
experimental design, 86–87
first generation, 86–87
food intake and weight gain, 87–88
limonoids and cholesterol, 90
litters, 90, 91*t*
second generation, 87
third generation, 87
weight data, 91*t*
Triacylglycerol (TG)
naringenin decreasing accumulation, 187
naringenin inhibiting synthesis, 192–193
Tumors. *See* Azoxymethane-induced rat colon tumorigenesis

U

Unnecessary worry, food and health concern, 258
UV-vis absorption spectroscopy, bioactive compounds, 11

V

Vascular inflammation, actions of polymethoxylated flavones (PMF), 193, 195
Vitamin C
  citrus, 2
  processing factors and citrus content, 9–10

W

Weight loss
  grapefruit, 8
  grapefruit consumption, 214, 215*f*
  insulin changes, 216*t*
  See also Metabolic syndrome
Worry, unnecessary, food and health concern, 258